Lecture Notes in Computer Science 3041

Commenced Publication in 1973
Founding and Former Series Editors:
Gerhard Goos, Juris Hartmanis, and Jan van Leeuwen

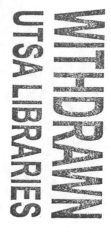

Constantine Stephanidis (Ed.)

Universal Access
in Health Telematics

A Design Code of Practice

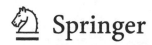 Springer

Volume Editor

Constantine Stephanidis
Foundation for Research and Technology - Hellas (FORTH)
Institute of Computer Science
Heraklion, Crete, 70013 Greece
E-mail: cs@ics.forth.gr

Library of Congress Control Number: 2005927142

CR Subject Classification (1998): H.5.2-3, H.4, C.2, K.4, K.8, J.3

ISSN   0302-9743
ISBN-10   3-540-26167-2 Springer Berlin Heidelberg New York
ISBN-13   978-3-540-26167-4 Springer Berlin Heidelberg New York

Springer is a part of Springer Science+Business Media

springeronline.com

© Springer-Verlag Berlin Heidelberg 2005
Printed in Germany

Typesetting: Camera-ready by author, data conversion by Boller Mediendesign
Printed on acid-free paper   SPIN: 11424628   06/3142   5 4 3 2 1 0

Preface

The Information Society is bringing about radical changes in the way people work and interact with each other and with information. In contrast to previous information processing paradigms, where the vast majority of computer-mediated tasks were business-oriented and executed by office workers using the personal computer in its various forms (i.e., initially alphanumeric terminals and later on graphical user interfaces), the Information Society signifies a growth not only in the range and scope of the tasks, but also in the way in which they are carried out and experienced. To address the resulting dimensions of diversity, the notion of universal access is critically important. Universal access implies the accessibility and usability of Information Society technologies by anyone, anywhere, anytime. Universal access aims to enable equitable access and active participation of potentially all citizens in existing and emerging computer-mediated human activities by developing universally accessible and usable products and services, which are capable of accommodating individual user requirements in different contexts of use and independently of location, target machine, or run-time environment. In the context of the emerging Information Society, universal access becomes predominantly an issue of design, pointing to the compelling need for devising systematic and cost-effective approaches to designing systems that accommodate the requirements of the widest possible range of end-users.

Recent developments have emphasized the need to consolidate progress by means of establishing a common vocabulary and a code of design practice, which addresses the specific challenges posed by universal access. IS4ALL is the acronym of the European Commission-funded Thematic Network (Working Group) "Information Society for All" (IST-1999-14101). IS4ALL is the first project that addresses in a systematic manner the task of consolidating and codifying available knowledge on universal access in the context of health telematics. The primary reason motivating the work of IS4ALL is the fact that universal access is a relatively new concept, frequently confused with more traditional approaches to accessibility. Secondly, it becomes increasingly obvious that prevailing conceptions (e.g., human-centered design), although useful, do not suffice to explicitly address universal access goals in the context of the Information Society. Thirdly, universal access is increasingly becoming a global quality attribute and a prominent factor of product/service differentiation in the public and private sectors. In this perspective, accessibility needs to be investigated beyond the traditional fields of inquiry (e.g., assistive technologies, landscapes, interior/exterior design, etc.) in the context of selected mainstream Information Society technologies and important application domains with significant impact on society as a whole, such as health, education and training, and public administration. There is, therefore, a genuine and compelling need to consolidate existing experiences into a body of knowledge, which can guide designers concerned with universal access through the various steps involved and provide concrete examples of good practice.

The domain of health telematics was selected in IS4ALL because it is a critical service sector, catering for the population at large, and at the same time involving a variety of diverse target user groups (e.g., doctors, nurses, administrators, patients).

These characteristics render it a complex domain, with an inherent diversity, and an ideal "testbed" for exemplifying the principles of universal access and assessing both the challenges and the opportunities in the context of the emerging Information Society. Such an objective entailed several challenges. Specifically, despite the increased research, academic and industrial interest in universal access in the recent past, the field requires further elaboration of the detailed knowledge necessary to practically apply universal access in the development of modern applications and services. The first and foremost evidence factor is the variety of conceptions about universal access. For instance, many researchers, typically in the field of assistive technologies, consider that universal access effectively entails a renewed interest in people with disabilities. From this perspective, it is claimed that an explicit focus on the needs and requirements of people with disabilities — who traditionally have been overlooked or underserved — will meet the objective of universal access. Others in mainstream sectors maintain that universal access is merely a matter of complying with existing principles and proven practices of user-centered design. On the other hand, others realize the need to improve prevalent user-centered design to encompass new methods of understanding user requirements and evaluating novel features of interactive software.

At the same time, previous research indicates that universal access in the context of Information Society applications and services comprises much more than incremental advances in each one of the dimensions implied by the above concepts. Indeed, it requires a better understanding of the users, which is a long-standing premise of user-centered design. However, users are no longer distinctly identifiable or easily studied. It also requires a better understanding of technology and use practices in a rapidly changing environment, but neither of these turns out to be an easy domain of study. The above considerations have motivated recent calls for revisiting existing theory, providing creative interpretation of design guidelines and establishing new engineering grounds, with the aim of extending the level and scope of current theory beyond keystrokes and task specifications to gain insight into novel computer-mediated human activities. This requires a retrospective on our experiences in the context of our expectations for the future of society and technology and a deep insight into the changes brought about by the radical pace of technological innovation, the modern and ubiquitous networking infrastructure and the proliferation of novel interactive devices. In addition, universal access cannot dismiss the changing execution contexts of tasks and the increasingly social nature of interaction.

IS4ALL has investigated the above in the context of health telematics, and has established bridges across various research communities, including usability engineering, human-computer interaction (HCI), assistive technologies, software engineering, software quality, industrial engineering, and the social sciences, in an effort to bring to the surface knowledge and best practices that can contribute to a better and more elaborate understanding of universal access. The application domain of health telematics was selected as a critical service sector in the emerging Information Society.

To achieve the intended objective, IS4ALL engaged in a data collection activity that aimed to unfold new requirements in health telematics and new or improved design processes and methods, which could be used to cater for the emerging requirements. The inquiry into health telematics was inspired by the scenario-based perspective into systems development and resulted in a rich set of representative scenarios depicting alternative patterns of use of electronic patient records. To this effect, the project involved a wide range of health telematics representatives working on health telematics research and development, everyday professional health telematics practices, regional health telematics networks, and end-users.

As for the methods, the project devised a common definition of what constitutes a 'method' and a 'process' of design. To this effect, a common template was compiled according to which all methods should be consistently described in terms of key features, such as the problem being addressed, the instruments and devices used, the process for using the device(s), inherent method assumptions, and method outcomes. This effort brought together, in a common format, knowledge (frequently tacit), that was previously hidden in practices of different design and engineering communities.

These methods, once consolidated, were validated and refined in the context of designated health telematics scenarios to assess relevance, practicality, and added value. The intention was to convey an insight into how each of the methods could be used in a practical design setting, as well as how each could be tailored to different organizational practices. The resulting experience and critical appraisal of the methods indicated the need to improve the method base with a view to establishing new design techniques to address unmet challenges.

This volume reports the most representative efforts of the IS4ALL consortium towards establishing a validated code of universal access practice. Although the book does not claim exhaustive analysis of relevant methods, it is worth noting that the methods presented share not only a common heritage, but also a common set of characteristics, aside from being oriented to interactive software design. First, they all are scenario driven, with the scenarios serving as an "engine" for directing and focusing the methods' activities. Second, the methods focus on documenting the rationale behind the design decisions made. In this way, the rationale serves as a knowledge base for existing and future decisions. Third, they all involve stakeholders so that multiple views of universal access quality are elicited, prioritized, and embodied in the systems being considered. Fourth, the methods can be tailored to the requirements and internal codes of practice of an enterprise or research group to ensure maximum benefit. Finally, the methods are compatible in the sense that a consultant, a quality assurance group, or a research team can select a specific portfolio of methods to guide their development process.

Constantine Stephanidis

Table of Contents

Part III   Design for All Methods and Their Application

Part I   Universal Access in Health Telematics

Chapter 1
Universal Access

Constantine Stephanidis[1,2]

[1] Foundation for Research and Technology – Hellas (FORTH)
Institute of Computer Science
Heraklion, Crete, GR-70013, Greece
cs@ics.forth.gr
[2] University of Crete
Department of Computer Science, Greece

Abstract. This Chapter provides an introductory account of Universal Access, identifies premises and highlights some of the reasons for attention being focused on Universal Access. The Chapter also provides a context for the work described in subsequent Chapters of the handbook.

1. Origins and Applications

The term Design for All refers to the conscious effort to consider and take account of the widest possible range of end-user requirements throughout the development lifecycle of a product or service. In many ways, universal design is not entirely new. Architects have been practicing it for several years now and have developed a common understanding, which is summarised in the following definition:

> "Instead of responding only to the minimum demands of laws, which
> require a few special features for disabled people, it is possible to
> design most manufactured items and building elements to be usable by
> a broader range of human beings, including children, elderly people,
> people with disabilities, and people of different sizes." Encyclopaedia
> of Architecture, Design, Engineering and Construction, 1989, p. 754

In recent years, there have been several applications of universal design in interior and workplace design (Mueller, 1998), housing (Mace, 1998), landscapes (Mace et al., 1991), etc. This is not to say, by any means, that the built environment we live in has been designed for all, but merely points to the fact that universal design is not specific to the Information and Communications Technologies (ICT) sector of the industry. However, the distinction that should be made is that, whereas the existing knowledge may be considered sufficient to address accessibility of physical spaces in a built environment, this is not yet the case with ICT, where universal design presents numerous challenges.

This Chapter is concerned with the challenges of Design for All in the context of Human-Computer Interaction (HCI), and with the design of interactive products and services in the domain of Health Telematics. HCI and Design for All have only

C. Stephanidis (Ed.): Universal Access Code of Practice in Health Telematics, LNCS 3041, pp. 3-8, 2005.

recently established reciprocal openings, leading to the formulation of new concepts and research agendas. Examples include the notions of Universal Access (Stephanidis et al., 1998; Stephanidis et al., 1999) and Universal Usability (Shneiderman and Hochheiser, 2001; Shneiderman, 2000), which now constitute core thematic areas in academic communities[1].

2. Universal Access

Universal Access in HCI, which is the strand motivating the present work, implies a conscious and systematic effort to advance proactive approaches (in terms of designated design processes, development tools, etc.) towards interactive products and environments that are accessible and usable by the broadest possible end-user population, anytime and from anywhere, without the need for additional adaptations or specialised (re-)design (Stephanidis et al., 1998; Stephanidis et al., 1999). It should be noted that the notion of Universal Access, as defined above, extends the previous conceptions of universal design by adding at least two dimensions of consideration. Specifically, Universal Access postulates explicit consideration, in the course of design, of the context of use and the platform and/or access terminal, in addition to users. In other words, if U, C and T represent a designated set of target user groups, envisioned contexts of use and technology platforms respectively, then Universal Access entails the consideration of a design space that is the Cartesian product UxCxT, as opposed to any particular subset. It follows, therefore, that the rationale behind Universal Access research in the context of HCI is typically grounded on revisiting some of the assumptions that have prevailed in HCI research and development efforts in the past two decades. In Chapter 1 of Stephanidis (2001c) these assumptions are summarised as follows:

- *The "average" typical user - in the context of the emerging distributed and communication-intensive information society, users are no longer the computer-literate, skilled and able-bodied workers driven by performance-oriented motives. Nor do users constitute a homogeneous mass of information seeking actors with standard abilities, similar interests and common preferences with regards to information access and use. In short, in the emerging Information Society and for the vast majority of modern applications (i.e., World Wide Web Services), conventional strategies will not necessarily help because the set of users of an application or service is*

---

[1] The term "community" is used in the present context to reflect the fact that research programmes on universal access and universal usability are scaling-up to obtain international recognition, having own and separate research agendas, technical and scientific forums (i.e., International Scientific Forum "Towards an Information Society for All" – ISF-IS4ALL, http://www.ui4all.gr/isf_is4all/ ; ERCIM WG UI4ALL, http://www.ui4all.gr/), international conferences, such as Universal Access in human Computer interaction (UAHCI) http://www.hcii2003.gr/thematic-areas/uahci.html and ACM Conference on Universal Usability (CUU) http://www.acm.org/sigchi/cuu/ and archival journals (i.e., International journal on Universal Access in the Information Society (UAIS) http://www.springeronline.com/journal/10209/about

unknowable, other than by statistical generalities, and the users have only indirect influence on developers or providers (Olsen, 1999). Instead, it becomes compelling that designers' conception of users should accommodate all potential citizens, including the young and the elderly, residential users, as well as those with situational or permanent disability.

- *The context of use - due to the unlimited business demand for information processing, the HCI community has progressively acquired a bias and habitual tendency towards outcomes (i.e., theories, methods and tools), which satisfy the business requirements and demonstrate performance improvements and productivity gains. However, since the early 1990s, analysts have been focusing on the increasing residential demand for information, which is now anticipated to be much higher than its business counterpart. Consequently, designers should progressively adapt their thinking to facilitate a shift from designing tools for productivity improvement to designing computer-mediated environments of use.*

- *Interaction devices & the "desktop" embodiment of the computer - the diffusion of the Internet as an information highway and the proliferation of advanced interaction technologies (e.g., mobile devices, network attachable equipment, etc), signify that many of the tasks to be performed by humans in the information age will no longer be bound to the visual desktop; New metaphors are likely to prevail as design catalysts of the emerging virtual spaces and the broader type and range of computer-mediated human activities. Arguably, these metaphors should encapsulate an inherently social and communication-oriented character in order to provide the guiding principles and underlying theories for designing more natural and intuitive computer embodiments. Consequently, the challenge lies within the scope of finding powerful themes and design patterns to shape the construction of novel communication spaces. At the same time it is more than likely that no single design perspective, analogy or metaphor will suffice as a panacea for all potential users or computer-mediated human activities.*

3. The Need for a Reference Framework

In the light of the above, it is argued that a prime Universal Access challenge is to provide a suitable methodological frame of reference to facilitate the objectives of understanding and designing for the global execution context of tasks. This involves the designer in a complex and iterative interplay between reflecting on prevailing practices (which may be sub-optimal) and envisioning anticipated or intended use (across a variety of contexts). The main departure from traditional design paradigms, especially those prevalent in HCI, amounts to the fact that whereas HCI designers are engaged in revising tentative designs within the realm of a specified design vocabulary (i.e., the visual embodiment of the desktop, interaction elements of some mobile devices such as PDAs), Universal Access designers increasingly need to articulate proposals which cross over the boundaries of a particular design vocabulary. In other words, Universal Access designers should seek to develop proposals to reflect how a particular task is executed by different users, under various conditions of use and using a variety of platforms or access terminals, as appropriate for a specific scenario of use. In this context, Universal Access designers are primarily engaged in the construction of new virtualities (i.e., novel concepts and tools for carrying tasks and activities), which need not necessarily follow prevailing rules of thumb or a designated set of design principles. This becomes evident when one considers some of the well-known and frequently acclaimed examples of application of universal design in landscapes (Mace et al., 1991), interior, exterior and workplace design (Mueller, 1998; Mace, 1998), and appliances (Rahman and Sprigle, 1997).

The issue therefore arises of identifying a reference frame that could inform and guide designers to pursue Universal Access in the context of HCI design. Experience from architectural or other engineering design disciplines may be useful for this purpose, but needs to be validated. On the other hand, prevalent HCI frames of reference, such as human factors and cognitive theories, have had little impact on the field, other than formulations of general principles and design guidelines. However, there are several factors impeding the use of such guidelines in the context of Universal Access. The first relates to the scope of currently available guidelines. By scope here, we imply the type and range of accessibility issues that can be adequately addressed by available knowledge and the kind of solutions that can be generated. The vast majority of the existing accessibility guidelines have been formulated on the basis of formative experimentation with people with disabilities. Despite their sound human factors content, in the majority of cases guidelines offer disability-oriented recommendations. Furthermore, their context-independent formulation, which is inherited from the context-free research protocol of the human factors evaluation paradigm, necessitates substantial interpretation before they can provide practically useful insight. Lack of structured and organised methods to facilitate interpretation, impedes even further their use.

Secondly, experience indicates that the engineering perspective adopted determines the outcome of guidelines interpretation. There are two such engineering perspectives (Stephanidis and Emiliani, 1999) briefly reviewed in Chapter 3. The first is rooted in the reactive protocol, whereby adaptations are introduced a posteriori to provide an alternative access system, used by specific user categories. In the context of Universal Access, such an approach is clearly inadequate due to the inherent complexity, and any short-term benefits are quickly outweighed by software updates, versioning, the radical pace of technological change, but also the short life-cycles of today's software products. The alternative is to formulate guidelines, resulting into systems that are inherently and by design accessible. In contrast to the previous alternative, the latter is more in line with Universal Access, since it entails proactive engineering practices to alleviate rather than remedy accessibility problems (Stephanidis, 2001a). However, with only few exceptions, it is claimed that the prevalent state of knowledge cannot facilitate such proactive accounts. Further research is needed to re-address the accessibility challenge in a more generic manner (i.e., Universal Access), which accounts not only for diversity in human abilities, but also for diversity in the technological environment and the emerging contexts of use. To this effect, the currently available accessibility guidelines offer a biased insight to HCI design, by prescribing desirable features to promote the case of accessibility by people with disabilities. However, Universal Access solutions, in the form of anyone, anywhere and at any time access systems, entail a thorough understanding of diversity, and generic approaches to address variety in: the target user community, including the disabled and elderly, as well as the technological environment (i.e., platforms, access terminals) and the contexts of use (i.e., desktop, mobile, nomadic). To this end, there is a compelling need to provide process-oriented guidance on Universal Access and develop methods that offer insights to, and take account of, the global execution contexts of tasks.

4. Methodological Frame of Reference

A possible approach to cope with the design complexity intrinsic in Universal Access draws upon action research and advocates the use of scenarios as minimal resources for design insight and evaluation (Carroll, 1995). In scenario-based design, which motivates the technical approach of IS4ALL, three phases predominate in the iterative process, and these relate to prevailing use, anticipated use and design rationale. Recent studies (Carroll, 2001) indicate that scenario-based design is becoming an increasingly accepted practice, due to several reasons; first of all, scenarios are cognitively sound and reusable; second, they offer a blending of empirical and analytical design perspectives; in this context, scenarios provide an integration of prevailing use patterns (resulting from the analysis of tasks as carried out today) and design envisionment (Carroll, 1995).

A particular track of scenario-based design builds on argumentation techniques to provide a basis for structuring the scenario analysis process. Argumentation as an approach to design is not new. In the context of software design, it amounts to the development of methodologies and notations that aim to improve the reasoning of designers. Rittel (1972) originated this approach in the Issue-Based Information System (IBIS) framework for argumentation. IBIS was a method developed by Rittel as a language and a graphical representation of the debate and negotiation, which is central to the process of tackling a particular class of problems called "wicked problems". IBIS made use of issues as a means for structuring argumentation. Options in IBIS reflect alternative design solutions to particular issues. Finally, arguments are used to formulate the pros and cons of the proposed solutions for a given issue. In recent years, the argumentation perspective was advanced further in the area of HCI, which lead to the development of additional frameworks and semi-formal notations (for a review see Carroll and Moran, 1996) for structuring arguments, communicating alternatives, documenting design reasoning and re-calling attention to HCI design problems.

IS4ALL pursues the above lines of research in the context of Health Telematics (Stephanidis and Akoumianakis, 2002). Specifically, the project adopts a technical approach based on a scenario-based perspective on systems development (Carroll, 1995; Carroll, 2001), and in particular on requirements engineering through scenarios (Jarke et al., 1998). Scenarios, in the context of IS4ALL, are perceived as narrative descriptions of computer-mediated human activities in a Health Telematics environment. The social setting of a Health Telematics environment may be bound to a clinic within the hospital, a ward within a clinic, or even to an end-user's business or residential environment. The scope of such scenarios is intended to be narrow and focused on specific issues.

Scenario analysis entails a process of extracting and developing scenarios for two primary purposes: first, to obtain a detailed insight into the Universal Access requirements relevant to Health Telematics, and second, to demonstrate the validity and applicability of the envisioned code of practice. These scenarios are being formulated around an agreed common theme, namely Electronic Patient Records. Scenario formulation is an iterative process. Initially, narrative descriptions of tasks, as carried out by actual users, are developed, and subsequently peer reviewed by health professionals or end-user communities. This peer review acts as validity check to ensure that the scenarios depict realistic and valid accounts of computer-mediated human activities in Health Telematics. In the course of this iterative phase, any system mock-ups, prototypes or other artefact that reveal aspects of the scenario's real execution context are taken into account. Once an initial formulation is compiled and agreed upon (by target users of the system being considered), scenarios are articulated in such a way as to unfold various perspectives relevant to Universal Access. Scenario articulation is primarily an argumentative process.

Chapter 2
Trends in Health Telematics:
Electronic Health Records in an Intelligent
and Communicating Environment

Georges De Moor

Ghent University
Department of Health Informatics and Statistics
De Pintelaan 185
Ghent 5k3 9000, Belgium
georges.demoor@UGent.be

Abstract. This Chapter provides a brief retrospective of how technological innovation affects and improves medical practices. It is claimed that Information Society Technologies (IST) will continue to foster radical changes in medical telematics provided that basic requirements such as quality, security, liability, interoperability, etc., become the prime design and development targets in eHealth. Moreover, as new technologies mature, Universal Access will increasingly become a predominant quality factor in medical informatics.

1. Introduction

Information and communication technology has benefited healthcare in many areas. It has allowed medical researchers to establish networks, share up-to-date information and create workflows in different geographic locations. Whereas they previously used to feel isolated in their work, they are now very much part of a larger medical research community.

Technology has also helped health administrators reduce costs, improve efficiencies, better communicate with employers and suppliers, and adapt quickly to their highly regulated and increasingly competitive environment.

The Electronic Health Records (EHRs) are of pivotal importance to any form of integrated healthcare delivery system. Physicians have embraced Information and Communication Technologies (ICT) to transmit and share mission-critical information, such as laboratory test-results, imaging data and patient records across the healthcare continuum, at any time and at the point of care. They are also seeing the benefits of Intranets, Extranets and the Internet as tools for prescription and prevention or for sending electronic lab test results to colleagues or, reminders to patients.

C. Stephanidis (Ed.): Universal Access Code of Practice in Health Telematics, LNCS 3041, pp. 9-16, 2005.

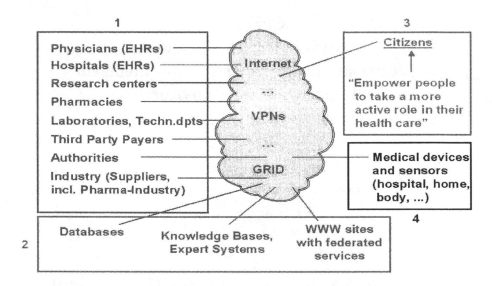

Fig. 1. Communication in e-Health: the Actors

However, not all physicians have been wholly convinced of the benefits that technology can bring to the consultation process. In the digital age, a patient and physician are required to sit down and access health networks, browse Internet sites and discuss possible remedies together.

Although physicians' offices, clinics and hospitals are bound to become Web-enabled, physicians are held back by the thought that the technology gets in the way of their proper work. Not only is the computer screen a physical barrier between patient and doctor, but the latter often feels that interacting with the computer takes away from the time they could and should be spending with the patient.

Fortunately for their patients, doctors carefully weigh a therapy against its potential risks and side effects. Many medical professionals view Information Technologies in much the same way: they are not prepared to use them until the benefits have been clearly proven. These benefits are now appearing, as doctors turn to technology to deal with, e.g., inefficient paper-based hospital systems, ever-expanding medical knowledge, and patients armed with website printouts about their condition. Supporting technology is becoming more powerful and less expensive.

At the same time citizens, are demanding a greater say and want to play a more important role in the management of their health. They want to be knowledgeable and participate in taking decisions that affect their health. This requires access to (part of) their health data as well as to the associated health information.

However, the full benefits of Electronic Healthcare (eHealth) will not be realised until there is widespread acceptance of ICT among all healthcare professionals across the board.

Next Generation Websites: "The Patients' Perspective"

- Access Internet resources for learning more about your health
- Schedule or reschedule an appointment
- Complete your own (hospital-) pre-admission forms
- Clear up billing issues
- Access (part of) any form of medical record
- Record your own personal health data
- Monitor prescription information
- Ask a physician a question
- Join a support group

(Issues : Quality, Security, Liability ...)

Fig. 2. Patient Empowerment and New Web Services

2. Mobile and Knowledge-Intensive Sector

As healthcare is a mobile and knowledge-intensive sector, many organisations today are looking for end-to-end wireless software solutions. A lot of processing power is being packed into new devices such as PDAs or PocketPCs, Tablet PCs and smart phones, allowing healthcare professionals to create new prescriptions or refill existing ones, access laboratory test results, dictate patient notes, and even take photographs of a patient's condition and email them to a colleague for a second opinion.

Only a few years ago, such wireless solutions were still regarded as risky, expensive and insecure, but they now have definitely matured from their research and development stage. The wireless revolution has been driven in part by new protocols for wireless networking, which set the interoperability rules so that users with ultra fast wireless modems can access different networks.

Using today's technology platforms and XML (Extensible Markup Language) Web services, healthcare organisations can create a seamless information environment that allows authorised parties to stay connected to their information base from any mobile device. They can operate with up-to-date information, on the Internet, on their networks, or on any other rich-client device.

The healthcare information systems are equally evolving and are becoming increasingly complementary. There are now legacy systems linked to Intranet systems and exchanging patient data through Extranets (VPNs), but also connected, through firewalls, to the Internet for accessing general content.

As healthcare organisations come to rely more heavily on electronic information systems, such as electronic medical records, they will need to increase the number of access points for staff to retrieve information. Installing and wiring workstations in different areas in a hospital or medical practice is expensive and disruptive. Wireless devices, on the other hand, tend to be less expensive than PCs and can be used at every bedside.

A great many tasks that were once performed with pen and paper can now be handled more efficiently with mobile devices. Hospital physicians can examine patients, tap their notes into a Tablet PC or some other device, and send a medication order to the hospital pharmacy via a wireless local area network. Even in an intensive care unit, computers can be connected without being tethered. It is because of scenarios such as these that healthcare professionals, who tended to be resistant to Information Technology, are now becoming the most enthusiastic proponents of wireless technology. Wireless systems disrupt established medical practice patterns far less than any other information system, and are in fact very much an extension of the physician's work.

3. Patient Oriented Healthcare

Errors made by physicians, pharmacists and other healthcare professionals are not necessarily caused by incompetence or recklessness, but often result from mistakes due to an overload of information within a complex and inefficient healthcare delivery system.

The healthcare sector is an information-intensive arena where it can be almost impossible to assimilate and relay all the information and make decisions in time-critical situations. When doctors reach for technology tools, rather than pen and paper, to write out prescriptions and patient notes, they reduce not only their paperwork but also the risk of medical errors and misplaced records. Technology can offer great benefit by making sure that the right information gets to the right people at the right time.

Technology can also be employed to prevent avoidable deaths from diseases that are not well diagnosed or monitored. For example, 150,000 Europeans die each year of heart disease complications that could be cured if recognised in time. The European Union is aiming to reduce that number by half within 10 years and then to close to zero by 2020. The European Union plans to achieve this with the help of improved monitoring through the use of technology. A number of European Commission sponsored research and development projects involve the development of portable devices with biosensors small enough to be worn as wristwatches. Patients with cardiovascular problems can wear the device and have their condition monitored continuously as the data are automatically transmitted to their doctor or hospital.

Everything is becoming intelligent and communication dependent. The next generation of healthcare technology will be one in which the computer is omnipresent. Though it will be ubiquitous, it will be unobtrusive and unnoticed–an interface with an invisible machine. Ultimately, the individual will trigger events that ICT services understand and follow up.

The combination of wireless technology and artificial intelligence will also help patients manage their own health. It will allow healthcare that used to be provided through practitioners and hospitals, to be gradually provided directly to the citizens and under their control.

Web portals also have tremendous potential in healthcare, offering personalised views of information aggregated from disparate sources. New technologies enable authorised stakeholders to access clinical information from remote locations through secure connections across the Internet to the hospital's private network. The information is then synchronised and displayed in a single visible, easy-to-read place. This is a big step towards enabling patients to maintain and control access to their personal, interactive health records.

As healthcare boundaries are fading and shifting, nobody knows what the interaction centre will be. Will it be the physician's website, the hospital's website, the patient's own health management site, an application service provider system, a medical portal, a search engine, or health service directories? The only certainty is that at present there is a trend from provider-oriented to patient-oriented healthcare.

4. Electronic Health Records: Trends

EHRs have always been considered the "Holy Grail" in health informatics and telematics: they are indeed at the centre of a multitude of eHealth applications and services.

Some of the expected benefits of health records being electronic include:

- the support of patient care and an improved quality of care;
- an enhanced productivity and a reduction of costs;
- the support of research (clinical, epidemiological, administration);
- a better privacy protection and security.

The current boundaries between the different types of EHRs (e.g., those held by physicians, nurses or even patients and healthy citizens) are fading away and their possible contexts of use are becoming rather complex. The latter is even more evident when considering the new services resulting from the merger of fields, such as medical informatics and bio-informatics (De Moor, 2003).

There is, in this context of communication and integration, a need to implement standards and policies that will ensure that distributed systems are able to interact with each other and share their data (De Moor, 1998). It is also understood that privacy legislation and security standards will have to be in place to ensure the protection of electronic records and the information they contain.

As the next generation of EHRs becomes life-long, multimedia, trans-institutional and multidisciplinary, they will inevitably be networked and virtual (hereby supporting more intelligent types of hyper-linking).

New access modes to records will naturally create new partnerships between different stakeholders. To grant access and to comply with existing security and privacy protection rules, new identification and authentication techniques will have an impact on accessibility and usability.

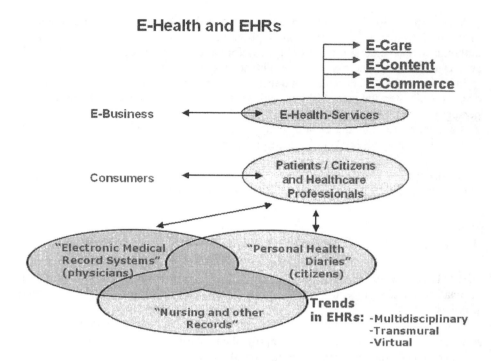

Fig. 3. Boundaries between EHRs are Fading Away

Achieving true interoperability is yet another challenge: it is critical for realising any new type of eHealth area. XML related standards (XML Schema, RDFS, OWL, etc) could hereby assist in enhancing the accessibility of health data.

Widespread interoperability is dependent upon the facility to interpret data correctly. Such correct interpretation of data requires that the meaning of the data (i.e., data semantics) be made available across applications. Capturing data structures, contents and meanings in a so-called ontology is the key step toward achieving healthcare-wide data interoperability. Natural Language Processing applied in medicine is making progress on the same basis.

New approaches should thus provide means to structure data in a machine-readable way to make independent applications communicate. Traditional XML technology is only one aspect of the total solution. Indeed, domain semantics are vital to interoperability and here RDFS (for simple semantic issues) and OWL (for more demanding ones) will most probably become some of the preferred approaches. Both RDFS and OWL are also languages with an XML syntax, but with increasingly more expressive formal semantics. Also ontology querying languages (OQL) are starting to emerge. Another important aspect is to come to a sound ontological theory on how classes, represented in an ontology, relate to the entities and processes within the real world (Ceusters et al., 2004).

All the above will enable machines to capture and exploit knowledge (cf. the linkage with Evidence Based Medicine related services).

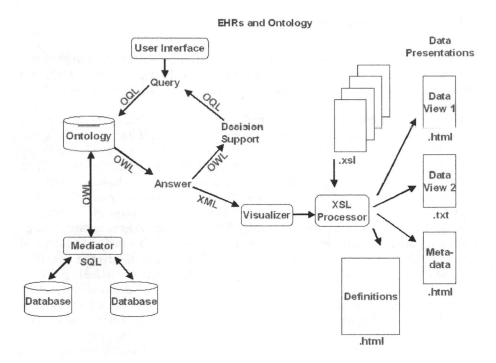

Fig. 4. The Importance of XML based Languages

The Semantic Web-like environments of the future will make content meaningful for intelligent search agents and other computer programs. As ontology and semantics relationships will continue to evolve, new expression modes will be needed to achieve more advanced and automatic maintenance mechanisms.

Last but not least, there is the promise of the emerging (Health-) Grid, which will allow to store, access and process large amounts of data by sharing resources and tools in a (virtual) distributed environment. Mass storage systems, high-end computational and other distributed Grid resources will become interlinked and, through intelligent middleware, will offer a series of new co-operative and collaborative services.

The first projects applying Grid technologies are covering such fields as medical imaging, sequence analysis, as well as database knowledge extraction (e.g., to provide guidelines to health professionals). Other collaboration examples will be the set-up of large clinical trials and the Grid interconnecting advanced diagnostic centres and health providers to make processes such as remote diagnosis possible.

The Grid will thus act as a seamless extension of the users' own workstations. As the Grid technology removes the barriers between local and remote resources, a whole range of communication scenarios will have to be re-analysed.

5. Universal Access and IS4ALL

Universal design is the term that refers to the design of interactive products and services, which respect and value the dimensions of diversity intrinsic to human capabilities, technological environments and contexts of use (Stephanidis et al., 1999).

The IS4ALL project concentrates on the European Health Telematics industry and seeks to develop appropriate instruments to facilitate approaching, internalising and exploiting the benefits of Universal Access in Health Telematics. The particular domain of Health Telematics of interest to IS4ALL is the user interaction with EHRs. In this context users comprise a broad and diverse community of humans interacting with segments of an EHR, and they include the medical community as well as other end-users (e.g., the chronically ill and in the future, healthy citizens also). Moreover, such interaction may be achieved by using different technological platforms (e.g., desktop machines, Internet appliances, mobile equipment), in a variety of contexts of use. More in particular, emerging interaction platforms, such as advanced desktop-oriented environments (e.g., advanced Graphic User Interfaces (GUIs), 3D graphical toolkits, visualisers) and mobile platforms (e.g., palmtop devices) that allow ubiquitous access to electronic data from anywhere, and any time, are expected to bring about radical improvements in the type and range of Health Telematics services. The accessibility, usability and acceptability of these solutions are key criteria for their success. To achieve its objective, IS4ALL has developed a comprehensive code of practice (e.g., enumeration of methods, process guidelines) that consolidates current knowledge of Universal Access in the context of IST, as well as concrete recommendations for emerging technologies.

Chapter 3
Towards a Universal Access Code of Practice in Health Telematics

Demosthenes Akoumianakis[1] and Constantine Stephanidis[1,2]

[1] Foundation for Research and Technology – Hellas (FORTH)
Institute of Computer Science
Heraklion, Crete, GR-70013, Greece
cs@ics.forth.gr
[2] University of Crete
Department of Computer Science, Greece

Abstract. This Chapter presents a consolidated overview of methods and techniques that can be used to advance Universal Access thinking in the design and development of interactive applications and services in Health Telematics. The results presented provide an overview of the IS4ALL "Code of Practice for Universal Access in Health Telematics", which is detailed in subsequent Chapters of the handbook. In particular, the Chapter describes the code of practice in terms of three main elements: (a) a process-oriented (macro-level) approach intended to define stages of a structured process towards Universal Access practice in Health Telematics, (b) a collection of micro-level methods which address specific technical targets across various stages of the above process, and (c) validation scenarios which exemplify the application of the code of practice in Health Telematics. The macro-level method builds upon the scenario-based perspective on systems development and unfolds stages involved in generating scenarios and devising scenario quality attributes relevant to Universal Access. Micro-methods cover a wide range of technical targets from requirements engineering for Universal Access to design representations, prototyping, evaluation and validation. The case studies intended to validate the IS4ALL results have been selected to reflect alternative access regimes to Electronic Patient Records. The Chapter concludes with a discussion and critical review of the implications of Universal Access for Health Telematics applications development, and with the identification of prominent challenges to be addressed through further research.

1. Introduction

IS4ALL aims to advance the principles and practice of *Universal Access* in IST focusing on the area of Health Telematics, and on emerging technologies shaping the nature and contents of this domain. The primary focus of IS4ALL is on the impact of advanced desktop and mobile interaction technologies on emerging Health Telematics products and services. Health Telematics, as a domain of application of Universal Access, offers a rich resource due to its explicit focus on catering for the population at

C. Stephanidis (Ed.): Universal Access Code of Practice in Health Telematics, LNCS 3041, pp. 17-35, 2005.
© Springer-Verlag Berlin Heidelberg 2005

large, thus involving a variety of diverse target user groups (e.g., doctors, nurses, administrators, patients), a rapidly increasing range of computer-mediated tasks, and a broad typology of contexts of use in which these tasks are executed (e.g., emergency situations, clinical settings, home-based care, etc). These characteristics render Health Telematics a complex domain - due to the inherent diversity - and an ideal "test bed" for exemplifying the principles of Universal Access, and assessing both the challenges and the opportunities in the context of the emerging Information Society. The specific objectives of IS4ALL have been elaborated elsewhere (see Stephanidis and Akoumianakis, 2002). For the purposes of this Chapter, it suffices to point out IS4ALL's principal technical target, which is the compilation of a validated code of practice to advance Universal Access thinking in Health Telematics. To attain this technical objective, IS4ALL seeks to provide design support at both the macro-level (i.e., a process-oriented protocol to explain to practitioners the steps and phases involved) and the micro-level (i.e., definition and examples of techniques to be used to attain specific targets, such as Universal Access requirements gathering, design, development, etc). The compound collection of validated macro- and micro-methods, along with the reference case studies, compile the IS4ALL Universal Access code of practice in Health Telematics.

The rest of this Chapter is structured as follows. The next section provides a contextual account of Universal Access in terms of its early connotations and of its meaning in the context of the present work, as well as of the research and development work that has been driving the prevalent Universal Access engineering methods. Then, the IS4ALL code of practice is described in terms of theoretical underpinnings, macro-level processes and micro-level methods. Finally, the Chapter provides insights to lessons learnt and discussion on the practicalities of the methods presented. The Chapter concludes with a summary and plans for future work.

2. Universal Access: Background and State of the Art

2.1 Conceptions and Engineering Perspectives

Two prevalent approaches, namely *reactive* and *proactive*, have emerged in the recent past to address the issue of accessibility. They are distinctively characterised by the timing of appreciating and responding to the problem of accessibility (Stephanidis and Emiliani, 1999), which in turn, gives raise to alternative engineering practices and corresponding solutions. In what follows, we will briefly review the baselines of each approach emphasising their relative merits and drawbacks in the context of accessibility.

2.1.1 The Reactive Approach

The first approach assumes a *reactive* perspective according to which accessibility is an a posteriori concern, remedied by developing add-ons or adapting the original implementation of a product or service to accommodate new requirements, as they arise. The reactive approach, which is the oldest and most explicitly related to disability access (Stephanidis and Emiliani, 1999), has given rise to several methods for addressing accessibility, including techniques for the configuration of input / output at the level of user interface, the provision of alternative access systems, such as screen readers for blind users, scanning techniques for motor impaired, as well as an extensive body of knowledge in the form of human factors and ergonomic guidelines (ISO TS 16071, Nicolle and Abascal, 2001; W3C-WAI guidelines[1]).

Experience with these techniques reveals several shortcomings which amount to fatal consequences for generic accounts of accessibility (Stephanidis, 2000a). Some of them emerge from the fact that reactive methods effectively facilitate the reproduction instead of the redesign of the dialogue, which in turn, requires extensive configuration of physical interaction parameters in order to be usable. Furthermore, there are inherent problems, which frequently cannot be overcome at the implementation level (e.g., cannot reproduce graphical images in a non-visual form). Most importantly, however, reactive methods – being programming intensive and lacking suitable tools to expedite development – exhibit no upward compatibility e.g., to new interaction technologies and terminals. These shortcomings have necessitated a revision of the reactive approach towards more generic accounts of accessibility, which is the premise of the proactive approach.

2.1.2 The Proactive Approach

The second and more recent approach is *proactive*, treating accessibility from the early phases of concept creation and design and throughout the development life cycle (Stephanidis and Emiliani, 1999; Stephanidis et al., 1998; Stephanidis et al., 1999; Stephanidis, 2001a). According to the proactive approach, designers need to invest effort in anticipating new / changing requirements and accommodating them explicitly in the design of the product or service in such a way as to allow for incremental design updates from the start. On the other hand, developers require tools offering extended facilities for the management of interaction elements and object classes (Savidis and Stephanidis, 2001b).

In the recent past, there have been several efforts aiming to promote proactive accounts of accessibility particularly in the context of Human Computer Interaction (HCI). For example, in the mid-90s the concept of *user interfaces for all* (Stephanidis, 1995), was the first systematic effort to provide a methodological and an engineering base for the development of universally accessible user interfaces. *Unified user interface development* (Stephanidis, 2001b), is the methodology proposed to facilitate this effort, while a collection of dedicated user interface software development tools (Savidis et al. 1997, Savidis and Stephanidis, 2001a) and design environments (Akoumianakis and Stephanidis, 1997) comprises the engineering instruments for realising user interfaces for all. Following the proposal of the *user interfaces for all* concept, and with the progressive move towards an Information Society, the notions of *Universal Access* (Stephanidis et al., 1998), *Information Society for all* (Stephanidis et al., 1999) and *universal usability* (Shneiderman, 2000) became prominent research topics and acknowledged thematic areas of research and development activities within academic communities.

Finally, under the cluster of proactive approaches, one should also acknowledge some early research and development activities, either at national or international

---

[1] http://www.w3.org/WAI/Resources/#gl

level, such as the FRIEND21 project (Ueda, 2001) funded by the Japanese MITI, the AVANTI project (Stephanidis et al., 2001) which was funded by the European Commission, but also recent industrial initiatives, such as Active Accessibility by Microsoft and Java Accessibility by Sun Microsystems (Korn and Walker, 2001).

2.1.3 The Problem to Date

For the purposes of the present work, a system is considered to be universally accessible if it can be accessed effectively, efficiently and with satisfaction by all authorised users, anytime and from anywhere, without applying other actions or means than those provided for this purpose for the software considered. This definition raises several implications summarised as follows:

- Universal Access is more than mere (low-cost) access.
- Universal Access assumes high usability.
- Universal Access means adaptation on behalf of the software.
- Universal Access entails not only user perceived qualities, but also features related to the development process.

Summarising the above, it is claimed that Universal Access requires an engineering base for unfolding, understanding and designing for the global execution context of tasks. To understand the global execution context of a task, one needs to cope with expected, foreseeable or likely changes, which can occur in the course of the task's execution. These changes, in turn, may be due to diversity in the target users groups, to alternative computational platforms hosting the executable task, but also to the physical environment in which a designated task is executed. It stands, therefore, to reason that designing for Universal Access is synonymous with designing for diversity or designing to cope with change.

Being able to explicitly foresee in advance and design a system so as it can cope with all possible changes in its execution context is probably a utopia. Consequently, the scope of a Universal Access code of practice should be the incremental construction of systems capable of undertaking the required context-sensitive processing to address and optimally respond to the changes taking place in their execution contexts. This assumes two prime responsibilities in the short to medium and long term. In the short to medium term, designers should proactively account for all those changes that can be identified and addressed in the course of design. For unforeseen changes, which may occur at a later stage as a result of changing user requirements, emergence of new computational platforms or novel contexts of use, the system's design should facilitate incremental updates so as to enhance its context-sensitive processing capabilities. In light of the above, the prominent challenge for Universal Access in the context of IST amounts to developing theory (e.g., models of global execution context of tasks) and engineering practices (e.g., design representations, tools, etc) towards designing to accommodate the global execution context of tasks.

2.1.4 The Focus of IS4ALL

In light of the above, IS4ALL set out to exemplify some of the above in the context of Health Telematics and in particular the area of Health Telematics concerned with access to Electronic Patient Records. Several clarifications need to be made before we outline the results of the project. First of all, the focus of IS4ALL is on the interactive manifestation (i.e., the user interface) of Electronic Patient Records and not the digital contents or the way in which it is structured, captured or represented. Second, the scope of Universal A considerations should span across a variety of issues including:

- *User-oriented aspects*, where users could vary in professional backgrounds (e.g., medical doctors, paramedics, patients), roles undertaken (e.g., administrative, data input, retrieval and diagnosis) and in physical capabilities (e.g., novices, elderly, patients with disabilities).
- *Interaction platforms* referring to the hardware and software elements of the computational environment in which a task is carried out (e.g., desktop terminals, PDAs, cellular phones).
- *Context-oriented* aspects indicating the alternative physical environments from which medical records may be accessed.

Third, IS4ALL did not consider issues related to security of data or unauthorised use, which, however, constitutes a critical issue in the context of Universal Access.

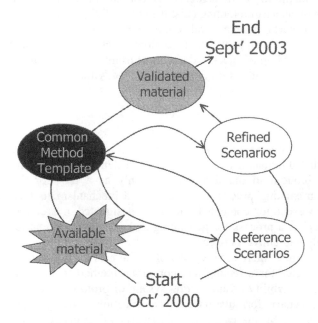

Fig. 1. Stages in IS4ALL methodology of work

Consequently, the emphasis is on engineering methods that can facilitate the design of Electronic Patient Records as interactive systems capable of performing context-sensitive processing to cope with changes in the execution contexts resulting from the three general categories of diversity identified above (i.e., user diversity, proliferation of interaction platforms and context variety). To attain its technical goal, IS4ALL engaged in a process (see Figure 1) to: (i) analyse and document accumulated knowledge on universal design and Universal Access, (ii) compile representative scenarios of Electronic Patient Records access to identify current use practices, and

(iii) devise methods to enrich the scenarios so as to depict designated Universal Access requirements (e.g., adaptability, scalability, platform independence, personalisation / individualisation, etc).

3. The IS4ALL Code of Practice on Universal Access

In the context of IS4ALL, Universal Access implies: (a) understanding how designated tasks are carried out by different users, across different interaction platforms and diverse contexts of use, (b) devising suitable artefacts for each relevant task execution context, and (c) building systems which can exhibit alternative interactive manifestation through context sensitive processing. IS4ALL has defined a technical macro-level approach, which is based on the scenario-based perspective on systems development (Carroll, 2001), and in particular on the use of dialogical techniques to advance a design practice which treats design as inquiry (Carroll and Rosson 1992) and inquiry as dialogue. At the core of our scenario-based process is an extended form of scenario retooling (Erskine et al., 1997), which is advanced through techniques for scenario screening and compilation of growth scenarios. The result is a set of techniques for using structured dialogue between stakeholders to increase designers' understanding of specific domains of users' work as well as to propose and define new execution contexts for the users' work activities.

3.1 Macro-level

Scenarios in the context of IS4ALL are perceived as narrative descriptions of computer-mediated human activities in a Health Telematics environment. In IS4ALL, scenarios are brought to the forefront, not only as a tool for documenting and reflecting upon existing practices, but also as a mechanism to foresee, study and understand new execution contexts for the tasks designated in a reference scenario.

Figure 2 depicts a process for generating and articulating scenarios to understand and gain insight into Universal Access.

As shown in Figure 2, there are a variety of techniques for generating scenarios. One important parameter for selecting an appropriate method to generate the reference scenario is the availability of an existing system or prototype. If a system is already available, then scenario formulation entails a reflection on designated tasks as carried out by actual users. In this case, the scenario should effectively document existing behaviours of end users. If the system is new, thus not available, then the scenario should act as a source for generating new user behaviours and unfold envisioned tasks to be supported. Once the scenario is agreed on, it then becomes the prominent resource for designing and evaluating concepts and tentative mock-ups. The design activities follow an analytical perspective influenced by design-space analysis techniques, retooled to facilitate an understanding of Universal Access. Initially, this implies an explicit account of the assumptions behind the scenario, which in subsequent stages are relaxed to envision how the scenario can be revised to accommodate novel execution contexts. This process of identifying assumptions and subsequently relaxing them is referred to as *scenario screening*, while generating new interaction styles suitable for the revised scenarios is referred to as compiling *growth scenarios* (Stephanidis and Akoumianakis, 2002). The rest of this section is devoted to reviewing some of the methods, which can be used in each of the three analytic steps depicted in Figure 2.

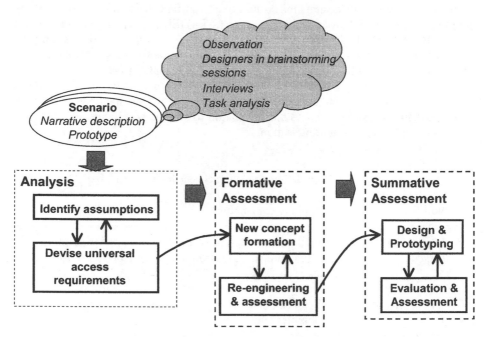

Fig. 2. Overall approach for working with scenarios

3.2 Micro-level

Various micro-methods have been defined to address specific design challenges posed by the process outlined above. All the addressed methods are *complete* in the sense of Olson and Moran, 1996. In other words, each one has been elaborated in terms of several features listed in Table 1.

However, a summary of representative micro-methods is depicted in Table 2.

The methods are represented by the rows in the table, while the three columns depict an elaboration of each method in terms of the basic criteria for complete design micro-methods proposed by Olson and Moran (1996), reproduced in Table 1. Further details on the development of each method and its application and validation in the context of Health Telematics are provided in the related Chapters as indicated in Table 2.

An important characteristic of the IS4ALL methods is their complementary nature in the context of a scenario-based inquiry. In practice, this is typically translated into portfolios of methods spanning all phases of development from requirements engineering to concept formulation, design of low- or high-fidelity prototypes and evaluation. For example, at an early stage the Universal Access Assessment

Workshop (UA^{2}W) method (Chapter 11, see also Akoumianakis and Stephanidis, 2003a) may be used to identify key Universal Access requirements (e.g., adaptability to different users, portability to different platforms) and to provide representative growth scenarios. To address some of these requirements and to realise the corresponding growth scenarios, the designer may choose from a suitable mix of methods to represent design mock-ups (e.g., unified user interface), develop prototypes (e.g., model-based techniques such as TADEUS, Chapter 18) and evaluate the results (e.g., MEdicSCORE, Chapter 19). In section 5 of this Chapter, we briefly comment on the criteria to be used when selecting methods, thus offering a basic guide as to how Health Telematics practitioners could make use of and exploit the methodology as well as individual methods. To this end, however, practitioners should note that the most effective and efficient use of the methods is through tailoring them to custom-practises and adaptation to suit the specific design tradition, processes and culture of an organisation.

Table 1. Template for micro-methods

Method feature	Example/ explanation
Problem being addressed	Requirements capture, artefact representation, capture design rationale, assessment of accessibility / usability, etc.
Device / technique(s) used	Representation technique, tool, checklist, design principles, etc.
Procedure for using the device	Structured sequence of inter-related phases.
Outcomes	Artefacts, scenarios of use or use cases, design templates, usability evaluation report, identification of accessibility problems, etc.
Assumptions	Prerequisites for using the method and which may relate to the availability of an artefact, availability of users, etc.
Examples	These are typically reported in the Chapters of Part C of this book in the validation case studies presented for each of the methods.

Table 2. Micro-methods

	Statement of the problem	Device (a tool, technique or model)	Statement of the nature of the result
Universal Access Assessment Workshop (*Chapter 11*)	UA²W sessions are held to: ○ Facilitate an insight into the current tasks in a reference scenario ○ Identify new plausible task execution contexts ○ Formulate growth scenarios	○ Scenario screening ○ Growth scenarios	○ Universal Access Assessment Form (UA²F) ○ Universal Access Quality Matrix (UAQM)
Non-functional Requirements Analysis (*Chapter 13*)	Drive interaction design providing the means for unfolding design options and building interaction design spaces.	○ Non-functional requirements as design drivers in design space analysis	○ Population of the NfRs hierarchy with clear indication of the specific NfRs considered and how they are intertwined. ○ A rich NfR-populated design space with mock-ups and low-fidelity prototypes accompanied by design rationale linking the various options to the NfRs hierarchy.

Requirements engineering

Design and development

	Statement of the problem	Device (a tool, technique or model)	Statement of the nature of the result
Unified User Interface Design (*Chapter 12*)	Fuse all potentially distinct design alternatives into a single unified for without requiring multiple design phases.	o Polymorphic task hierarchy	o Polymorphic task hierarchy o Styles of interaction o Interface adaptation rationale
Multimodal interfaces (*Chapter 17*)	Provide a design approach that makes it possible to create interfaces interpret multimodal input data and generate multimodal output	o A generic architecture based on a five-layer software model.	o Generic multimodal user interfaces
Model-based development (*Chapter 18*)	Develop design representations which allow the development of role-adapted user interfaces	Models & design representations of: o Users o Tasks o Interaction o Domain	o Design models and representations o User interface specification o Prototypes of role-adapted user interfaces
Participatory Methods (*Chapter 21*)	Gain insight into the context of use of an artefact or the way in which tasks are performed by end users and allow user-involved and consensus-based design of systems to be used by different end-user communities.	o Short visits to end user sites o Questionnaires o Interviews o Brainstorming o User Trials o Task analysis	o Rich empirical data sets useful for design teams and evaluators

Evaluation

	Statement of the problem	Device (a tool, technique or model)	Statement of the nature of the result
Screening (*Chapter 14*)	An inspection-based technique which seeks to identify potential barriers to use (according to filters) in a scenario and develop proposals to eliminate them	o Accessibility filters o Heuristics o Design criteria or principles	The filtering grid, which consolidates: o Set of Universal Access filters o Universal access problem descriptions o Rationale for new artifacts
W3C-WAI Content Accessibility Auditing (*Chapter 15*)	Ensure accessibility of WWW content for people with disabilities	o Guidelines o Checkpoints o Priority levels	o Accessibility problems o Possible corrective actions o Conformance level A, AA, AAA
Usability inspection (*Chapter 16*)	Find usability problems in the design	o Cognitive walkthrough o Feature inspection o Heuristic Evaluation	o Usability report which includes findings (i.e., potential usability problems) and recommendations for fixing them.
MedicSCORE (*Chapter 19*)	Provide a multifaceted and holistic framework for the design and evaluation of electronic health records (EHR)	o Expert screening o User observation	o A list of strengths and weaknesses of the evaluated EHR. o A problem severity rating
Standards Adherence and Compliance (*Chapter 20*)	How standards can provide a structured instrument for summative evaluation of Universal Access in the case of Health Telematics	o Audit o ISO standards	o Specification of context of use o Specification of usability o Determination of consistency / compliance with criteria o Revised system or product

4. Reference Scenarios and Validation

To validate the methods and to consolidate the experiences into a code of practice, IS4ALL compiled reference scenarios. All reference scenarios are related to accessing Electronic Patient Records, but they reveal alternative usage contexts. Thus, there are scenarios addressing access to medical records by doctors on duty moving around in the ward of a hospital, members of a hospital's administration department, surgeons in (or preparing to enter) the operating theatre, paramedics attending to an emergency situation with an ambulance, patients accessing parts of their medical record from a residential environment, etc. In all cases, the objective has been to make use of the methods described earlier to analyse, revise and extend the initial formulations of the scenarios, so as to address designated Universal Access challenges.

Thus, there have been studies addressing the *accessibility* of selected parts of a system by using the W3C Content Accessibility Guidelines (Chapter 15, see also Burzagli and Emiliani, 2003), the *adaptability* of a system to different user roles (e.g., view of medical record by pathologists, paramedics, administrators) by applying model-based approaches to user interface development (Chapter 18, see also Stary, 2003), the *usability* of a system by making use of heuristics and feature inspections (Chapter 16, see also Karampelas et al., 2003), and *patients' access* to medical data using participatory analysis methods (Chapter 21, see also Stroetmann and Pieper, 2003).

In total, sixteen validation case studies carried out in the course of the project cover a range of typical concerns facing Universal Access practitioners. They can be summarised in terms of their intended focus and contribution, as follows:

- *Articulating Universal Access quality attributes*: When starting a new project recognising that adaptability, scalability, platform independence, ubiquitous access are important qualities to be addressed, then *Non-Functional Requirements (NFRs)* analysis can provide an explicit focus on these quality attributes highlighting how they are intertwined. Moreover, the technique can help identify user, software and accessibility requirements, thus facilitating informed choice of critical system parameters, such as the architecture (Chapter 13).

- *Understanding the global execution context of a task (or scenario):* When there is no system but a design concept, then UA^2Ws can help define shortcomings in the design concept, envision new contexts of use, which the initial design concept should aim to facilitate and define new design concepts by consensus. In cases where a system is already available, UA^2Ws can be also used to facilitate a consensus-based analysis and the compilation of growth scenarios illustrating system extensions towards Universal Access (Chapter 11).

- *Mapping requirements to analytical design representations*: When requirements are specified and detailed design work is being undertaken, then *Unified User Interface Development* can help develop design representations, map representations of artefacts, develop a design rationale and foster incremental design updates (Chapter 12, see also Savidis and Stephanidis, 2004a). The usefulness of this method has been demonstrated using an extract of the MediBRIDGE/C-CARE reference scenario and building polymorphic task hierarchies to allow access to a patient's record users with different access rights using different interaction platforms in different contexts.

- *From design representations to model-based prototyping*: When there is a system to be improved, then *model-based development* can help build quick mock-ups, test mock-ups with end-users, identify usability problems and revise accordingly the initial prototypes. This was validated using the TADEUS model-based development environment and an Austrian Health Telematics scenario (Chapter 18, see also Stary, 2003), focusing on populating the TADEUS models and subsequently using these models to generate role-adapted user interfaces. The user roles considered were those of an administration assistant, a paramedic in a ward responsible for updating a patient's medical record following an operation, and that of a doctor. In all cases, TADEUS generated alternative user interfaces for accessing the patient's medical record depending on the user's role and corresponding interests, task sequence and access rights.
- *Focusing on accessibility and usability:* When there is an explicit requirement for accessibility then the *W3C-WAI Content Accessibility Guidelines (WCAG) Audit* can provide useful guidance on what is to be done during design, the shortcomings to be corrected as well as specific accessible design recommendations. As an example, a typical WCAG Audit was designed and carried out to assess the accessibility of specific parts of the Health Telematics information system in Pisa, Italy, focusing specifically on the parts of the system available through the World Wide Web. The audit concentrated on Web elements such as text, table and images to identify shortcomings in the current implementation as well as to provide recommendations and prototypes of improved accessibility (Chapter 16, see also Burzagli and Emiliani, 2003).

5. Experience, Feedback, and Lessons Learnt

All methods briefly described above have been validated in at least one reference scenario, while the results of the validation have been widely presented to the Health Telematics community in the course of six IS4ALL seminars and four consolidation workshops with invited experts from the field. One prominent issue raised during the assessment of these methods with field experts relates to the choice of methods and the criteria, which need to be kept in mind to facilitate informed choice. In this section, an attempt is made to address precisely this issue in an effort to provide guidance to Health Telematics practitioners.

5.1 Scope of the Methods

The methods of the IS4ALL code of practice and their corresponding validation case studies cover a wide range of issues related to the various phases of software development. In the context of the project, they have been used for one or more of the following purposes:

- Early in the development life cycle, either to elicit requirements or to facilitate concept formation and low-fidelity prototyping.
- During design to facilitate the development of design representations and design rationale.

- In the context of a user-involved prototyping stage, facilitating computer-mock-ups of low-fidelity artefacts compiled in the course of early requirements engineering or concept formation.
- During development to provide support for adaptable user interface development.
- As formative design instruments in the course of design to assess progress or obtain end user feedback before committing to a final design concept.
- To provide instruments for summative evaluation of high-fidelity prototypes or a system as a whole.
- Establishing benchmarking instruments for long-term process or product improvement strategies.
- Assessing adherence and compliance to process- or product-oriented standards and thereby claiming accreditation.
- Choosing appropriate development tools or selecting an architectural abstraction suitable to the system's intended purpose and scope of use.
- Evaluating compliance to accessibility guidelines related to a particular user group or category of users.

Table 2. Scope of the IS4ALL methods

Phase	Target	Technique/method
Requirements gathering	Quality attributes	*NFRs Analysis*
		UA^2W
	User interface requirements	*Unified User Interface Design*
		Participatory methods
Concept formation & design	Low-fidelity prototypes	UA^2W
		Screening
		Participatory methods
	Design representations	*Unified User Interface Design*
		Model based development
	Design rationale	*Unified User Interface Design*
		UA^2W
Prototyping and development	User-adapted interfaces	*Model based development*
	Accessible user interfaces	*Multimodal Interfaces*
		Unified User Interface Design
Evaluation	Formative	*Usability Inspection*
	Summative	*Standards compliance*
		MedicSCORE
	Accessibility	*WCAG Audit*

Table 3 summarises the above and provides a guide for choosing a method depending on the intended purpose and phase within a project. It should be noted that there are no absolute measures of comparing the methods or assessing their potential value and contribution. Much depends on project-specific details (e.g., scope of the project, development phase, resources), management practices (i.e., commitment to

Universal Access versus opportunistic interest), and on the competence of the practitioners and their previous experience in the use of the methods. In the following section, we provide some insight into how the above may influence the choice of methods based on one's own experience in the use of the methods in various circumstances and design cases. However, our discussion is only illustrative of the considerations to be addressed and thus it should not be interpreted as an absolute guide towards selecting design methods. In general, the ultimate choice will depend on the relative weighting factors assigned to the various influencing parameters.

5.2 Criteria to Be Considered

Selecting an appropriate portfolio of methods to facilitate Universal Access will have to take into account a range of considerations. Some of them are of a general nature, while others are specific to the project in which the methods are to be applied. In what follows, we provide a brief account of both these categories of factors indicating plausible options based on the experience accumulated in the course of the IS4ALL project.

5.2.1 Scope of Universal Access Deliberations

Scope of Universal Access entails an understanding of the dimension of Universal Access relevant to the project. For example, the intended scope of Universal Access may be to facilitate:

- *User-adapted* access to a system by different categories of users, including elderly and people with disabilities; in this case, designing for diverse user groups should be the prominent criterion for selecting design methods.
- *Context-adapted* access to the system so as to allow access to the system's functionality across different contexts of use using alternative access devices and media; in this case the prominent criterion for selecting methods is its capability to capture diverse contexts of use and platform independence.
- *Platform* independence so as to allow the system to scale up or down so as to become usable across different platforms; in this case the relevant criterion is to use development methods (e.g., such as TADEUS), which provide inherent support for platform abstraction and integration.

Alternatively, it may be the case that the project seeks to introduce Universal Access features into a pre-existing system. In this case, Universal Access forms a methodological approach towards re-engineering of the initial system. However, there may be limiting constraints posed by the original implementation which may be binding conditions and difficult to overcome. Such constraints may be related to the development and implementation level and the corresponding tools that have been used to realise the system. For instance, the system's architecture may be such that it seriously inhibits the system's portability. This makes re-engineering based on Universal Access with the intention to build a platform-independent system rather expensive, if indeed possible.

The above indicate that prior to any effort aiming to address Universal Access in the context of a specific project, it is important that the design team invests considerable time to identify the scope of Universal Access and to establish relevant criteria, which will influence the selection of appropriate methods.

5.2.2 Gaining the Commitment of Management

Another issue that is likely to influence the choice of methods is the commitment of management to Universal Access. As in the case of usability engineering, the higher the commitment of management the more complete and involved the design process will be. Completeness of the design approach means that the design team will pay the attention needed to all stages of design and make use of suitable methods to facilitate the objectives of each stage. In the context of the IS4ALL Universal Access code of practice, this may entail a choice of user-based or participatory methods to gather functional and non-functional requirements (e.g., UA^2Ws), more demanding design techniques (e.g., Unified User Interface Design) to facilitate artefact representations and mock-ups, and advanced prototyping tools (e.g., TADEUS) which allow quick prototyping of design concepts and assessment of end-users' feedback regarding the system being developed. However, all these methods incur a cost, as they do not constitute typical design practice in prevalent software development paradigms.

Absence of management commitment to Universal Access will most likely hinder the willingness of the design team to engage in analytical design and explore plausible options. In this case, the Universal Access inquiry is likely to be limited in scope, resulting in ad hoc selection of methods. It is therefore important for the design team to realise and, if necessary, seek to obtain management commitment to Universal Access, as this is likely to act as catalyst and a driving force of design activities. Nevertheless, to gain this commitment, the design team should be able to justify the technical approach towards Universal Access, the claims made on resources as well as the expected / resulting benefits.

5.2.3 Competence of the Design Team

Finally, effective use of Universal Access methods requires some special skills, which should be available in the design team. These skills are typically method-specific. For example, seeking to assess compliance to a standard requires knowledge of the standard in question and experience in auditing. Similarly, assessment of the system's accessibility will require experience in using and interpreting accessibility guidelines, competence in the use of tools for carrying out such assessments and knowledge of the limits of these tools. However, one can expect that such skills will be available to the design team or could be easily acquired through external sources.

In addition to the above, there are methods, which can be effectively used only by specialised designers possessing detailed knowledge of certain design domains. Examples of such methods include the UA2W, non-functional requirements analysis, screening artefacts and model-based development methods for prototyping. Effective use of these methods typically requires prior experience in planning and conducting the design inquiry and the capability to synthesise results of analytical inquiries. Moreover, the experience gained through the IS4ALL seminars reveals that training to use these methods in practical settings is important and necessary for designers to gain competence. Such training sessions do not need to be extensive but they do require detailed planning and execution to allow designers to gain hands-on experience in the use of specialised instruments for conducting the method. For instance, completing a Universal Access Assessment Form (A2F) or compiling the Universal Access Quality Matrix (UAQM) require an understanding of the UA2W method, the processes involved and the way in which the designer can move from the concrete to the abstract level.

6. Universal Access Versus Prevailing Practices

From the discussion thus far, and the experience gained throughout the project, it becomes evident that Universal Access introduces several challenges to software development practices. Some of them are intrinsic to the aims and objectives of Universal Access and thus require dedicated research efforts by the Universal Access engineering community. Others however are compliant with on-going efforts in Human Computer Interaction and Software Engineering, thus establishing a potential for common ground and cross-disciplinary contributions. In this section, we recapitulate some important implications of Universal Access and relate them to prevailing engineering practices. Our intention is to show that, although Universal Access remains a viable goal in software development, it will require substantial extensions or refinements in prevalent practices before industry can fully capitalise the benefits of Universal Access.

Table 4 provides a summary of such implications by contrasting premises of prevailing practices (mainly in HCI) against premises pertaining to Universal Access design. The table seeks to convey the shift (along various criteria) that is necessitated by a commitment to Universal Access. Some of these shifts are substantial but possible, given the current state of knowledge and the accumulated know-how, while others require additional research to become viable and feasible. Specifically, today there are methodologies addressing NFRs both in terms of underlying processes needed to attain designated goals corresponding to NFRs (Mylopoulos et al., 1992; Barbacci et al., 1995; Barbacci et al., 2002; Bass et al., 1998), and in terms of measurable product attributes, such as for example adaptability (Subramanian and Chung, 2003). Nevertheless, their relevance to Universal Access or their refinement to facilitate Universal Access targets is still pending. On the other hand, there are issues raised in the table, which are still in a research phase and the only evidence is through experimental laboratory prototypes. This is the case for most of the transitions described under the development and implementation category.

With regards to HCI design, which has been the primary focus of the present work, it is important to acknowledge that Universal Access necessitates a blending between traditional and new methodologies, which can result in new design methods, tools and engineering practice. The prominent target should be the commitment to an analytical perspective to unfold insights regarding the global execution context of (a set of) tasks. Then, the engineering challenge amounts to the management of design spaces (e.g., the broad range of styles and the accompanying rationale), which must be appropriate or plausible for alternative execution contexts. Managing complex design spaces entails, enumerating plausible alternative styles, justifying their role in the design space, relating them to the global execution context of the associated task, specifying conditions for style initiation and termination, style re-engineering, etc. As

Table 3. Assessment of Universal Access versus the traditional paradigm

Phase	Criterion	Traditional paradigm	Universal access design
Requirements engineering	Scope	Capturing the data and the functions a system should support	In addition to the traditional scope, emphasis is on non-functional requirements (NFRs) such as adaptability, scalability, platform independence, usability, etc.
	Approach	A variety of techniques for data-, function- or object-oriented analysis, e.g., entity-relationship diagrams, data flow diagrams, object-oriented models	Goal-oriented driven by NFRs to complement traditional approaches
Design	Focus	Generating a single artefact that meets the designated requirements	o Exploration of design alternatives to address the NFRs and analysis of trade offs
	Unit for dialogue design	Physical interaction objects	Abstract interaction object classes
	Outcome	Single artefact depicting physical user tasks	o Collection of alternative task structures (as opposed to a single interaction object hierarchy) represented by multiple dialogue styles o Accompanying rationale for each task structure and style
	Representation	Interaction object hierarchy	o Abstract object classes o Rationalised design space
	Process	User-centred design	Enumerate – Retool – Rationalise cycles
Development & implementation	Implementation model	Programming as the basis for generation of the run-time environment of the system	Generation of run-time environment by compiling an abstract specification
	Premise of run-time code	Making direct calls to the platform	Linking to the platform
	Platform independence	Generalisation across platforms belonging to a certain class (e.g., GUI window managers)	Platform abstraction mechanism which mediates between the specification and the target platforms
	Platform utilisation	Multi-platform environments	Multiple toolkit environment

discussed earlier, some of the above require new methods to address the corresponding challenge, while other challenges may be facilitated by refinement and extension of existing methods.

7. Concluding Remarks

In the previous parts of this Chapter we have overviewed and summarised recent efforts in the direction of consolidating current design practices on Universal Access and constructing a validated code of practice to guide designers in identifying Universal Access challenges and subsequently planning and devising appropriate processes and methods to cope with them. Our account of the topic has not been exhaustive, but rather illustrative of the type of methods considered appropriate for Universal Access and the way in which specific challenges can be addressed. However, one can draw some conclusions regarding the contributions of the present work and the future research that is needed.

The contributions of the IS4ALL project to advancing Universal Access and closing the gap between Universal Access engineering and prevalent practices are three-fold. First, we have tried to define the scope of the Universal Access inquiry, as an effort towards understanding and designing for the global execution context of tasks. Second, the project has compiled for the first time a collection of design-oriented methods, covering the major phases of HCI design, such as requirements gathering, design and evaluation, emphasising their contribution to the aforementioned challenges. Finally, the designated methods have been validated to assess their practical application to allow Universal Access insights in the context of specific reference scenarios from the domain of Health Telematics and in particular access to Electronic Patient Records. The above three types of contributions constitute the IS4ALL code of practice for Universal Access in Health Telematics.

As the code of practice is an on-going effort, future work focuses on studying additional methods and refining some of the concepts. With regards to new methods, future work should focus on emerging techniques related to the use of biometrics to enhance adaptive behaviour and security, as well as multi-modal techniques. One particular dimension of methods-oriented work, which needs additional attention, is related to providing tools, which ease the task of developing universally accessible systems. Another issue requiring further work is developing a comprehensive benchmarking framework for Universal Access. The work conducted so far has reviewed and pointed out desirable Universal Access properties of interactive software, but clearly further research is needed in the direction of establishing a complete and effective benchmarking framework comprising qualitative and quantitative process- and product/service-oriented measures of Universal Access.

In conclusion, it is important to note that Universal Access engineering as presented in this handbook is not necessarily a niche methodology relevant to a particular type of interactive system or service. On the contrary, it is presented as a mainstream design philosophy of potential use to all modern interactive software systems destined to incremental evolution. However, the distinctive property of the proposed method, as compared to other approaches to software evolution, is that it focuses primarily on non-functional qualities and the interactive properties of a system.

Part II Reference Scenarios

Chapter 4
The HYGEIAnet Reference Scenario

Demosthenes Akoumianakis[1] and Constantine Stephanidis[1,2]

[1] Foundation for Research and Technology – Hellas (FORTH)
Institute of Computer Science
Heraklion, Crete, GR-70013, Greece
cs@ics.forth.gr
[2] University of Crete
Department of Computer Science, Greece

Abstract. This Chapter describes a reference scenario that has been extracted from current practices regarding the use of Electronic Patient Records in Greece, and in particular in the Regional Health Network of the Region of Crete (HYGEIAnet). At the time of writing, HYGEIAnet is one of the most complete and mature regional health telematics networks in the country. Nevertheless, HYGEIAnet is in continuous refinement and expansion through national and European funding. Consequently, the present Chapter does not aim to present the state of the art developments in HYGEIAnet, but rather to convey a particular instance in the network's development life-cycle as perceived by IS4ALL.

1. Electronic Patient Record of HYGEIAnet

1.1 Background

HYGEIAnet is a Regional Health Telematics Network of the Region of Crete (Tsiknakis et al, 1997). In its current form, HYGEIAnet implements a variety of applications and services intended to facilitate a continuum in health care provision. Some of these services are explicitly focused on the use of Electronic Patient Records, and to this extent they are of particular interest to IS4ALL. In what follows, some specific interaction scenarios are described that have been taken from daily activities of healthcare professionals interacting with the Electronic Health Record (EHR) services of HYGEIAnet.

1.2 Interaction Scenarios

Date: Tuesday, September 4th, Dr Fred reviews the Electronic Patient Record of N. Stathiakis.

C. Stephanidis (Ed.): Universal Access Code of Practice in Health Telematics, LNCS 3041, pp. 39-45, 2005.
© Springer-Verlag Berlin Heidelberg 2005

- Following last night's notification by the Local Service Center, Dr Fred logs on to HYGEIAnet Electronic Patient Records service from his office in the University Hospital of Heraklion.
- Dr Fred requests from the system to present demographic data about the patient N. Stathiakis, who was admitted last night into the hospital. Dr Fred wishes to have an overview of the patient's demographic data and health condition before visiting him in the clinic.
- The system responds to the request and presents two screens in sequence (see Figure 1 and Figure 2) regarding demographics.

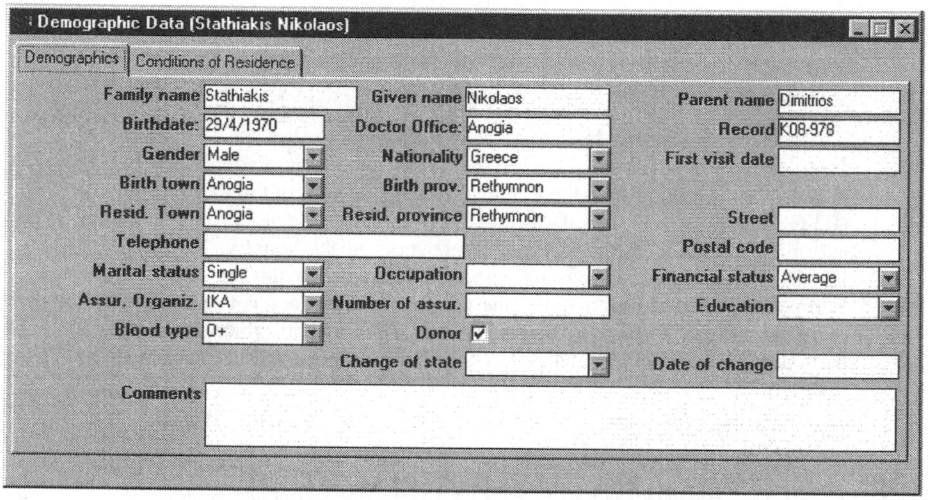

Fig. 1. Demographic information about the patient

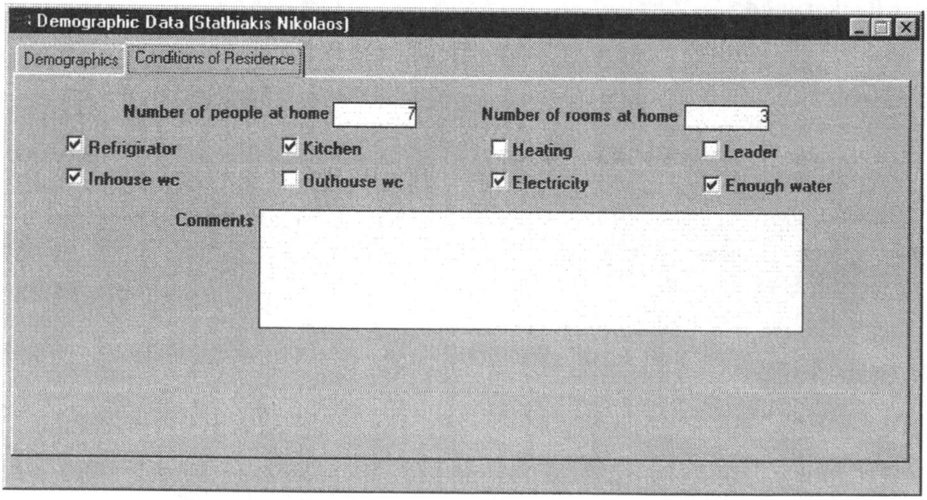

Fig. 2. Demographic information about the patient (Cont.)

- Having reviewed the data, Dr Fred decides to further query the system to find out the clinical history of the patient. He therefore issues queries based on clinical exams (see Figure 3), diagnosis (see Figure 4) and recommended actions (see Figure 5).
- To obtain a more accurate overview of the patient's medical condition, Dr Fred decides to consult the HYGEIAnet Electronic Patient Record History service.
- The system responds to the request presenting the patient's history (see Figure 6) and related diagnosis (see Figure 7)
- From last night's briefing, Dr Fred was informed that the patient suffers from asthma and that this was the cause of his recent admission to the hospital. To obtain an insight into the patient's past treatment, Dr Fred requests to review the patent's previous drug treatment for asthma. The system responds with the screen of Figure 8.
- Having obtained a sufficient insight about the patient's history, past treatment and current conditions, Dr Fred decides to visit the patient in the clinic.

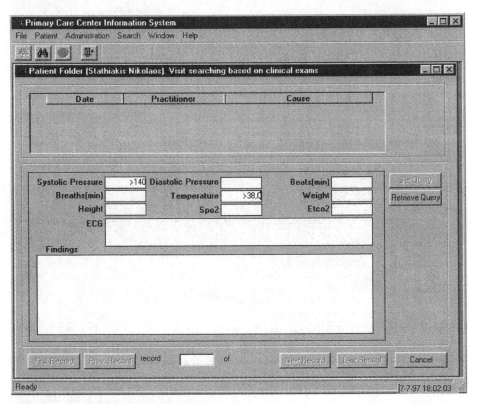

Fig. 3. Search based on clinical exams. In the example illustrated above the criteria set are Systolic Pressure > 140 and Temperature >39.0

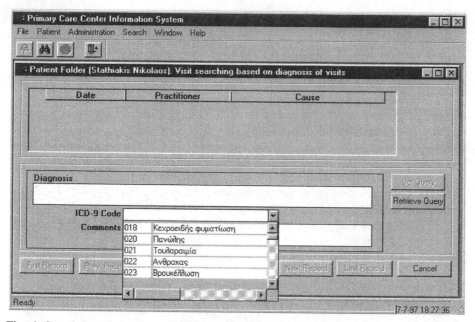

Fig. 4. Search based on diagnosis. Here the search is driven by setting the ICD-9 Code by making a choice from a drop-down listbox

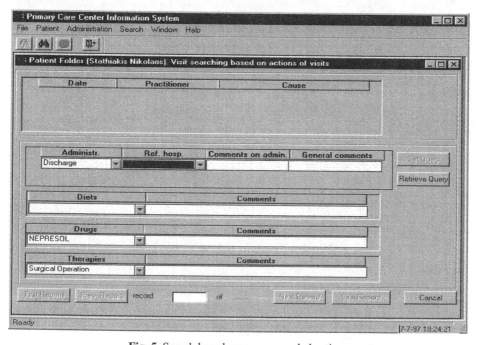

Fig. 5. Search based on recommended actions

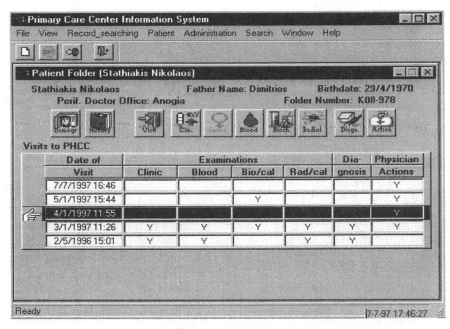

Fig. 6. Extract from the patient's history

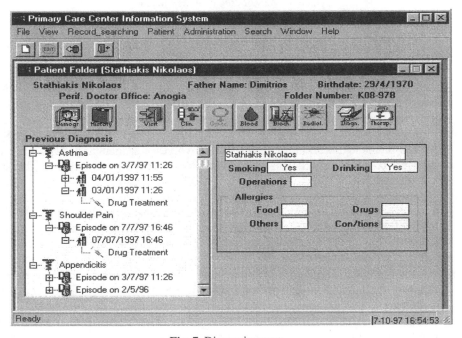

Fig. 7. Diagnosis screen

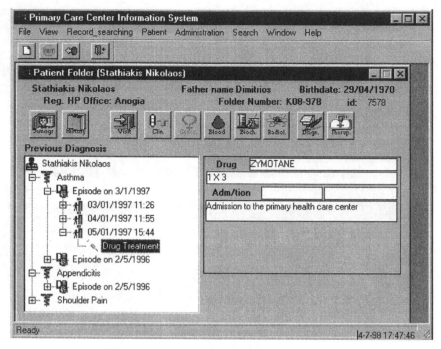

Fig. 8. Review of drug treatment for asthma

2. Concluding Remarks

Having briefly reviewed how Dr Fred carried out the designated tasks of reviewing demographics of a patient or searching the Electronic Patient Record using various criteria, the issue of how this scenario links with the aims and objectives of IS4ALL is being reviewed. Following the project's methodology, as reported in Part A (Chapter 3) of this handbook, working with scenarios involves a sequence of steps, such as identifying potential breakdowns and envisioning new design alternatives through scenario screening.

Identifying breakdowns is an analytical step that involves a conscious effort to unfold, record and reflect upon explicit and implicit claims or assumptions embodied in the original scenario. For example, by inspecting (parts of) the current implementation of the user interface to the integrated electronic health record of HYGEIAnet, one can derive several implicit assumptions, such as the following:

- The user interface is designed for a particular delivery medium (i.e., a conventional desktop machine) and computing platform (i.e., Windowing Graphical User Interface).
- The user interface is designed for professional users with fine spatial control, fine eye-hand coordination, ability to pull and push targets, ability to initiate movement on demand, etc.
- The user of the system can only carry out the designated tasks from a stationary point (i.e., office).

If some of these assumptions were to be relaxed, then the designated artefacts of Figures 1-5 would no longer suffice to provide the means to carry out the tasks. Thus, any Universal Access methodology should provide answers to the following non-exhaustive set of questions:

- How can the system be re-engineered so that it can be delivered through the web (changing the delivery medium)?
- How can the system be re-engineered so that it can be accessed from a radically different computing platform, such as a mobile phone or a palm device?
- How can the interactive experience of the user be improved by perhaps introducing new interaction techniques?

The above provide only indicative examples of the type of requirements, which should be addressed when designing universally accessible systems. However, any new requirements do not make the existing system obsolete, at least this need not be the case. On the contrary, our claim is that Universal Access involves an extension in the patterns of use of a designated system, so that the re-engineered system is able to respond to changes in its execution context, irrespective of the reason of their occurrence (i.e., different users, alternative physical or social contexts of use, new interaction devises and access terminals). From this perspective, Universal Access introduces a particular view on software evolution, rooted in a new design philosophy, which emphasizes the concept of designing to accommodate the global execution context of a system's tasks. In Part C of this handbook, specific methods and their validation using the HYGEIAnet Electronic Patient Record service are being described to shed light into aspects of re-engineering that remove designated obstacles and expand the scope of a reference system to encompass novel requirements, some of which have been briefly outlined above.

Acknowledgement

The authors would also like to explicitly acknowledge the co-operation with the Center for Medical Informatics & Health Telematics applications (CMI-HTA) of the Institute of Computer Science, Foundation for Research and Technology – Hellas. The CMI-HTA Laboratory is the developer of HYGEIAnet.

Chapter 5
The SPERIGEST Integrated System

Pier Luigi Emiliani and Laura Burzagli

Consiglio Nazionale delle Ricerche
Istituto di Fisica Applicata "Nello Carrara"
Via Panciatichi, 64
Firenze 50127, Italy
{p.l.emiliani, L.Burzagli}@ifac.cnr.it

Abstract. In this Chapter, a scenario is presented that constitutes an example of healthcare delivery based on the Italian SPERIGEST information system. SPERIGEST was a national initiative, supported by the Italian Ministry of Health for the management of healthcare of patients mainly affected by cardiovascular diseases, and deals with clinical and administrative aspects. The scenario reflects various aspects of SPERIGEST, including sharing of information amongst autonomous clinical information systems and web-based management of patient medical records.

1. Background

SPERIGEST was developed to integrate different heterogeneous sources of patient data, supposing that for each specialised category of clinical information (i.e., diagnostic instrumental labs, nurse activities, etc) a subsystem was in charge of data treatment. Integration between subsystems was obtained by means of a network backbone and software interfaces, connecting each data source to a central database devoted to collect relevant clinical and administrative information. At the same time, this information is distributed to external environments, other than the entire World, through an Internet network interface.

The whole system has been in use since 1999 in many clinical structures and it has been tested on thousands of in and out patients. A campaign of General Practitioner education is in progress to promote the use of this system in all aspects of patient's care. In the scenario reported in this Chapter, focus is on clinical practice, rather than on administrative or demographic aspects, due to the greater relevance of this process in patient care.

Not all the tasks described in this scenario are covered by the current SPERIGEST version. Therefore, the scenario is intended as a realistic view of what is available today and what can be actually done with the present information technology for the overall management of healthcare.

C. Stephanidis (Ed.): Universal Access Code of Practice in Health Telematics, LNCS 3041, pp. 46-55, 2005.
© Springer-Verlag Berlin Heidelberg 2005

2. Scenario

2.1 Patient's Sign and Symptoms, Tuesday March 19th

Mrs. Arca Loretta is a 62 year-old patient, suffering from chronic stable angina, treated with medical therapy (nitro-derivates and beta-blockers). After dinner she suffered from chest pain refractory to sublingual nitrates. She decided to make a telephone call to Dr. Dalmiani, her General Practitioner (GP).

2.2 General Practitioner Visit, Tuesday March 19th

Dr. Dalmiani received Mrs. Arca's telephone call at 22:30 and, having heard the patient's symptoms, he decided to perform an immediate home visit. Before leaving home, Dr. Dalmiani connected his palm-PC (see Figure 1) to Internet with a GPRS interface and, selecting Mrs. Arca among his available patients, recalled clinical data from the SPERIGEST Network. Driving to the patient's home, his palm-PC, which in the meanwhile had received the requested data, informed Dr. Dalmiani, through its speech processor, about the patient's history (e.g., previous cardiological visits, patient latest events, currently prescribed medical therapy, etc).

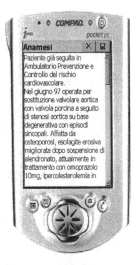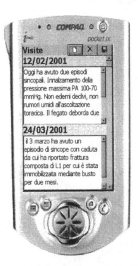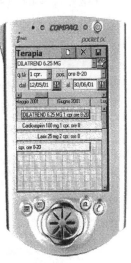

Fig. 1. Dr. Dalmiani's palm-PC data

Dr. Dalmiani arrived at patient's home at 22:55, and after examining her, performed a 12 leads EKG with his portable EKG device connected to his palm-PC. As the obtained exam results were ambiguous, Dr. Dalmiani decided on an immediate transfer to an emergency unit, suspecting a myocardial infarction. An ambulance was called to transport the patient to the Hospital.

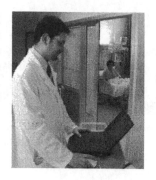

2.3 Cardiology Ward Admission, Tuesday March 19th

During the patient's transport to the local Hospital in Pisa, the Hospital Information System received an admission request from Dr. Dalmiani and started the request of clinical data from the SPERIGEST network. Data concerning Mrs. Arca were integrated with the GP's latest patient's status update.

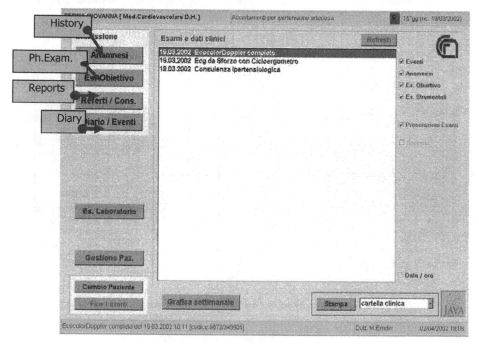

Fig. 2. Electronic medical record view

After patient admission at ICU department at 23:45, the cardiologist on duty, Dr. Emdin, looked at the patient history and latest events on his Electronic Medial Record (EMR, see Figure 2), developed using WEB technology (Java, HTML). In the EMR, the basic function for consultation is the time-oriented representation of patient parameters, care events and examinations. Then Dr. Emdin performed a 12 leads EKG that showed a well-defined anterior ischemia (Figure 3). He decided to start a nitrate e.v. infusion that led to a complete regression of angina symptoms.

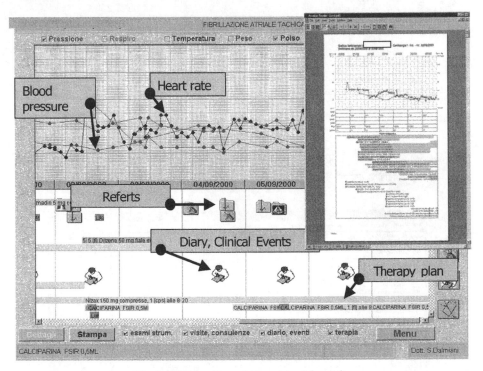

Fig. 3. EKG results and Chemistry lab results

A blood sample was drawn and sent to the chemical lab for myocardial necrosis markers (CK MB, troponine, myoglobin) evaluation. Blood sample parameters were sent back to the EMR, and the cardiologists, consulting Lab results (Figure 4), excluded the diagnosis of Acute Myocardial Infarction.

The next morning, the cardiologists decided to plan a set of instrumental examinations: echocardiography and coronary angiography. They sent directly from the EMR the exam requests to the labs in charge, and notified the nurse system for patient preparation. Exam executions were confirmed with the exact data and time from each lab subsystem, and clinical data were transmitted to the lab physicians to allow a comprehensive characterisation of the patient under test. In the meantime, the nurse unit was collecting bioumoral data and continuously updating the central system's database (Figure 5), and therefore the EMR of the patient.

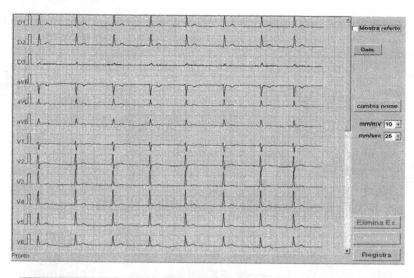

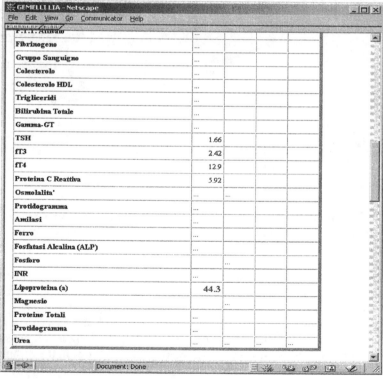

Fig. 4. Graphical trace of bioumoral parameters (on screen and printout)

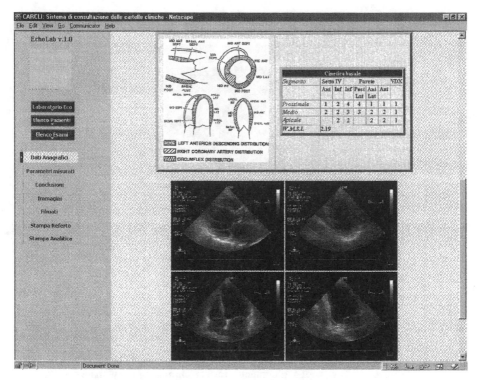

Fig. 5. Web view of echocardiography results

The echocardiography, executed on Wednesday morning, March 20th, reported a reduced ejection fraction to the cardiologist (Figure 5). A text report and relevant images were recorded and sent back to the ward EMR. On Thursday, March 21st, an angiography reported of a trivasal coronaropathy (Figure 6), and cardiologists decided on a surgical consult. Most significant images of the stenotic coronaries were extracted from the angiographic film and transmitted to the clinical central database, thus being available also to other physicians for remote consulting.

2.4 Surgery Consultant, Thursday March 21st

As requested by the cardiologist, the cardiac surgeons of Massa Hospital evaluated the clinical case through the use of a WEB connected EMR, looking at the patient's history, EKG, echocardiography and coronarography film executed at Pisa Hospital. The surgeon Dr. Bevilacqua suggested a CABG procedure (LIMA>LAD, SAPH>OM1, SAPH>PDA) on an urgent basis. He wrote a text report (Figure 7) describing the patient's diagnosis, and sent it to the cardiologists in Pisa for patient transfer.

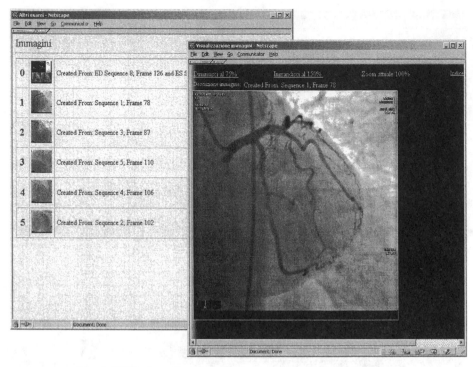

Fig. 6. WEB view of angiography's results, chromatography images

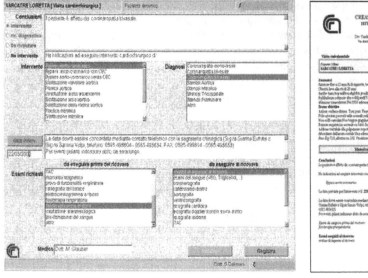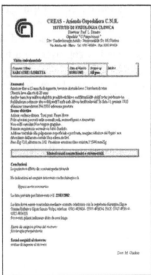

Fig. 7. Surgeon report

2.5 Massa Hospital, Friday March 22nd

Massa Hospital nurses arranged everything for patient arrival at 9:30 in the morning. During the patient's transfer to Massa by ambulance, 60 Km away from Pisa, a ward clerk at Pisa Hospital completed the discharge letter and notified the surgeons of the patient's latest events. At patient arrival at Massa Hospital, Dr. Glauber, the surgeon on duty, admitted Mrs. Arca to the Sub Intensive Cardio-surgical unit and a bar-code identification bracelet was attached to the patient's wrist. The surgical procedure was scheduled for the same afternoon.

2.5.1 Anaesthesiological and Surgical Procedures, Friday March 22nd

At 14:30, the patient entered the Operating Room n°3. The local OR informative system recognised the patient through the identification bracelet and started recording events: arterial blood and central venous pressures were invasively monitored, together with 4 leads EKG, arterial oxygen saturation, and end-tidal carbon dioxide level (Figure 8). Anaesthesia was inducted and maintained with fentanyl and propofol infusion. CABG surgery was performed using a standard technique with the institution of extracorporeal circulation and cardioplegic heart arrest. The procedure was uneventful and at the end of the procedure the patient was transferred to the surgical ICU. The material used during the procedure was recorded and discharged from local storage, associating each item with the patient by bar-code identification bracelet. Significant clinical information collected during the procedures by monitors and anaesthesiologists were sent to central EMR and Clinical Registry System.

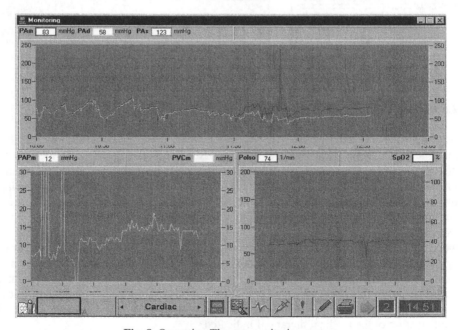

Fig. 8. Operating Theater monitoring system

2.5.2 ICU, Friday March 22nd

The operating surgeon compiled the operation report in ICU, just after patient arrival (Figure 9, left side). During patient monitoring, both the operating surgeon and the anaesthesiologist filled in the patient data registry with the postoperative course parameters and evaluation, partially obtained directly from the Operating Theatre information system Figure 9, right side). The ICU period was uneventful and the next day the patient was discharged from ICU and transferred to a sub-intensive unit for health care course completion.

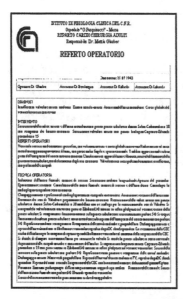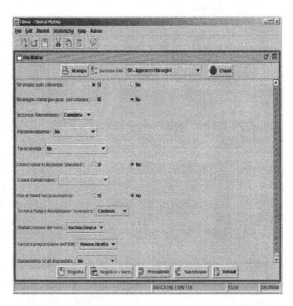

Fig. 9. Text report and Clinical Registry

2.6 Patient Discharge and Follow-Up, Friday March 29th

At patient leaving, a discharge letter (Figure 10) was composed automatically with the information collected at each step of the diagnostic and therapeutical pathway (patient history, etc). This letter was transmitted electronically also to Dr. Dalmiani, General Practitioner of Mrs. Arca, for updating his local clinical records and for guaranteeing the continuity of the home health care of the patient. Structured diagnoses were compiled for DRG classification, with a list of the most significant procedures executed during patient stay; these data, among others related to the patient discharge, were communicated to the Administrative system and to the National Health Security system for patient recovery reimbursement.

At hospital discharge, a follow-up appointment was automatically booked and reported in the discharge letter. The follow-up visit implies a complete physical examination, chest X-ray and echocardiography assessment and an eventual modification of the medical therapy if indicated.

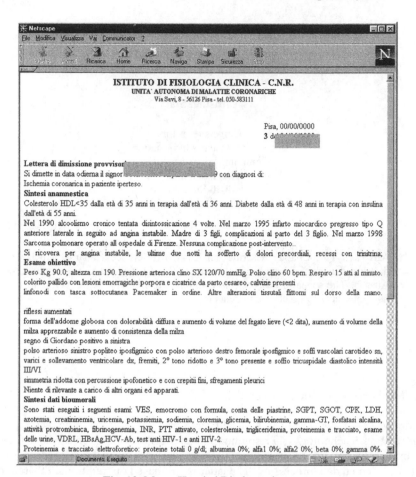

Fig. 10. Massa Hospital Discharge letter

Chapter 6
The Barmerzige Schwestern Reference Scenario

Christian Stary

University of Linz
Department of Business Information Systems
Communications Engineering
Freistaädterstraße 315
A - 4040 Linz, Austria
christian.stary@jku.at

Abstract. This Chapter describes an Austrian reference scenario, which was developed as part of a subcontract between IS4ALL and the University of Linz, Austria. The scenario has been used to validate model-based development of user interfaces to Electronic patient data.

1. Context

1.1 The Health Telematics Provider

Barmerzige Schwestern is a healthcare provider which operates innovative Information Technology (IT) solutions in upper Austria. Over the last few years, several shifts have been made, namely from data-driven to function-driven towards patient-oriented data processing. The latter is still based on traditional IT-architectures that are currently adapted to follow the acquired business processes from the perspective of patients rather than functional units or roles from the provider.

1.2 Current Practices

The defined business processes are the core processes of the Barmherzigen Schwestern. They can be decomposed into distinct classes, which comprise the medical, care-taking, and logistic activities with respect to patients (records), namely admission, anamnesis, diagnosis, therapy and discharge (see Figure 1).

In the present work, a (business) process is intended as a set of logically arranged tasks that are executed to achieve a defined set of results. Such a process is characterised by the following properties:

- There are internal or external customers for whom the set of results has to be achieved.
- A process involves more than one organisational unit – it is a cross-border activity.
- Each process results in information or physical objects.

C. Stephanidis (Ed.): Universal Access Code of Practice in Health Telematics, LNCS 3041, pp. 56-63, 2005.
© Springer-Verlag Berlin Heidelberg 2005

- A process might involve activities at the management, as well as at the operational level.

From the perspective of Universal Access in Health Telematics, those cases where patient data are accessed or manipulated by different users or users in different functional roles are of particular interest. Therefore, the current focus is on representative processes that involve several different user roles, such as the ward and medical experts. However, a generic process of the provider can be defined based on the process classes mentioned above (Figure 1).

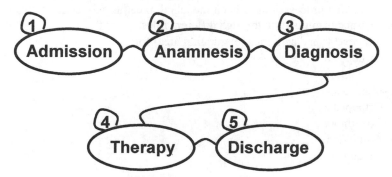

Fig. 1. A Generic Process for Health Care Provider

Each process can be decomposed according to the organisational units and the generic activities performed in the respective unit. Figure 2 depicts such decompositions for two process elements, namely Admission and Therapy.

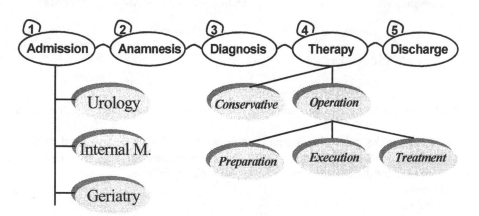

Fig. 2. A Sample Decomposition of Generic Processes for Health Care Provider

In order to obtain a detailed insight into the preparatory and execution phases of these processes, additional information is needed about.
- The activities that have to be performed to achieve a certain result.
- The flow of control between the activities, in terms of loops, sequences, etc.

- The use of goods and material including IT-support, in terms of documents, forms, etc.
- The information required to successfully accomplish a certain task.
- The events leading up to a task.
- The functional role (i.e., responsibility for task accomplishment).
- Interfaces between organisational units and roles.
- States of persons (in our case patients), objects (e.g., patient data), products or services (e.g., treatment) along the different phases of task accomplishment.

The following processes have been modelled, meeting the requirements of patient data access and manipulation through different roles:

- External events and activities (extramural area) for:
  - Orthopedia
  - Coxathrose
- Hospital area
  - Orthopedia
  - Coxathrose
  - Admission
  - Diagnosis

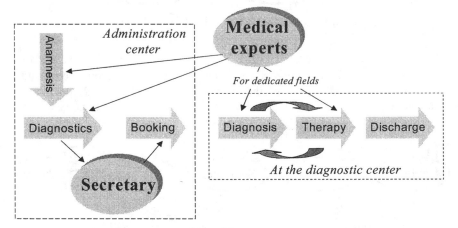

Fig. 3. Role-specific Access and Manipulation of Patient Data at the Barmherzige Schwestern

The process design of the organisation is shown in Figure 3. It is evident that a deviation from standard processes for healthcare providers has occurred. The list of sub-processes for the Barmherzige Schwestern looks as follows:

- Admission
- Anamnesis
- Initial Diagnostics and Continuous Diagnosing
- 'Booking', i.e., Initiating relevant in-house sub processes leading to care and treatment
- Therapy
- Discharge

Figure 3 depicts the role-specific access for the secretary and the medical experts for the sake of organisational efficiency. The processes have been modelled in the German version of ARIS (for details see Stephanidis, 2003). For further processing, they have been translated to English and transformed to a textually compressed form. However, the raw data are required to communicate with the staff and to avoid misconceptions about the organisation and content of work. For the sake of accuracy, the support systems are listed, user roles, tasks, and problem domain data as originally provided, together with their translations.

1.3 Current Technology

This section provides a summary of automated data processing support at the site of the Health Telematics provider in Austria. In what follows, details of the technical infrastructure, as well as some of the forms that have been mapped on SAP screens, are presented.

1.3.1 Operating System
Server: Windows NT 4, Clients: Windows 95, Windows NT

1.3.2 Database Management
Oracle (Version 7 and up)

1.3.3 Standard Software
Microsoft Office 97, Internet Explorer, Outlook
Herold phone directory
Railway schedule

1.3.4 Software
Work plan, Pschyrembel-encyclopedia, Austria-Codex

1.3.5 Software Solutions
Patient Accounting medico//s (Systema)
Controlling SAP R/3
Patient Administration Systema
Laboratory Support Systema
Diagnosis Support Systema
PACS-System Siemens

1.3.6 Meierhofer MCC (Medical Control Center)
Configuration tool
Anaesthesia-Documentation (ISOP-ANA)
Operation-Planning (ISOP-PLAN)
Operation-Documentation (ISOP-OP)
ISOP-View

1.4 Forms and Artefacts

The form in Figure 4 is filled in when a doctor or a member of staff awakens patients, following an operation.

Aufwachraumprotokoll

Schmerzinfusion	Dipidolorschema

bei Rückfragen:

Infusionsvorschlag für den AWR:	Ringer-Lsg	POLsg.	HÄS
Laborkontrollen im AWR:	BB	BZ	K

Besonderheiten für den AWR:

Vigilanz:	wach	auf Anruf weckbar	nicht weckbar
Haut:	rosig	blass/kühl	shivering
Schmerzen:	keine	mäßiger	starke

übernommen von: Sr./Pfl.   Um

Arzt

∀	B D	
A		
●	P	
⇩	entleert	
M	mit Sog	
O	ohne Sog	
K	geklemmt	

SaO₂
O₂-Gabe L/min

Harn
DRAIN I
DRAIN II
DRAIN III
Erbrechen
Verband

mg i.V.
mg i.V.
mg i.V.
mg i.V.
mg i.V.
mg i.V.

Labor:
Uhrzeit:
Ery
HB
HKT
Plt.
NT
PTT
AT₃
BZ
pH
BE
pCO₂
pO₂
SaO₂
STB
K⁺

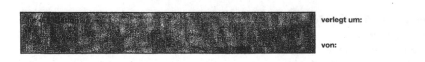

verlegt um:

von:

Fig. 4. Post-operation form

The form in Figure 5 is filled in throughout the operation by anaesthetists.

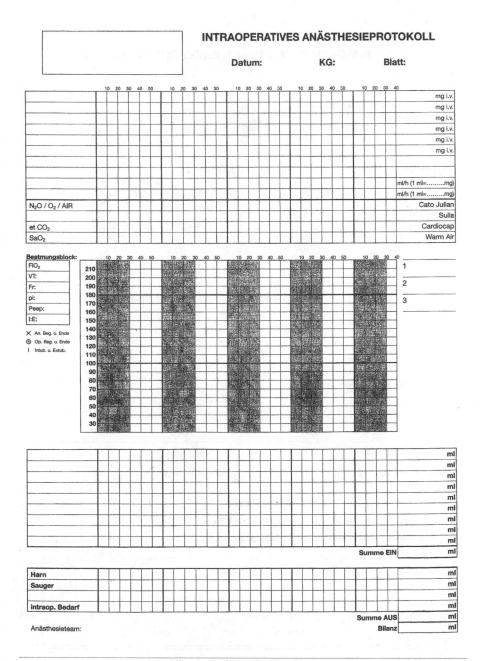

Fig. 5. During-operation form

The two-page form in Figure 6 contains all data required for an operation. It is completed prior to the actual operation.

PRÄOPERATIVES ANÄSTHESIEPROTOKOLL

Krankenhaus der Barmherzigen Schwestern Linz
Betriebsgesellschaft m.b.H.
Abt. f. Anästhesie und Intensivmedizin
Leiter: Prim.Dr.E.Oman

Diagnose: **geplante Operation**   **am**

Besonderheiten aus Status und Anamnese:

Größe: cm, Gewicht: kg

RR:

Allergie:

Medikamente:

Ery	Thr	**EKG**	**THORAX-Rö.**
Hb	NT		
Hkt	PTT		
Leuko	AT3		
Na	U		
K	Kr	**BGA**	**LUFU**
BZ	CHE		

KONSILIUM / spezielle Untersuchungen:

Aufklärung erfolgte über:

Patient: ASA 1, 2, 3, 4, 5   Wahleingriff   dringlicher Eingriff   Notfall

○ **der Patient ist anästhesiologisch zur OP freigegeben**

○ **der Patient ist freigegeben, wenn folgende Befunde OB sind**

○ **Rücksprache nach Einlangen folgender Befunde erforderlich**

                                 Unterschrift

Dauermedikation am OP Tag:

Prämedikation: zu verabreichen am   um   tel.

                   verabreicht um   durch:

POSTOP.DIAGNOSE / OP. ART   OP-TEAM:

Airway Management: Maske   Larynxmaske   Tubus   DLT   fiberopt. Int.   Jet Vent.

Venöser Zugang:

Cavakatheter: V. subclavia L / R V.jugularis int. L / R V.femoralis L / R	**Zeit:** ~	**Signum:**
P A Spirale Modell G		
LA J / N		
Arterielle Kanüle: A.radialis L / R		
LA J / N P		
SpinalAn: L /L LA J / N P E B Nadel G		
EpiduralAn: / P E B Punktionstiefe.................................cm		
Hautniveau.......................................cm		
Testdosis:.........ml Carbostesin......%		
Caudalblock: Nadel: ml Carbostesin %		
Periphere Nervenblockade:		

HÄMODILUTION:		Stk. Vollblutkonserven			
MAT: Sammelvolumen:		ml	Retransfusionsvolumen		ml
Sammelbeginn:					
	Bg ok		Bg ok		Bg ok
	Bg ok		Bg ok		Bg ok
	Bg ok		Bg ok		Bg ok
EK1	Bg:	BST ok	EK6	Bg:	BST ok
EK2	Bg:	BST ok	EK7	Bg:	BST ok
EK3	Bg:	BST ok	EK8	Bg:	BST ok
EK4	Bg:	BST ok	EK9	Bg:	BST ok
EK5	Bg:	BST ok	EK10	Bg:	BST ok

Fig. 6. Two-page Operation Summary form

Chapter 7
The ClinicCoach Reference Scenario

Elizabeth Hofvenschiöld and Frank Heidmann

Fraunhofer
Institute for Industrial Engineering (IAO)
Nobelstrasse 12
Stuttgart D-70569, Germany
{Elizabeth.Hofvenschiold, Frank.Heidmann}@iao.fhg.de

Abstract. This Chapter describes a reference scenario that has been extracted from current practices regarding the use of Electronic Patient Records (EPR) in Germany, and in particular the ClinicCoach application developed by the company HIG Coachit. The application is an EPR (or otherwise described as an Electronic Health Record - EHR) and was first implemented in the Accident Surgery Department of the Kassel Clinic on August 24th, 2001. Before the test run was initiated, the developers spent nine months observing the everyday tasks of the hospital staff in the ward. The development process was user-centred and continues iteratively. Nurses, doctors and other medical professionals have direct access to the developers and can communicate any issues that may arise from using the EPR. These in turn are analysed and adjustments or changes are made on the system accordingly.

1. Introduction

ClinicCoach runs on a Personal Digital Assistant (PDA) and on a PC. The operating system used for the application is the Palm OS and the chosen PDA for the Kassel Clinic is a Handspring. The primary patient data is gathered with the PDA whilst the hospital staff moves around and visits patients. They can then synchronise their devices on a special station so that the gathered data is sent to the PC and any new data (from other PDAs) on the PC is sent back to the device. The synchronisation process takes about nine seconds and it is recommended to be done every few hours so as to reduce the risk of data loss and ensure the timeliness of the data.

The scenario described in this Chapter is based on a small ethnographic study of one of the accident surgery wards at the Kassel Clinic. The ward used six PDAs – nurses and other professionals used three, doctors used two units and one unit was assigned to the 'Dienstzimmer' or the ward's office. The ward is divided into areas, which are represented by the colours blue, red and green. The scenario discussed below is based on the observations made on the green team.

C. Stephanidis (Ed.): Universal Access Code of Practice in Health Telematics, LNCS 3041, pp. 64-68, 2005.

1.1 The Start of a Shift

The beginning of the shift starts with an update of the patients' conditions and any other matters that need to be discussed. Members of the previous shift report on their experiences to the new shift members. Whilst doing so, the reporting staff brings in the PDAs that they used for recording their data. They describe their findings from memory but also continually refer to the PDAs for certain important facts, such as increased temperature or change in medication. The listening members of staff make notes on a patient list that is printed out before the meeting.

After the meeting, which takes about forty-five minutes, the staff disperses and the lead member of each team picks up a PDA and synchronises it on the docking station. The PDAs are then ready for use and the lead member of each team logs in (see Figure 1).

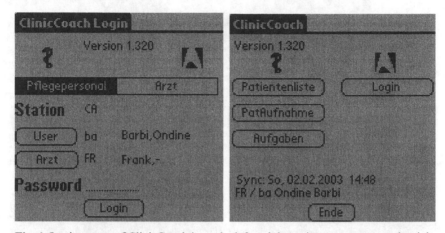

Fig. 1. Login screen of ClinicCoach is on the left and the main menu screen on the right

1.2 Recording and Checking Data

The green team's nurse, Anna, makes sure that her work trolley is ready and sets off with her assistant, Lena, who also has a work trolley loaded with fresh bed linen. Before Anna visits her first patient, she calls up the patient's records on the PDA and checks the details (e.g., type of medication and when it should be given, when the temperature should be taken). She then proceeds with her tasks and asks the patient how he is feeling.

After Anna and Lena complete their tasks, Anna confirms that she has done what was required and sometimes has to add a new item to the list if the patient required further assistance (see Figure 2). She does this by clicking on the task in a list and checking it off. For example, if a patient has to be given ice twice a day, then the data on the patient's record will show: Ice 2x daily 1-1-0- (see Figure 3). If Anna is on the morning shift and she and Lena have just given the patient some ice, she can click on the 1-1-0- where she is given the option to check off the task. She chooses the first 1 and after doing so, the data on the screen now reads: Ice 1+1-0-. Anna does this for all completed activities and if she is busy collecting medicine or speaking to a doctor, Lena can use the application and tick off the tasks performed.

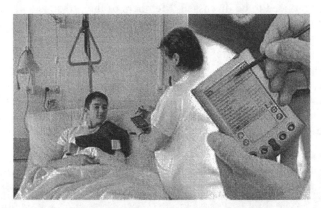

Fig. 2. Nurse recording patient data on her PDA, which is running the ClinicCoach application (picture provided by HIG Coachit)

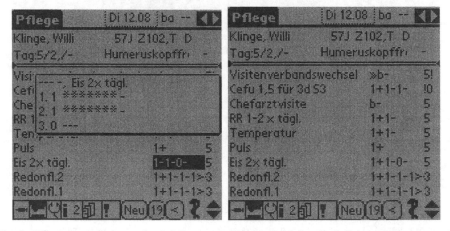

Fig. 3. When Anna clicks on the 1-1-0- next to 'Eis 2x tägl.' (ice 2x daily), a window pops up and she can choose the first line of asterisks to confirm that she has done the task. The second screen shows the confirmed task and now it reads 1+1-0-

ClinicCoach also allows Anna and Lena to record new patient information. For example, a patient's blood pressure must be measured twice a day. Anna measures the blood pressure and shortly afterwards enters the value into the PDA. The EPR also allows the hospital staff to add medications or change the medication plan of a patient. There is also a function to indicate if the addition or change is a regular or irregular one (e.g., medication to be given every day or every second day).

1.3 Synchronising the PDA and Printing Out Information

Once nurse Anna and her assistant Lena are finished with their patient rounds, they proceed to the ward's office to synchronise the PDA and do any other administrative duties they might have. The PDA is placed in the synchronisation station and the data is transferred between the PC and the mobile device. Once the data has been uploaded, any member of the staff can see the green team's input. This is also the time when Anna or Lena can print out any charts they might need or lists of information for the doctors. However, it is also possible for Anna to view graphs on the PDA (see Figure 4). Hardly any data can be input directly into the PC; it is essentially a viewing device and printing server for the data collected on the PDAs.

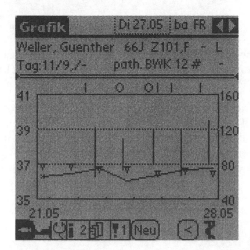

Fig. 4. Screen showing a patient's temperature history over a period of six days

After synchronisation, it is time to write the patient reports (see Figure 5). Nurse Anna decides to sit outside because of the nice weather, and brings the PDA with her. She comments that the PDA is much lighter than the previous device used for recording patient data, i.e., forms attached to metallic clipboards, and that PDA enables her and her colleagues to work outside if they wish to do so. Anna then proceeds to 'write' the records for each patient she saw during her round. She does so by using the available screen keyboard; however, it is also possible to enter information using the scribble field of the PDA.

2. Concluding Remarks

The scenario presented here does not describe the full range of ClinicCoach's functionalities. Rather, it serves the purpose of illustrating the types of interactions that the application supports. The dynamic nature of the EPR and the iterative development process have made it acceptable to all members of staff in the accident

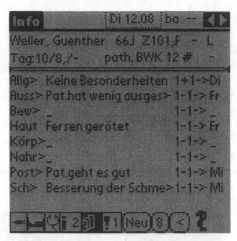

Fig. 5. The screen shows comments on the different aspects of a patient's care. Nurse Anna can write her patient reports from here by clicking on the terms on the left hand side

surgery ward described in this Chapter. The user-centred approach continues and any issues that the staff have with ClinicCoach are directly presented to the developers, who solve the problems and meet the requirements of all the stakeholders. This iterative design process is highly recommendable for the development of truly accessible and ultimately acceptable Health Telematics applications.

Chapter 8
WardInHand – Mobile Access to EPRs

Salvatore Virtuoso

TXT e-Solutions SpA
via Frigia 27
20126 Milano, Italy
salvatore.virtuoso@txt.it

Abstract. This Chapter describes a reference scenario that has been extracted from the IST-funded WardInHand project (IST-1999-10479). The scenario depicts access to electronic patient data by professionals (i.e., doctors and other medical staff) in a ward of a hospital, using an iPAQ device. The scenario, as described below, provides only an extract of possible tasks and activities enabled by the WardInHand prototype. The designated tasks have been selected to suit the aims and objectives of IS4ALL. Other tasks, such as setting and initiating workflows, are deliberately excluded from the current version of the scenario.

1. Introduction and Context

WardInHand is an acronym for "Mobile workflow support and information distribution in hospitals via voice-operated, wireless-networked handheld PCs", a European Commission funded IST project (IST–1999-10479) that was started in January 2000 and was completed in spring 2002. Participants were three IT companies (TXT e-solutions, Italy; BMT, UK; and RT, Greece), the Department of Informatics and Information Sciences - University of Genoa (Italy) and three Healthcare organisations as end-users (the Department of Endocrinology and Metabolism – University of Genoa, Italy; Corporaciò Sanitària Clinic – Barcelona, Spain; and Staedtische Kliniken Offenbach, Germany).

WardInHand aims to support the day-by-day activities of doctors and nurses within a hospital ward by providing a tool for workgroup collaboration and wireless access to the patient's clinical records. The project is based on accessing the information system from the patient's bedside through a PDA client. WardInHand is not intended to replace or compete with Hospital legacy systems, but to complement them. It exchanges information with existing tools, updates data in real time and makes them available to doctors and nurses, adding mobility and ubiquitous computing as new dimensions to currently available Hospital Information Systems.

C. Stephanidis (Ed.): Universal Access Code of Practice in Health Telematics, LNCS 3041, pp. 69-76, 2005.
© Springer-Verlag Berlin Heidelberg 2005

1.1 The Objectives and the Approach of WardInHand

The problem addressed by WardInHand is to significantly reduce the inconveniences of paper handling and repeated transcriptions during the process of delivering healthcare services to patients in a hospital ward. Processes associated to services delivered in a hospital involve a large amount of information collected from the patient, exchanged by the several actors concerned, filed for legal purposes, etc. Examples are prescription of analysis and collection of the results; prescription, execution and monitoring of treatments; coordination among doctors and nurses performing and monitoring treatments; exchange of information between the department and the other units of the hospital (lab services, logistics, etc.). Most often, the processing of this information is based on paper, with subsequent transcriptions made by different actors in different places at different times. In other industry sectors, such as the manufacturing industry, the effort to minimise losses in efficiency and quality intrinsic to this kind of practice has long since led to the adoption of real time data collection and production tracking systems, which gather data at the time and the place where it is generated and organise the flow of information with limited human intervention.

In a traditional environment, clinical information is often recorded on paper documents (the clinical record) and notes are taken on notebooks by nurses while doctors conduct their visit tours, and then transcribed to other paper files for planning treatments, exams and drug distribution. The result is often inefficient, as this activity drains valuable time from the hospital personnel. Additionally, it can also introduce errors and inaccuracies, either due to the transcription process or to the fact that the information is not updated in real time.

Even when systems for electronic records management exist, manual input and transcription is not eliminated. Moreover, such systems are often located in fixed positions within the wards, forcing people to move there for data entry and data retrieval, leading to errors, omissions, duplication of information and adding huge overloads to doctors' and nurses' work.

In WardInHand, the entire process is centred around the patients' clinical records, and involves activities such as retrieving information about the patients, including results of analysis, monitoring its progresses, prescribing treatments, executing and monitoring them, etc. It also comprises activities such as: exchanging information among doctors, among nurses and between doctors and nurses; co-coordinating and synchronising activities; ensuring that the necessary drugs and consumables are available when needed, etc.

The need for transcription is then virtually eliminated by providing the Hospital personnel with direct access to information at any time and in any place, by using PDAs as well as their desktop systems.

In summary, the major objectives of WardInHand are:
• To increase the quality of the services provided by the hospitals to patients, by: reducing the possibility of error in data transcription; enforcing quality and safety standards; providing better and more timely information to Healthcare professionals; and improving the control of access to clinical information and of task execution responsibility.

- To reduce costs by increasing the productivity, through less time spent in low added value activities, as well as more efficient team communication and synchronisation.
- To increase the satisfaction of the Hospital's personnel.

1.2 The Architecture

In a scenario where WardInHand is installed, doctors and nurses are equipped with personal handheld PCs linked via wireless networks to a server. The server maintains in a repository all clinical records and all relevant information about patients in the ward, including results of tests and clinical analyses, etc. The server is connected through the Hospital's intranet to other hospital systems, such as systems running in the analysis labs, treatment rooms or the logistic department.

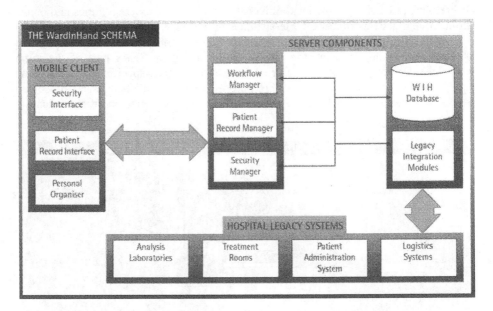

Fig. 1. General system architecture

Figure 1 illustrates the client-server architecture of WardInHand. The functional modules included in the client (left) just show that users access the corresponding functional modules on the server (right), as the design has been intentionally made to support "thin clients", for security reasons and to ensure application longevity.

Handheld PCs and desktop systems – as long as they are connected to the intranet - completely replace traditional paper-based management of clinical records, allowing, e.g., doctors to access and update information on the patient status, to prescribe drugs, treatments and clinical analysis, etc. Data is transmitted to the server in real time, allowing other doctors or nurses in the ward to always get the most up-to-date information.

The server runs a workflow application, which, based on the information collected triggers actions updates a "personal organiser" of each doctor and nurse, automatically assigning and scheduling tasks for them. Nurses use handheld PCs to confirm that treatments have been performed, so that clinical records of patients are updated in real-time. Doctors and nurses are also allowed to exchange informal messages and information via an internal E-mail service available via handheld PCs, regardless of their location in the hospital unit.

2. PDA Access to Electronic Patient Records

2.1 Login

Dr Fred has just arrived at the local university hospital from external duties and is just about to visit patients in a ward. He switches on his PDA and runs the WardInHand system that has recently been installed on all PDAs within the hospital. The system asks Dr Fred to log-in using the screen shown in Figure 2. As part of the login procedure, Dr Fred selects the preferred language and then specifies the user name and password (see Figure 3). For this purpose, the system displays an on-screen keyboard which allows Dr Fred to type in text by selecting characters from a selection panel.

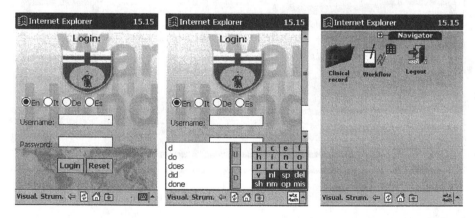

Fig. 2.   Fig. 3.   Fig. 4.

Dr Fred is now logged in and the system displays the applications currently available, namely clinical record and workflow, as shown in Figure 4

.

2.2 Applications Overview

Dr Fred has now entered the ward and has selected the "Clinical record" application of the WardInHand system. By this time, he is also facing his first patient. The system lists patients by name, their current location in the ward (i.e., the bed) and their system identification number (see Figure 5). Dr Fred can either define a new record or can ask the system to download available information about a patient from the legacy system. Dr Fred asks the patient for his name and then selects his clinical record.

The doctor has selected the patient and the system previews the applications related to a particular patient, namely clinical record, personal data, physiological signs, treatments, tests, admission, workflow tasks and logout (see Figure 6). Dr Fred selects the "Personal data" application from the main applications panel. The system responds by presenting a list of options (Figure 7). Dr Fred previews the patient's personal (Figure 8) and family anamnesis (Figure 9).

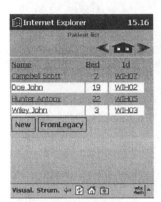

Fig. 5.

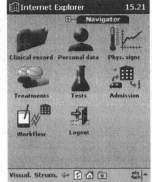

Fig. 6.

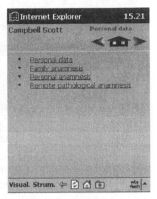

Fig. 7.

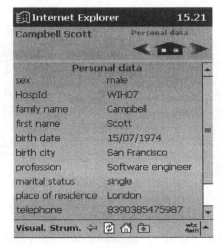

Fig. 8.

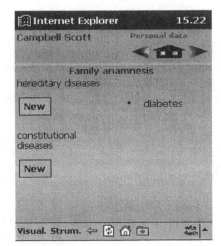

Fig. 9.

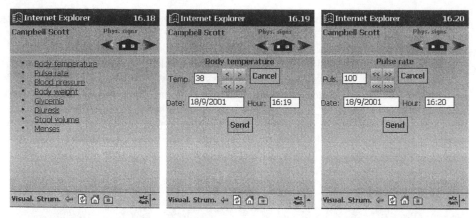

Fig. 10.   Fig. 11.   Fig. 12.

2.3 Updating the Patient Record

Having reviewed the patient's personal data, Dr Fred returns back to the main applications panel and then selects the "Physiological Signs" application. The system responds by listing the options shown on the screen of Figure 10. Dr Fred asks the nurse nearby to take the body temperature of the patient. Then, he selects the relevant option from the previous screen. He enters the body temperature and the date and time of the measurement (Figure 11). Subsequently, Dr Fred asks the nurse to take the pulse rate of the patient and enters the value and the date and time of the measurement (Figure 12).

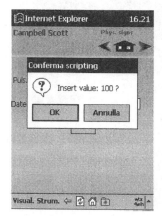

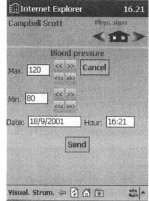

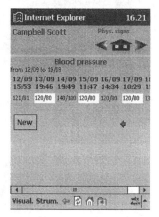

Fig. 13.   Fig. 14.   Fig. 15.

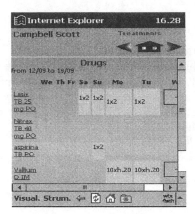

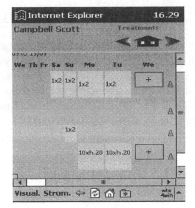

Fig. 16.   Fig. 17.

The system asks the user to confirm the pulse value before storing it in the system (Figure 13). Then Dr Fred asks the nurse to take the blood pressure of the patient and then he updates the patient record by entering the blood pressure value, the date and time of measurement (Figure 14). The system updates the blood pressure history of the patient and presents the results to the user (Figure 15).

Dr Fred now wishes to review the drugs already prescribed. The system presents in Figure 16 and Figure 17 the results as follows. In the first column there is the name of the drug, along with details such as dose and type of administration, in the top row there is the date. The yellow boxes indicate how many units and how many times a day (ex. 1 tablet twice a day). The '+' button is used to extend the prescription for the following day (this is a common practice in the hospitals). The 'A' is used by the nurse to record that the drug has been given (today).

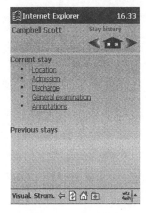

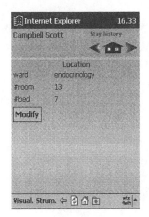

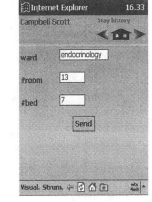

Fig. 18.   Fig. 19.   Fig. 20.

2.4 Reviewing the Patient's Stay History

Dr Fred would also like to review the current stay history of the patient. From the main applications menu he taps on "Stay history". The system responds (see Figure 18) by presenting details of the current stay as well as an option to access previous stays in the ward. From the previous screen Dr Fred taps on "Location" and the system responds by presenting information about the ward, the room number and the bed where the patient resides (Figure 19). In case of change of the patient's location, "Modify" can be used to designate the new location as in Figure 20.

3. Concluding Remarks

The previous extract of activities carried out with the WardInHand system is obviously not exhaustive. Rather, it serves the purpose of indicating the kind of interactions that the system supports. What is important to note however, is that the WardInHand scenario involves a wide range of universal access challenges, which are related not so much to the target users of the system, but mainly to the way in which information is presented and accessed. For instance, one can easily imagine that certain functions offered through the PDA could also be delivered via a WWW-based information system and carried out at another point in time (e.g., prior or after visiting the patient in the ward). Additionally, one can consider a variety of issues related to alternate styles of interaction.

Chapter 9
Patients and EHRs Tele Home Monitoring Reference Scenario

Michael Pieper[1] and Karl Stroetmann[2]

[1]Fraunhofer - FIT
Schloss Birlinghoven
Sankt Augustin 53754, Germany
michael.pieper@fit.fraunhofer.de
[2]empirica
Oxfordstr. 2
D-53111 Bonn, Germany
Karl.Stroetmann@empirica.com

Abstract. This scenario focuses on patients as users of Electronic Health Records (EHR) relevant information. The concrete field of applications is telemonitoring at home, a field where many new approaches and devices are showing up on the market in various countries, an indication of the perceived relevance and market potential of this type of patient involvement. After an introduction to key aspects of patients as users of EHRs, we describe the main application scenario. Generic considerations of telemonitoring at home, as well as the concrete context and application, the telemonitoring equipment presently in use, and screen shots of EHR patient data as seen by the physician (which will later be used for evaluation and validation purposes of patients' access to their vital data) are presented and discussed. We conclude with a vision of the empowered patient using his EHR data to improve his medical condition and quality of life.

1. The Shifting Healthcare Paradigm and Home Care

1.1 The Patient-Centred Healthcare Paradigm – A New Definition of "Patient"

The traditional health care model is based on a highly structured, hierarchical delivery system dominated by physicians and with patients as mere receivers of health services, which are usually provided by public or government institutions - with strict boundaries between local/GP services and stationary services in hospitals. This model is shifting towards a new paradigm accepting the citizen/patient as a self-determined individual.

The new paradigm of *patient-centred, seamless* healthcare processes requires - when taken seriously - the full involvement (as much as reasonably possible) of citizens in all aspects of healthcare and during all stages of the healthcare value chain, from health information and prevention all the way through to rehabilitation and long-

C. Stephanidis (Ed.): Universal Access Code of Practice in Health Telematics, LNCS 3041, pp. 77-87, 2005.

term care. Such a paradigm also implies that the term "patient" is reinterpreted towards meaning "citizens concerned about their health or the health of their friends and relatives".

Under the new paradigm, citizens/patients are self-determined individuals with their own wills and aspirations, which may differ from what a doctor or nurse requests or expects from them, or what best medical practice, and guidelines suggest as optimal treatment in a given situation. This relates to the patient's own definition of quality of life which might imply, e.g., for severely chronically ill patients, a shorter, but from their point of view, more fulfilling life.

Additionally, the patient is a person who is well informed about his/her own illnesses or chronic disease, and discusses with health professionals the optimal treatment path and the interventions best suited to his/her situation. There are already today cases of patients suffering, e.g., from rare diseases, who exchange information and experiences through the Internet and who quite often are much better informed than medical professionals.

In such a context, the patient is part of a real dialogue, and is no longer only the recipient of information from a physician or a nurse. This collaborative model needs to be further developed towards a "tria-logue" model involving also the support network of the patient (spouse, other relatives, informal carers) and a "multi-logue" model (involving formal and community carers, paramedical supporters, social workers) to provide a comprehensive health and social/psychological environment with the primary objective to preserve health and, only as a second option, to treat diseases.

1.2 Rationale for Scenario Selection – Patient Communication and Home Care Lead to Better Medical Outcomes

Home care is a prime example to demonstrate the new paradigm of collaborative and collective organisation of healthcare. All industrial societies are ageing. This has profound socio-economic and health sector implications (Stowe, 2001a), underlined, e.g., by the dramatic increase of the old age dependency ratio - the ratio of the number of people aged 65 and over to the number of people between the ages of 15-64 - from 2000 to 2030 (85% and more in France, Germany, Italy and the UK; more than 100% in Japan) (Stowe, 2001b). As a consequence, an increasing number of older and very old people will suffer in the future from chronic diseases.

To cope with the resulting challenges to our societies, telemedicine and e-health applications hold promise to provide better care, and support independent living (Porteus and Brownsell, 2000). In parallel, the costs per service can be expected to decrease (Wootton, 2001). Research has shown that improved communication with patients, and the possibility for them to remain in an environment they are familiar with and comfortable in, leads to better medical outcomes and, at the same time, improves the quality of life for older people (Stroetmann and Erkert, 1999).

For patients who are actively involved by their physicians in the healthcare delivery process, better results were experienced (Miller, 2001). Patients of doctors who give more information and engage in more positive talk report higher satisfaction and compliance, better recall and understanding, and more favourable health status ratings and clinical outcomes (Hall, Roter and Katz, 1988). At the same time, distrust is reduced, as well as the likelihood of complains, disputes and even lawsuits (Mechanic, 1998). On the other hand, in this context, ethical and legal implications, such as the patients' privacy and security concerns, including a fear of third party access to electronically recorded health and medical data, need to be taken into account (Stanberry, 2000).

1.3 Patients and Universal Access

Why access by patients to their health records is a Universal Access issue? As discussed above, many patients are already today highly interested in accessing their health data, e.g., via their EHR, and various empirical research results strongly support this (Stroetmann and Stroetmann, 2002). For individual and social (improved medical outcome, quality of life, empowerment of patients) as well as economic reasons (pressures to contain costs in the health system; ageing of our societies), strong support for this concept is expected in coming years. A pressing issue, which at this stage needs policy attention, is what we term the "medical divide". A quite considerable portion of the population, particularly many older, disabled and frail people, those with no or little education and/or on low income, people who have been disappointed by what they find (or cannot find) on the Internet, and who are not interested in e-health services, will be left out of these developments and cannot or will not participate in the benefits and advantages of e-health, unless user-friendly interfaces and design-for-all features are fully taken account of. Creativity, innovations and support are needed to integrate such patients, to progress towards a true Information Society for all, and to ensure cohesion and equality in access to medical and health services.

2. Reference Scenario: Patients, Their Context and Tasks

The scenario reported in this Chapter is based on a real application situation. The Chapter will, therefore, describe such an application and discuss the related medical issues from the point of view of the patient, introducing the measurement devices presently in use and describing the tasks of the patients. Subsequently, activities carried out at the nephrologist's office will be reported, and screen shots of patient vital data from their EHR will be presented.

2.1 The Application Situation

Our reference scenario is built around patients suffering from End Stage Renal Failure (ESRF) being treated by continuous ambulatory peritoneal dialysis (CAPD), and who, at the same time, also suffer from high blood pressure. End-stage renal disease (ESRD) (or end-stage renal failure - ESRF) is the stage in chronic renal disease in which renal replacement therapy, dialysis or kidney transplantation, is needed to sustain life. ESRD is generally an irreversible state. When being treated by continuous ambulatory peritoneal dialysis (CAPD), the patient empties a fresh bag of dialysate into the abdomen. After 4 to 6 hours of dwell time, the patient returns the dialysate containing wastes to the bag. The patient then repeats the cycle with a fresh bag of dialysate. CAPD does not require a machine; the process uses gravity to fill and empty the abdomen. A typical prescription for a CAPD patient requires three or four exchanges during the day and one long overnight exchange when the patient sleeps. The dialysate used for the long overnight exchange may have a higher concentration of dextrose, so that it absorbs wastes for a longer time.

In what follows, we consider two designated categories of tasks, namely those carried out by patients at home and those carried out by professionals in the office.

2.2 Activities Carried Out by Patients at Home

Patients carry out tasks that enable measurement of certain vital signs on a daily basis. The vital signs measured are described below.

2.2.1 Body Weight
Being obese increases the risk for many diseases, especially heart disease, stroke, cancer, and diabetes. In addition, for conditions like severe heart diseases and for dialysis patients, increasing body weight is a very important indicator of a beginning decompensation, which is a highly critical situation. Cardiologists regard changes in weight as one of the most relevant vital signals for their chronic patients. In PD patients, attainment of target weight is based on clinical indicators.

2.2.2 Blood Pressure
Blood pressure is expressed in millimetres of mercury, or mm Hg. The systolic blood pressure is the top number of a blood pressure reading. This shows the maximum pressure in the blood vessels as the heart contracts and circulates blood throughout the body. The diastolic blood pressure is the bottom number of a blood pressure reading. It shows the lowest pressure in the blood vessels between heartbeats, when the heart is at rest. Both high blood pressure (hypertension) and low blood pressure (hypotension) are indications of a condition that might necessitate a medical intervention. High blood pressure is also called the silent killer. Chronically high blood pressure can cause blood vessel changes in the back of the eye (retina), thickening of the heart muscle, kidney failure, and brain damage. This condition is considered a (high) risk factor for the development of heart disease, peripheral vascular disease, stroke and kidney disease.

2.2.3 Pulse Rate
The pulse rate is the number of times a person's heart beats in one minute. The pulse rate can give important information about overall health and fitness, and is usually measured as part of a physical exam. Whenever a person has an appointment with a healthcare provider, the pulse rate is measured routinely. An irregular pulse often indicates an electrical problem in the heart. This may be normal for a given person or may indicate a life-threatening problem. For example, irregular pulse rates can be due to a heart attack or enlargement of the heart. Pulse rate is usually measured concurrently with blood pressure.

2.2.4 Electrocardiogram – ECG (1-lead to 12-lead)

An electrocardiogram, also called an ECG, is a graphic record of the heart's electrical activity. Healthcare providers use it to help diagnose heart disease. They can also use it to monitor how well different heart medications are working.

Though 9- to 12-lead ECGs can be taken at home, a 1-lead ECG (a so called rhythm strip, which reliably shows abnormal rhythms such as arrhythmias or dysrhythmias) can be much easier performed and more simply applied by lay persons.

Other information may concern:

- The patient's medication compliance and feedback on this to both the patient himself and the physician, and
- General information on the disease, its treatment procedures and options and lifestyle information and training material.

Users of all this information and data can be

- The physician or nephrologist looking after the patient
- The patient directly
- Family members or informal carers
- Formal carers or nurses

2.3 Presently Used Measuring Devices

For the described requirement and assessment tests, a modular set of TeleCare measurement devices has been being used. These measurement units have single-button or no-button operation. Each device is equipped with a radio transmitter, capable of sending the measured information reliably to a Home Hub. This eliminates the need to cable patients' living quarters, and also provides a degree of freedom to move the devices within the home.

The model of use for this equipment is based on automatic, not patient-initiated, data transmission.

Once the patient has completed a measurement, for example blood pressure, the data are automatically transmitted to the Home Hub. The Home Hub is a microcontroller communication link that uses TCP/IP, MSCHAP, plus encryption to send the data over conventional phone lines to an ODBC database, located in a hospital or other secure setting. No additional user interaction is required to enter the data into the database, or to match it with a patient.

The NT server, running a standard SQL database and a web server, automatically collects incoming patient data, presents it to the database for entry, and allows care providers with the appropriate authorisation to review the data as web pages via Intranet, or secure virtual private Networks.

Special attention was devoted to the fact that most patients are frail or elderly. The patients units therefore need to be unobtrusive, very simple to use, and robust. Special features of the physiologic measurement devices are:

- Large displays and numbers making it easy to read the measurements
- Only one button to run measurement
- Voice and light prompts to support required behaviour
- Battery powered to allow mobile use at home
- Fully automatic data transmission (no patient interaction required)

- No wiring between measurement devices and the home hub
  Examples of the three measurement devices are depicted in the following pictures.

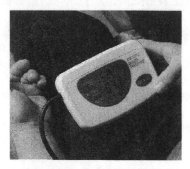

Fig. 1. Blood pressure

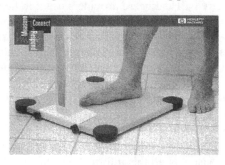

Fig. 2. Scalemeasurement

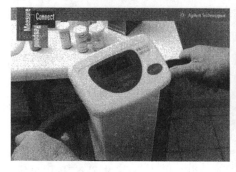

Fig. 3. Scale

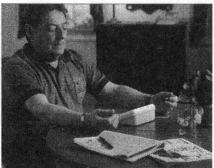

Fig. 4. Rhythm strip device

The scale (Figure 2, Figure 3) offers a very large, low profile platform (easy to step on), and a column with hand bars to hold on to, as well as voice announcements.

2.4 Context of Use for the Home-Based Tasks

The context of use from the patient's point of view is presently only the patient's home, usually a corner in the bedroom, or, in large homes/apartments, a separate room. If the bathroom is large, it may also be a small table/corner there, and during the day some of the measurements can also be taken in the living room or at a dining table. PD requires a considerable amount of supplies which are also heavy (e.g., dialysate) and may be stored in a separate room, the basement or elsewhere.

Before breakfast, the first task of the patient is to step onto the scale; he is "asked" by a synthetic voice to stand still (which is also indicated by a light on the display) for about 5 seconds (he/she may, of course, use the handle to keep balance without affecting the measurement result, which is particularly important for frail people) till the scale "talks" to him (and also provides a flashing light signal on the display) and tells him to step off the scale. Afterwards, the scale "tells" the patient his weight and this value is also displayed. The volume of the synthetic voice can be adjusted by a separate key. The data is automatically transmitted to the home hub underneath the telephone.

Next, the patient attaches the cuff of the blood pressure device to his upper arm with a Velcro fastener, presses a large, round button on the front of the device, and then the device automatically pumps the cuff, allows the air pressure slowly to decrease and takes the necessary measurements (systolic and diastolic pressure, pulse rate), displays these data and also transfers them automatically to the home hub.

Then the patient attaches the two leads of the rhythm strip to his wrists, pushes a button on the measurement device, waits for about one minute, and takes the leads off. The device has no display to show the ECG, but it automatically transmits the data to the home hub.

All of these vital data are then automatically, without any action on the part of the patient, transmitted via the home hub and his telephone dialling into an "800" number to the server at the nephrologist's office or in a hospital or community care centre. Without action on either side, the vital data are added to and integrated into the EHR of the patient. In other words, the EHR is updated every time the patient takes new measurements.

In addition to taking these measurements, the patient has to empty his abdomen and allow the dialysate containing wastes from his blood to return to the bag by attaching the catheter implanted in his belly to the bag. After this, the patient fills his abdomen again with a fresh bag of dialysate. The bag with the waste is weighed on a small scale and the result recorded by hand on a piece of paper.

The exchange of fluid is usually repeated for another three times every day, and each time blood pressure and pulse are measured as well, but not weight and ECG.

Presently, input of patient data is made by the physician for those data and information collected during the visit of the patient to the ambulatory clinic or office of the nephrologist. In addition, in our scenario, vital data are measured in the described manner by the patient using telemonitoring measurement devices that automatically record and transmit the measurement data via a telecommunications connection. This is a new form of input made possible by telemonitoring technology.

Target users for the reference scenario are presently those high-risk PD patients where changes in blood pressure (hypertension which is difficult to adjust) and weight (i.e., patients who have problems with their fluid balance - either the filtration is too low or they tend to drink too much) can be expected to occur within a short time period. It is estimated that for about 10% of all present (German) PD patients, close monitoring would be medically indicated. When the system becomes available permanently and for general introduction, it can be expected that the market potential will be considerably expanded: Perhaps 10% to 20% of all new (hitherto haemo) dialysis patients may then, in addition, qualify for PD treatment. Presently, their unstable health requires close monitoring which is only assured when they have to visit the dialysis clinic three times a week (PD patients: usually once a month or every six weeks).

Beyond this, any patient who would benefit significantly from closer telemonitoring such data at home or while moving, particularly patients with a severe heart disease, qualify as target users in future.

2.4.1 Activities Carried Out at the Nephrologist's Office

The nephrologist's office is equipped with web-technology based service software, which allows review of a patient's medical condition. Simply by clicking on a patient's name, his or her individual record is accessed. On the standard interface, the physician sees the graphical trend of the patient's weight and, in tabular form, all other data measured. To have a closer look at any data or combination of data, he can click on the relevant buttons on his screen to select them, request a graphical presentation and adjust the time period reported on. These data can, if preferred by the medical staff, also be presented in tabular form. Additional files for medical history, laboratory results, medication régime etc. are available.

For security and privacy reasons, presently no external access to the server in the physician's office is possible. However, various screen shots of anonymous patient data as recorded by the system based on the telemonitoring data transmitted were obtained. In the following, they are presented and briefly explained. In principle, these data are already today also available to patients in printed form from their physician, and they could easily be made available via Internet technology.

Figure 5 shows a simple diagram of weight measurements for one month as a full screen without any other information:

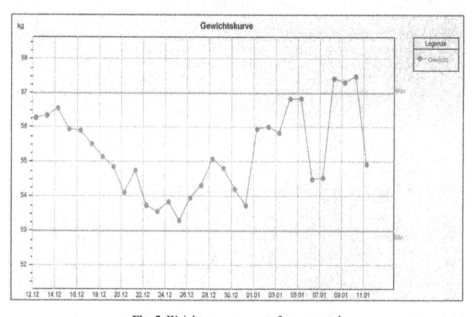

Fig. 5. Weight measurements for one month

Figure 6 depicts are more complicated graphical design showing three measurement values over two weeks in parallel:

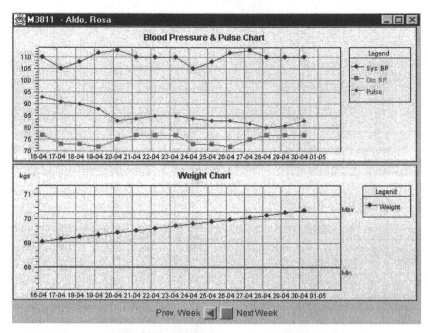

Fig. 6. Combination of blood pressure, pulse and weight chart on one screen

A further degree of complexity is shown in Figure 7.

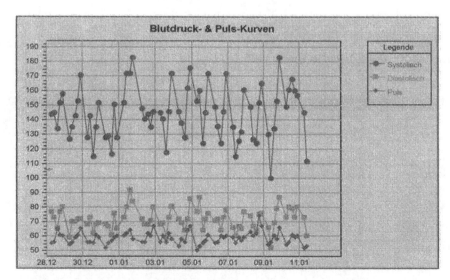

Fig. 7. Blood pressure and pulse values, measured four times a day for two weeks

As an alternative, a tabular presentation of these values was also offered to the patients as seen in Table 1:

Table 1. Blood pressure and pulse values, measured four times a day for six days

Trends für

Telefon: Alter: 56 Jahre   Pat.-Nr.: Dias 1

Datum	Gewicht		Sys/Dia(Mitt)		Puls	
22.07.2001	95.8 kg	10:56	161 / 92 (150)	00:44	75	00:44
			170 / 97 (155)	10:58	66	10:58
			159 / 90 (136)	13:44	69	13:44
			156 / 93 (131)	18:27	66	18:27
21.07.2001	95.8 kg	10:45	148 / 88 (119)	00:55	78	00:55
			155 / 92 (138)	10:46	68	10:46
			155 / 87 (107)	12:36	73	12:36
			156 / 84 (132)	16:52	72	16:52
20.07.2001	95.20 kg	10:47	165 / 92 (144)	20:56	69	20:56
			163 / 92 (147)	00:44	72	00:44
			152 / 96 (129)	10:49	72	10:49
			156 / 87 (126)	13:16	72	13:16
19.07.2001	94.87 kg	10:13	146 / 85 (118)	21:15	80	21:15
			159 / 91 (130)	00:51	76	00:51
			150 / 92 (137)	10:16	68	10:16
			151 / 91 (134)	13:04	66	13:04
18.07.2001	94.33 kg	10:14	156 / 89 (137)	17:16	68	17:16
			154 / 88 (136)	21:45	69	21:45
			160 / 94 (131)	00:59	72	00:59
			156 / 95 (134)	10:17	70	10:17
17.07.2001	95.20 kg	11:08	145 / 92 (124)	13:58	65	13:58
			153 / 90 (132)	19:11	66	19:11
			184 / 98 (143)	11:10	67	11:10
			145 / 90 (120)	13:16	69	13:16
			152 / 90 (121)	17:37	68	17:37
			152 / 87 (127)	21:37	75	21:37

Finally a representation of a 16 second rhythm strip (one-lead ECG) with a minor irregularity was selected as shown in Figure 8.

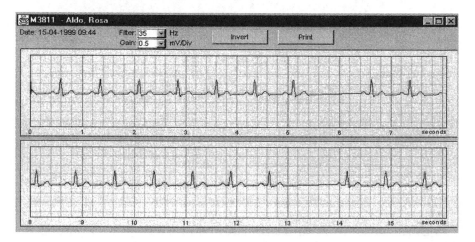

Fig. 8. 16 second rhythm strip (one-lead ECG)

3. Concluding Remarks

Experience with chronically ill patients engaged in the above reference scenario as well as reports in the literature (Cimino et al., 2001) show that patients having access to their vital data by whatever means are in a much better position to monitor their environment, their behaviour, their diet and their own compliance with medication. Both medical outcome and quality of life improve, and the patients feel more in control of their own health. Therefore, as a logical extension of such considerations, the need arises to identify ways and means to ensure that all those patients who want access to their EHR obtain information on those data which are of prime relevance for them and which they are able to interpret and translate into meaningful action to improve, or at least to stabilise, their physical and mental health status.

Chapter 10
MediBRIDGE / C-CARE: Remote Access to EPRs

Georges De Moor[1] and Louis Schilders[2]

[1] Ghent University
Department of Health Informatics and Statistics
De Pintelaan 185
Ghent 5k3 9000, Belgium
georges.demoor@UGent.be

[2] MediBRIDGE nv-sa
rue du Bourdon 100
1180 Brussels, Belgium
louis.schilders@medmail.medconf.be

Abstract. This Chapter describes a reference scenario that has been extracted from current practices regarding the use of Electronic Patient Records in Belgium, and in particular the C-CARE services as hosted by MediBRIDGE. The scenario has been provided by the IS4ALL member MS-HUGe in collaboration with MediBRIDGE.

1. Background

MediBRIDGE was founded in 1994 by the major actors in Belgian Health Care and became the first Healthcare Telematics Service Provider in Belgium. More than 19.000 users rely on MediBRIDGE to exchange their daily patient correspondence.

1.1 MedSERVE Service

The MedSERVE service has been developed to exchange patient related information between Medical Professionals. Basically MediBRIDGE provides completely secure unattended data transfer from Hospitals and Medical specialists to General Practitioners. At the sender's site the information produced by the host system (Hospital Information System, Departmental Information System, Electronic Healthcare Record System, etc) is captured automatically. All this information is sent in one communication session to the MedSERVE servers. At the receiver's site, upon receipt of information, procedures are provided to prepare the received data for automatic integration in the host EHCR system. Since the transfer involves personal medical data, the system guarantees watertight security, confidentiality and data integrity. It is based on asymmetric data encryption, including a digital signature. An intelligent interface sub-system allows MedSERVE to cooperate with virtually any system installed in the GP's practice.

C. Stephanidis (Ed.): Universal Access Code of Practice in Health Telematics, LNCS 3041, pp. 88-96, 2005.

1.2 MedIMAGE Service

The MedIMAGE application offers the possibility to import medical images produced by a wide range of imaging modality applications. It is possible to export the images as well as the examination report in XML format, taking into account the specificity of the target medical application. The collaborative working features (based on internet technology) offered by the MedIMAGE application allow Healthcare Professionals to discuss cases on-line whenever required. Representative /educational data can be transported to an Image Reference Database for further consultation / teaching.

1.3 C-CARE Service

The Service Continuous Care (C-CARE, see Figure 1) allows General Practitioners on duty, Pharmacists and Emergency Hospital Departments – with the citizens' consent – to access essential clinical data in a geographical area. A "Permanent Referral Letter" is automatically exported (periodically or on a predetermined trigger) from distributed EHCR systems (held by GPs, specialist clinics, hospitals, etc) towards a central server.

The information held in this server is accessible to authorised users only (healthcare professionals, pharmacists or the citizens themselves) – duly authenticated – through a web-browser or a normal telephone set (or cellular phone / GSM). Information is always presented according to the user profile, in such a way that each user receives only the appropriate information, presented in the most suitable way for the most relevant data to be grasped at a glance. The service will implement the concept of Integrated Care on a local – regional basis by means of industry standards in ICT (XML, XSL, Text – to – Speech, etc).

2. Accident on the Road

2.1 At the Scene of the Accident

The Ambulance arrives at the scene of the accident. The paramedic obtains the patient's ID and transmits the ID to the Emergency department. In case a physician is present, he can contact the C-CARE voice server.

2.2 At the Emergency Centre

The physician on duty connects to the web-based C-Care server (Figure 1), clicks on the C-Care logo and obtains immediate access to the patient's data according to his/her access rights.

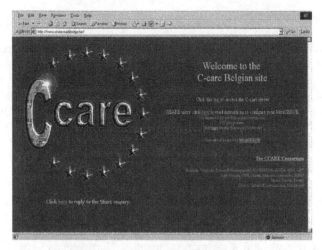

Fig. 1. The Web-based C-Care server

2.3 The C-CARE Service

The physician enters his username and password and clicks on the "Log In" button (see Figure 2). The server assesses his access rights and accordingly grants access to the service. The physician enters the patient's identification data - patients are identified uniquely. The medical record becomes available, and the system presents a summary table (see Figure 3).

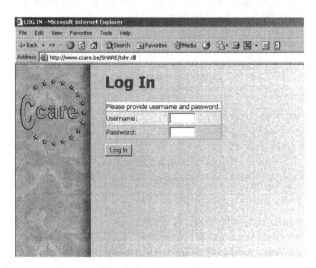

Fig. 2. Login screen

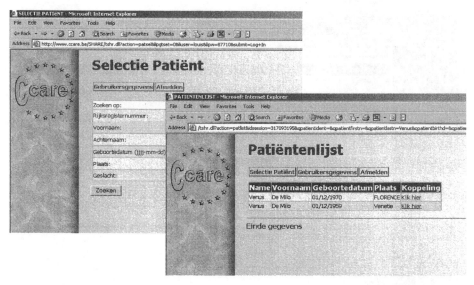

Fig. 3. Searching for a patient and presenting the medical record

The physician reviews the available patient's information according to his/her access rights (see Figure 4). The following rubrics are displayed when available, including administrative data, medication, allergies, medical antecedents, medical evaluation, vaccinations, etc.

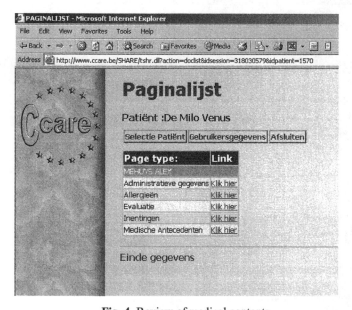

Fig. 4. Review of medical contents

The physician consults the allergy data (Figure 5) and alerts the ambulance if necessary.

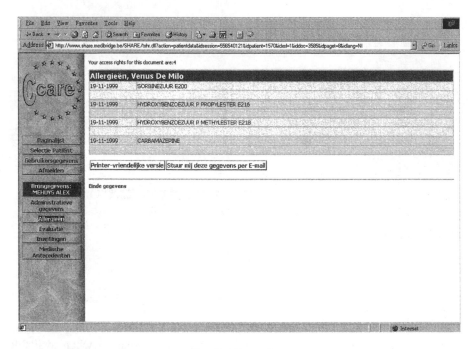

Fig. 5. Allergy data

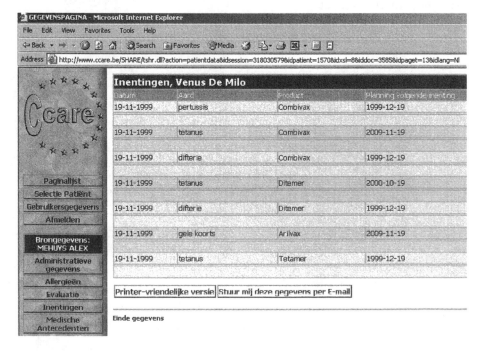

Fig. 6. Medication list

Then the physician consults the medication data (Figure 6) and accordingly alerts the ambulance if necessary (e.g., contra-indications). The medication list provides a first impression of the patient's health-care status.

The physician consults the vaccination data (Figure 7) and checks, for example, the date of the last tetanus vaccination.

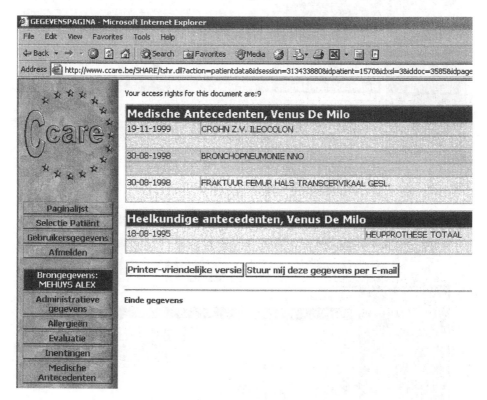

Fig. 7. Vaccination data

In a similar fashion, the physician consults the medical antecedents. The system provides coded data (ICD-9/ 10) and a description (pathology + treatment) as shown in Figure 8).

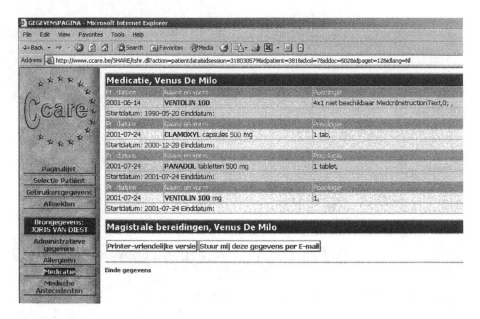

Fig. 8. Medical antecedents

The physician consults the evaluation data: Risks, Diagnoses (see Figure 9).

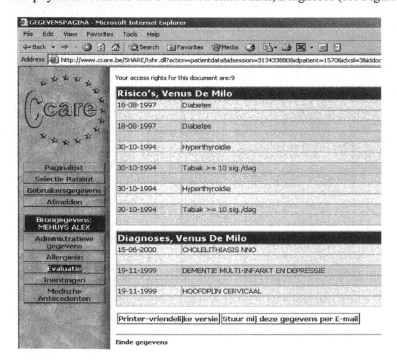

Fig. 9. Risks and diagnosis screen

Using the "transmit" button, the selected item is transferred to the physician device. He receives the data automatically on his system (see Figure 10), which can be a portable device (PDA / Mobile Phone).

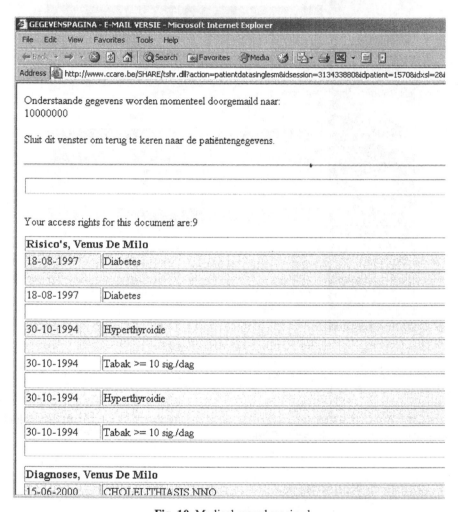

Fig. 10. Medical record received

2.4 The Patient Arrives at the Hospital

The normal procedure starts. The E&A does not waste time collecting information from/about the patient. Quality of care is improved substantially. Clinical patient data are available wherever necessary.

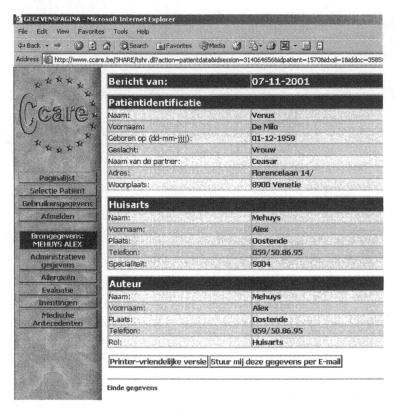

Fig. 11. Medical record of patient

2.5 Verification of the Patient's Administrative Data

The nurse verifies the patient's administrative data available on the system, which displays an overview as shown in Figure 11.

3. Concluding Remark

It is important to note that the above reference scenario depicts only parts of the MediBridge service functionality that explicitly relates to the C-CARE project. Additional features, not addressed in the current reference scenario, include recent efforts to update the service platform so as to facilitate a more systematic account of universal access.

Part III Design for All Methods and Their Application

Chapter 11
The Universal Access Assessment Workshop (UA²W) Method

Demosthenes Akoumianakis[1] and Constantine Stephanidis[1,2]

[1] Foundation for Research and Technology – Hellas (FORTH)
Institute of Computer Science
Heraklion, Crete, GR-70013, Greece
cs@ics.forth.gr
[2] Department of Computer Science
University of Crete, Greece

Abstract. This Chapter describes the Universal Access Assessment Workshop (UA2W) method and how it was validated in the context of a design case study. The Chapter first describes the method in terms of the problem addressed, the devices and instruments used, the procedure for using the devices, and the outcomes and assumptions. Then, it presents a case study and describes the application of the method in the context of WardInHand reference scenarios (Chapter 8). The Chapter concludes by briefly discussing experience in the use of the method and some lessons learnt.

1. Introduction

Universal Access in the context of IST-based applications and services entails a thorough understanding, on the part of the design team, of the global execution context of an application's designated tasks. At any time, the execution context of a task can be considered in terms of three basic elements, namely the user, the platform used to provide the computational embodiment of the task, and the context in which the task is executed. A simple way to gain an insight into the global execution context of a task is to hold constant any one of the three parameters and to consider variations in the others. Nevertheless, the ultimate design space of Universal Access UA, given a set of users U, a range of interaction platforms P and a set of alternative contexts of use C, is contextually defined as the Cartesian product $UA=\{U \times P \times C\}$.

The above conception of Universal Access poses several questions regarding the design processes needed, the appropriate methodology and the related instruments to be employed in order to facilitate insights to Universal Access and provide tangible outcomes in the course of Human-Computer Interaction (HCI) design. Some of these questions challenge basic assumptions of HCI design as formulated and practiced over the past two decades (see Chapter 1), while others raise implications on the use and application of specific methods and techniques. For example, one of the basic assumptions or principles of user-centred design is "know the user". This became a primary focus with the advent of human-centred processes in the period where users

C. Stephanidis (Ed.): Universal Access Code of Practice in Health Telematics, LNCS 3041, pp. 99–114, 2005.
© Springer-Verlag Berlin Heidelberg 2005

of interactive computer-based applications were office workers, with specific objectives and performance characteristics. However, with the advent of the Internet and the WWW, users are no longer homogeneous in the conventional sense, and do not carry out tasks of the same type and scope. Additionally, the devices that have become available enable new patterns of use in ubiquitous contexts. Thus, the conventional desktop is increasingly being complemented by a range of network attachable devices, such as mobile phones, PDAs, etc. As a result, in the emerging paradigm design, should be diversity-centred rather than user- or technology-centred.

This Chapter describes a technique that can be used to elicit requirements for Universal Access and provide early design insights towards an understanding of the global execution context of the tasks of a designated system. The technique offers several structured instruments, which are briefly introduced and discussed. Using these instruments, the design team can formulate design concepts, develop low-fidelity prototypes, record their rationale and reach consensus on envisioned system use and non-functional quality attributes.

2. The Universal Access Assessment Workshop

2.1 Problem Being Addressed

The UA^{2}W is a participatory inquiry aiming to provide an argumentative context for reflecting upon existing practices and envisioning future interactive experiences. The central theme in UA^{2}W sessions is unfolding and understanding the global execution context of a system's tasks. This implies an early involvement in exploratory design activities, in an effort to unfold diverse requirements, emerging use patterns as well as alternative access regimes, which may be required. In the past, software engineering and human computer interaction tackled these problems from distinct perspectives leading to a growing body of knowledge on adaptable and adaptive systems, personalisation, user modelling, etc. Despite recent progress, further research is needed on design methods, which could form the ground for a normative design cycle focused explicitly on gaining insight into the global execution context of tasks. In what follows, an attempt is made to present UA^{2}W as a complete micro method (in the sense of Olson and Moran 1996) which serves this purpose.

2.2 Device / Technique(s) Used

2.2.1 Overview
UA^{2}W is a technique which seeks to bring together early in the design phase as many stakeholders as possible to identify the type and scope of Universal Access requirements for a particular product or service. From this perspective, the UA^{2}W is essentially a participatory technique in which experts, end users, or representatives of end users may be invited to participate. A UA^{2}W is always organised by an analyst and may be tuned in such a way as to facilitate a variety of targets, including critical

design reviews, artefact re-engineering, design rationale, etc. Accordingly, the devices or instruments used may vary.

Two main techniques or instruments are central to the conduct of UA²W, namely scenario screening and growth scenarios (see also Chapter 14). Both mechanisms serve the purpose of extrapolating (some of) the Universal Access design considerations relevant to a particular reference scenario (see Figure 1).

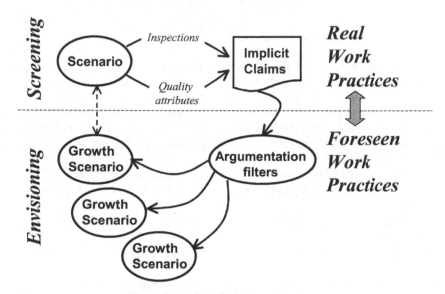

Fig. 1. Scenario articulation mechanisms

2.2.2 Scenario Screening

Scenario screening assumes the availability of artefacts for review and discussion. It entails a structured process whereby implicit or explicit assumptions embedded in an artefact and related to the intended users, the platform used to implement the artefact and the context of use, are identified and documented. Typically, scenario screening is a group activity initiated and guided by an analyst. Participants may include representatives of end user communities, project managers, developers, etc. Thus, screening is best organised as a collaborative activity in which participants converge to obtain a common understanding of what is at stake by identifying implicit or explicit assumptions in the reference scenario.

2.2.3 Growth Scenarios

In a subsequent phase, these assumptions are relaxed to facilitate envisioning and generation of new artefacts through compiling growth scenarios. Growth scenarios assume a slightly different approach in the sense that they are instruments for envisioning rather than reflection. Growth scenarios are formulated as a result of argumentation based on the identified assumptions in the reference scenario. Argumentation of this kind may be facilitated through posing and addressing critical design issues or questions, such as:

- "What if … the task was to be carried out by another user?"
- "What if … the task was to be carried out through an alternative device?" etc.

Through such argumentation, the group reaches consensus on the new task execution contexts relevant, which, in turn, is documented as growth scenarios comprising narrative description of envisioned activities and corresponding artefacts in the form of mock-ups or low fidelity prototypes.

2.3 Procedure for Using the Device

It is important to mention that the UA^2W need not be a one-off event. Instead, it may take place several times to provide the required materials and design insight. Specifically, in cases where the resources are available, at least one UA^2W should be devoted to scenario screening, followed by a separate UA^2W targeted towards the compilation of suitable growth scenarios. It follows that planning and organising the UA^2Ws needed for a particular project is important and may act as a catalyst for subsequent phases.

To this effect, critical organisational aspects to be addressed include:
- Ensuring appropriate stakeholder participation and that all participants understand the process
- Making design documentation materials self-explanatory and available to all participants
- Setting appropriate targets (in each stage of scenario screening, or growth scenario compilation)
- Making effective use of resources (time, participant competences, etc).

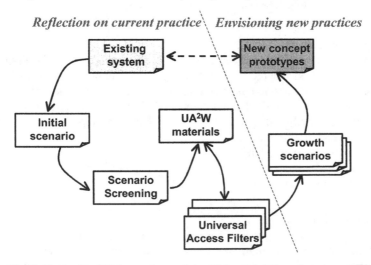

Fig. 2. Cycles in planning and organising Universal Access Assessment Workshops

Schematically, the iterative character of UA^2Ws together with the various outcomes involved in the process are depicted in the diagram of Figure 2 and described below.

The procedure to be followed depends on the purpose of the UA²W, whether scenario screening or compilation of growth scenarios. These two options are briefly described below.

2.3.1 Procedure Followed for Scenario Screening

The first step is usually a preparatory activity carried out by the analyst, and entails the development of a reference scenario. Scenario formulation is an iterative process. Initially, narrative descriptions of tasks, as carried out by actual users, are developed, and subsequently peer reviewed by health professionals or end-user communities. This peer review acts as a validity check to ensure that the scenarios are realistic and valid. In the course of this iterative phase, any system mock-ups, prototypes or other artefacts, which reveal aspects of the scenario's real execution context, are taken into account. Once a tentative scenario is formulated, the analyst selects the participants of the UA²W, who are subsequently invited to take part.

In the second stage, designers present the use case or reference scenario, with appropriate paper or computer-based mock-ups of a system in use, to the participants of the UA²W. During this stage, any questions about the system in use are addressed and all participants obtain a common understanding about the current system, how it is used, as well as any problems that may be encountered.

The third stage is devoted to consolidating the filters to be used for screening the scenario. For this purpose, the analyst may decide to propose an extract of relevant filters from the list of Universal Access Filters compiled by IS4ALL (see Chapter 13 on "Screening Artefacts"). Alternatively, the analyst may ask the participants to select the filters. In any case, at the end of this third stage, the group should have a clear view of what criteria are to be used to facilitate screening. This kind of roundtable assessment may be carried out for a pre-specified period of time or until participants identify a manageable set of relevant filters. At the end of the third stage, the UA²W may be considered complete and the analyst usually reports back to the participants the agreed materials and invites participation to the next UA²W, which will seek to develop growth scenarios based on the filters used during screening.

2.3.2 Procedure Followed for Compiling Growth Scenarios

Compiling growth scenarios usually follows the screening exercise. This time the procedure to be followed when conducting the UA²W is somewhat different from the previous case. Specifically, following a brief overview of the screening phase (i.e., outline of reference scenario and designated set of Universal Access filters), the group engages in a process where each filter is elaborated and associated with a growth scenario. For each filter, participants develop proposals that satisfy the filter and propose tentative design mock-ups to justify their propositions. Usually, low fidelity prototyping techniques are used for this purpose, such as paper and pencil, drawings on a white board, etc. Any questions that may be raised regarding the proposed artefacts are addressed until agreement is reached. This process is iterated for as many filters as the set designated during the screening phase, and until the workshop chair has elicited all the necessary information substantiating the reference scenarios.

At the end of the UA²W, the workshop chair consolidates the findings into a designated set of growth scenarios and fills in a form referred to as the Universal

Access Assessment Form (UA^2F). Finally, a summative account of the growth scenarios is captured in the Universal Access Quality Matrix (UAQM).

2.4 Outcomes

The primary outcomes of UA^2Ws include the Universal Access Assessment Form (UA^2F), growth scenarios and the UAQM. Each one is briefly described below.

2.4.1 Universal Access Assessment Form
The results of a UA^2W are documented in the UA^2F depicted in Figure 3.

Artefact:	
Functional Unit:	
Style:	

Objectives:

Functional Description Overview:

Universal Access Issues:

Issue Id.	Issue Description	Priority (H/M/L)	Constraint

Claims:

Constraints / Dependencies:

Functional / Operational Assessment:

Fig. 3. Outline of UA2F

2.4.2 Growth Scenarios

As already pointed out earlier, for each entry in the UA^2F, the design team develop a corresponding growth scenario. A growth scenario is a narrative description depicting the envisioned use of the system. In contrast with the initial reference scenario, a growth scenario may be shorter, targeted and supported by low-fidelity prototypes. In essence, it should provide all needed information for prototyping to take place.

2.4.3 The Universal Access Quality Matrix

All growth scenarios are subsequently consolidated and documented in a more abstract template referred to as the UAQM, illustrated in Figure 4. In summary, the primary outcomes of a UA^2W include several instances of the UA^2F, screening criteria if the UA^2W is organised to facilitate scenario screening, and growth scenarios if the UA^2W is organised to facilitate envisioning and the UAQM.

2.5 Assumptions

The technique assumes the availability of tentative reference scenario, supported by narrative description of how design mock-ups or system components are actually used.

Root	Quality Attribute	Attribute parameter	Question
Adaptability	... to users	... who are novice	
		... who are experienced	
		... with disabilities	How can the task be carried out by a user with gross temporal control
			How can the task be carried out by users with reduced eye-hand coordination
	... to platforms	... such as the desktop	
		... such as public terminal	
		... such as a cellular phone	What kind of navigation control is needed
			What's the structure for WAP pages
	... to context	... such as public building	Is device emulation needed?
		... such as a train	

Fig. 4. Example of the UAQM

3. Case Study: The WardInHand Prototype

The following case study is motivated by an early version of the WardInHand prototype. The first exposure to the aims and objectives of the WardInHand system was in October 2000 during a workshop between designated Health Telematics projects funded by the EC's IST Programme. Following the initial preliminary contact, WardInHand and IS4ALL organised another meeting, shortly after the first stable WardInHand prototype was available. The meeting was organised as an informal walkthrough of the current prototype. During the demonstration, the product's intended purpose, target users, as well as type, range and scope of supported tasks were described and an agreement was reached according to which WardInHand would provide the necessary materials to compile a representative scenario of use of the system.

3.1 Developing and Refining the Scenario

In an attempt to define a preliminary resource for design deliberations, a scenario was drafted, and it was subsequently confirmed by WardInHand representatives that the designated description provides an accurate account of the system's intended use in real practice. The scenario built upon the prototype implementation of the WardInHand system and addressed all possible tasks that a professional user can carry out as part of his/her daily activity plan. This resulted in a fairly substantial design document.

To facilitate the aims and objective of the case study, the scenario was split into smaller, more manageable parts. One of these sub-scenarios concerned access to, and navigation in, the patient record database that is described in the following section. The scenario described below is an extract from the larger WardInHand use case. The choice of the designated tasks to study was based on the outcomes of the usability evaluation of the system, which revealed high frequency of certain activities. Indeed, from the system's demonstration, it became obvious that the tasks of searching for patient records, and reviewing patient data were both carried out very frequently and prone to user error. Based on the above, the scenario selected for investigation is depicted in Exhibit 1.

Exhibit 1: Access to a patient records

- Dr Fred is preparing for his morning visit to the patients in the ward of the hospital. To assist him, he makes use of his iPAQ to access the WardInHand service, which was recently installed in the hospital.

- As part of the login procedure, Dr Fred selects the preferred language and then specifies the user name and password. For this purpose the system displays an on-screen keyboard which allows Dr Fred to type in text by selecting characters from a selection panel.

- Upon successful login, the system presents the user with the main applications menu (see Figure 5a). By this time Dr Fred is now by the bedside of the first patient.

- WardInHand has already listed patient records (see Figure 5b) and the doctor asks for the patient's name to select the corresponding record.

- Once a particular patient record is selected then the doctor can initiate a range of tasks from the menu of Figure 5c, such clinical overview, admission details, treatments assigned, examinations ordered etc.

It should be noted that the tasks designated in Exhibit 1 depict actual use of the system during a demonstration session. To reduce the scope of the case study, we chose not to address tasks such as login procedures, even though their usability in the current implementation could be improved. Instead, we focused on frequently re-occurring tasks, such as searching and reviewing patient records (see Figure 5a, b). In particular, the interaction with the dialogue of Figure 5c, may take place several times for each patient. Finally, it is worth pointing out that the designated tasks are associated with container object classes, which raise the issue of effective and efficient navigation within the containers.

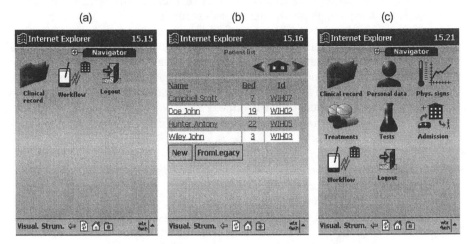

Fig. 5. WardInHand screens to accessing a patient record

3.2 Preparing and Conducting the UA²Ws

As already pointed out, the UA²W can be organised with the intention either to filter out aspects of the scenario which limit Universal Access (i.e., scenario screening) or to envision future use and to develop design proposals in the direction of Universal Access (i.e., growth scenarios). Ideally, the development of growth scenarios should follow and respond to a thorough phase of scenario screening.

3.2.1 Scenario Screening

Scenario screening may take several forms, depending on the intended purpose. For instance, it may be conducted as a co-operative inspection of a product using an agreed set of heuristics. Alternatively, it may involve a few experts assessing the product's compliance with standards or a designated guideline reference manual. In any case, it is intended to provide an inter-disciplinary forum for exchanging knowledge, perspectives and experiences.

The screening process assumes an agreed set of criteria or design heuristics against which the product is assessed. The content and scope of these instruments may vary depending on the aims of the exercise. For the purposes of this case study, we have made use of filters as a mechanism to support argumentation about a tentative design.

Filtering helps the team explore explicit or implicit assumptions, which determine or limit the use of the product. In many ways, filters are similar to questions used by other analytical HCI design techniques, such as Design Space Analysis and QOC (MacLean et al., 1991). The difference is that filters, as used in scenario screening, assume the availability of a prototype. The fidelity of the prototype is not of critical importance, so long as the prototype conveys the intended concept and provides a reference for discussing intended use. In this regard, filters can provide a useful instrument in unfolding aspects of the design, which prompt Universal Access insight. Nevertheless, filtering is unlikely to generate design solutions. Rather, it is intended to facilitate the identification of potential problems or breakdowns, which can then be addressed in a subsequent phase, through growth scenarios.

Identifying a suitable set of filters to unfold Universal Access insight is far from trivial. This is partially due to the lack of consolidated knowledge on Universal Access, but also due to the misunderstanding that is usually associated with the term. In the context of the present work, the term Universal Access implies the development of an interactive service that can automatically facilitate access to any authorised user from anywhere and at anytime.

Our baseline, which is rooted in previous work, is that Universal Access entails two prime concerns, namely:

- Understanding the global execution context of tasks
- Managing the design of artefacts suitable for different execution contexts

Filtering facilitates the former target, while growth scenarios are intended to assist in attending the latter. Thus, the filters to be used should aim to facilitate an understanding of the global execution context of the tasks involved in the scenario. Our previous work in this area indicates that the execution context of task is determined or influenced by three distinct categories of design parameters, namely:

- The intended users
- The computer platform used to execute the task
- The context in which the activity takes place

The WardInHand prototype was implemented on an iPAQ, and was to be used by authorised users. Therefore, a doctor wishing to review a patient's examination results at a certain point in time from his/her office or from another location outside the hospital (i.e., home), and accordingly refine the treatment or prescribe additional medication, or schedule a task for a colleagues the following day, could not do so. With such thinking in mind, the Universal Access Filters that immediately emerge as relevant are (at least) the following:

- How can (relevant parts of) the system be used from outside the ward (i.e., the office or the home)?
- How can (relevant parts of) the system be refined to offer the service over a different platform (i.e., the WWW)?
- How could (relevant parts of) the system be refined to be accessible by an authorised motor-impaired patient?

Addressing separately or in combination design concerns such as the above, new execution contexts are unfolded, either for the entire system or relevant parts of it. In this manner, iteratively, one can gain a detailed understanding of the global execution context of the system's tasks so as to fulfil the intention of Universal Access.

It is important to note that each cube (or alternative execution context) in the matrix necessitates separate treatment and design consideration, which may give rise to further refinement. For instance, a WWW version of WardInHand may facilitate access to the system by authorised users at home (i.e., patients or professionals). This makes individualisation a predominant concern, which, in turn, may necessitate further refinement of the designated execution context to facilitate access by different categories of authorised users (i.e., people with disabilities, elderly, novices, experts, etc). From the above, it becomes apparent that understanding a task's global execution context is far from a trivial task, since the parameters that become potentially relevant grow in type and range. The outcome of the filtering process is documented in the UA^{2}F (see Figure 6).

Artefact:	Mock-up listing all the tests ordered for the patient
Functional Unit:	Ward of the clinic

Style: Currently the system runs on an iPAQ

The style is depicted in the mock up shown in the following figure

Objectives:

We would like to make the service accessible over the Web for authorised users.

Functional Description Overview:

No change

Universal Access Issues:

Issue Id.	Issue Description	Priority (H/M/L)	Constraint
1	Adaptability to different user groups	H	Blind, motor impaired and able-bodied users
2	Scalability to different platforms	H	Desktop, PDAs and Kiosks
3	Context-sensitive	H	Ubiquitous

Claims:

Growth scenario 1	How can the task be performed over the Web
Growth scenario 2	How can the task be performed using an alternative interaction technique such as scanning, suitable for users with motor impairments
Growth scenario 3	How can the task be performed through an auditory input modality

Constraints / Dependencies:

Not known yet

Functional / Operational Assessment: Not yet available

Fig. 6. Example of the UA2F

3.2.2 Growth Scenarios

For each of the designated filters appearing in the "Universal Access issues" section of the UA^{2}F, a growth scenario can be developed to provide a reference context for the issue (or challenge) being addressed. A core target in the development of growth scenarios is the generation of revised or new artefacts, which relax some of the assumptions embedded in the initial prototype. During this phase, participants should be solely focused on crafting creative design solutions and should not be encumbered with aspects such as implementation cost, time to market, availability of resources to realise the design, etc., or any other factor which may pose constraints on the development process. This relieves participants from the temptation to settle for obvious design solutions, or emulating existing poor design, when novel and more powerful ones may be within their grasp.

A number of representative growth scenarios have been developed, depicting WWW and WAP phone prototypes of some of the relevant artefacts. For example, Figure 7 depicts an example of how the WWW-based system could realise the task of searching for a patient. Moreover, Figure 8 depicts a WWW style augmented with scanning[1], which allows a patient with a motor impairment to enter medical data and to update the electronic patient record. For more details on the design and implementation of the scanning technique, see Stephanidis, Paramythis, Sfyrakis, & Savidis (2001).

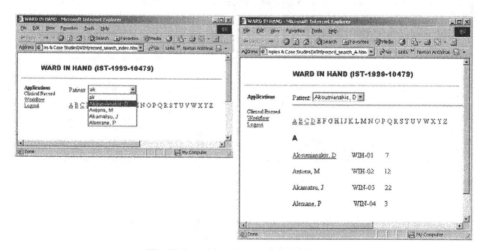

Fig. 7. Searching for a patient in the ward

The mock-ups depicted above were developed in an effort to address the Universal Access issue "adaptability to different user groups" (see Figure 6), and in particular to

---

[1] As indicated in the figure, the virtual keyboard in automatic scanning mode is used to allow the motor-impaired user to carry out text editing (i.e., to enter a value for the text edit fields of the user interface).

enable access for users with motor impairments who are familiar with the use of binary switches and hierarchical scanning of interaction elements[2].

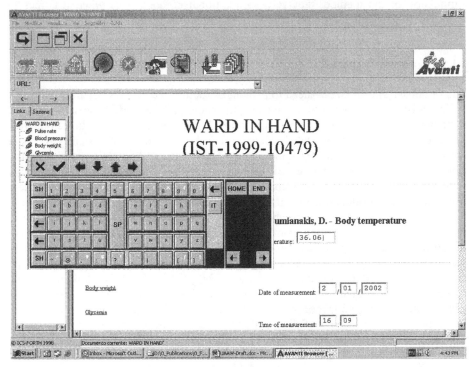

Fig. 8. Patient's medical entry using an augmented WWW style accessible via the AVANTI browser

4. Discussion and Lessons Learnt

The UA^{2}W is a technique, which shares common grounds with some prevalent HCI design methods, particularly within the cluster of participatory action research and collaborative inquiry methods. Links also exist with recent developments in the field of software engineering and the study of non-functional quality attributes (see Chapter 13). Nevertheless, the specifics of the technique (i.e., its strong orientation towards scenario-based design, the instruments for articulating scenarios, either through screening or by compiling growth scenarios), distinguish it from other similar approaches. As with other similar proposals, the UA^{2}W assumes a number of pre-requisites, including:

- Sufficient preparation on behalf of the organisers
- Availability of a working (reference) scenario

---

[2] As a clarifying remark, it should be noted that the mock-up of Figure 8 depicts an interactive session through an instance of the AVANTI Browser (Stephanidis et al., 2001).

- Agreement and commitment of participants towards using the instruments of scenario screening or filtering and compilation of growth scenarios

As discussed below, the above ingredients although necessary, for a successful application of the method, they rely on additional competencies when it comes to implementing design decisions.

4.1 Organiser's Preparation

The organiser(s) of a UA^2W need to plan and structure the activity. Critical decisions in this effort are the choice of participants, the choice of the working scenario and the sequence in which the scenario articulation instruments are to be employed. Regarding participants or stakeholders in the UA^2W, it is important to ensure representatives of different users, including current users and potential users resulting from a future implementation of growth scenarios. This will guarantee clear statements on requirements and underlying rationale for building Universal Access features into the product or service. Moreover, participants need to be informed about the overall process, the success check points and the stages involved, in order to facilitate a seamless transition from scenario screening to the compilation of growth scenarios. Circulation of suitable documents and support materials is important. Such documentation may include the agenda of the UA^2W, the reference scenario (if available), design documentation forms (i.e., UA^2F, the UAQM). In addition, a whole range of issues, which appear as prominent success factors in other participatory action research and collaborative inquiry efforts (i.e., democratic decision making, sympathy and appreciation of different perspectives, conflict resolution, time spent, etc) need to be taken into account when planning and executing a UA^2W.

4.2 Working (Reference) Scenario

The choice of the reference scenario turns out to be very important. A successful scenario must be an extract of a realistic system, described in a manner conveying actual rather than intended use. One important consideration relates to the nature and scope of the reference scenario, which should make it amenable to Universal Access considerations. For some systems and corresponding scenarios, Universal Access may not be a suitable cause of action. For instance, an application running on a conventional computer in an operating theatre and intended to be accessed by the surgeon in the course of an operation is less likely to be amenable to Universal Access considerations than a community service which by definition should be accessed by all authorised users, anytime and anywhere. It is therefore critical to choose a suitable reference scenario and to define the scope of the intended intervention. Our experience with the WardInHand prototype shows that in order to eliminate potential problems, but also to speed up the conduct of the UA^2Ws, the reference scenario needs to be agreed upon and confirmed by end users. Ideally, this is an activity, which should take place prior to the UA^2W, since it may involve several iterations and in some cases may be time consuming. If this is possible, then the draft reference scenario should be documented, circulated and presented to the UA^2W participants.

4.3 Using the Instruments

Familiarisation with the prime instruments used during UA²Ws, namely scenario screening (or filtering) and growth scenarios, is also important to yield useful results. As already pointed out, scenario screening should precede the compilation of growth scenarios, so that the latter builds upon the outcomes of filtering. It is important to underline that the objective of the filtering exercise is not to exhaustively list all design parameters that influence the accessibility of a system. Instead, the target is to enumerate a relevant sub-set, and consequently devise the corresponding execution contexts for a designated set of the system's tasks. Accordingly, it may be argued that Universal Access is not to be measured only with regards to the outcomes of design, but, perhaps more importantly, in terms of the design processes engaged and the extent to which these processes allow for incremental updates and refinements.

5. Concluding Remarks

This Chapter has described a participatory method and two analytical design-oriented techniques that have been developed and refined in the context of the IS4ALL project. Both the method and the techniques seek to facilitate an understanding of the global execution context of a designated set of tasks, and thereby contribute towards a design code for practicing Universal Access. We have used these instruments to guide design work in the context of one of the IS4ALL reference scenarios, namely WardInHand, and several conclusions can be drawn from this experience. First of all, the entire approach makes several demands upon the analyst. Some of these relate to preparatory steps, such as finding the appropriate peers to become engaged in screening and growth scenario compilation, while others relate to the conduct of the screening phase. Specifically, it turns out that the choice of argumentation (Universal Access) filters is significant, as well as critical for the outcomes of the entire re-design activity.

As a general guideline, designers should seek to work on argumentation filters which cover, according to relevance, the three aspects which determine the execution context of a designated set of tasks, namely the target users, the platform and the context of use. A possible way to approach the task is to start with relevant non-functional quality attributes, and incrementally derive a set of argumentation filters. For example, a non-functional quality attribute is "scalability" to another platform, which may lead to argumentation filters regarding the delivery medium of an application or a service. Another approach is to formulate argumentation filters by consulting assessment manuals or human performance criteria.

Examples of such argumentation filters are the following:

- "How is the task performed by a user who can perform alternative reliable control acts, such as movement of one / both hands, directed eye-gaze, head movement, movement of lower limbs, vocalisation, etc?"
- "How is the task performed by a user who cannot push and pull targets, or cannot isolate finger movement, or cannot initiate movement on demand, or does not have fine spatial control?"

In a similar fashion, one can devise argumentation filters on the basis of terminal- or platform-specific issues. Representative examples include: locating and accessing the terminal, card systems, keypads, typefaces and legibility, touch screens, screens and instructions, external features, labels and instructions, operating instructions, etc. Nevertheless, irrespective of the type or source of the designated set of argumentation filters, growth scenarios need to be tightly linked to this set. This does not imply that there should be a growth scenario for each respective argumentation filter. Rather, growth scenarios may relate to several filters. By implication, designers should aim for a few representative growth scenarios, which satisfy the conditions of usage set by the argumentation filters.

Chapter 12
Applying the Unified User Interface Design Method in Health Telematics

Anthony Savidis[1], Margherita Antona[1], and
Constantine Stephanidis[1, 2]

[1]Foundation for Research and Technology – Hellas (FORTH)
Institute of Computer Science
Heraklion, Crete, GR-70013, Greece
{as, antona, cs}@ics.forth.gr
[2]University of Crete
Department of Computer Science, Greece

Abstract. This Chapter presents an application of the Unified User Interface Design method in the context of Health Telematics. Towards this end, the Chapter first outlines the fundamental objectives, conceptual framework, design process and outcomes of the Unified User Interface design method. Subsequently, the Chapter presents selected fragments of an experimental case study based on: (i) introducing into the MediBridge C-Care scenario elements of user, context of use and interaction platform diversity, and (ii) conducting the Unified User Interface Design process for such a scenario and delivering its outcomes through the use of a support tool.

1. Introduction

Universal Access implies the accessibility and usability of Information Society Technologies (IST) by anyone, anywhere, anytime. One of the main challenges in this context is the design of computing technologies accessible and usable by users with different abilities, needs, requirements, preferences and skills, including disabled and elderly users, in different contexts of use and through different technological platforms.

The Unified User Interface development methodology (Stephanidis, 2001b; Savidis and Stephanidis, 2004b) has been proposed as a complete technological solution for supporting universal access of interactive applications and services. Unified User Interfaces convey a new perspective into the development of user interfaces, providing a principled and systematic approach towards coping with diversity in the target user requirements, tasks and environments of use.

The notion of Unified User Interfaces has originated from research efforts aiming to address the issues of accessibility and interaction quality for people with disabilities (see Stephanidis and Emiliani, 1999). Subsequently, these principles were extended and adapted to depict a general proposition for HCI design and

C. Stephanidis (Ed.): Universal Access Code of Practice in Health Telematics, LNCS 3041, pp. 115-140, 2005.
© Springer-Verlag Berlin Heidelberg 2005

development, and were intensively tested and validated in the course of large development projects (Stephanidis et al., 2001; Stephanidis et al., 2003).

From a user perspective, a Unified User Interface can be considered as an interface tailored to personal attributes and to the particular context of use, while from the designer perspective it can be seen as an interface design populated with alternative designs, each alternative addressing specific user- and usage-context- parameter values. Finally, from an engineering perspective, a Unified User Interface is a repository of implemented dialogue artifacts, from which the most appropriate are selected at run-time according to the specific task context, by means of an adaptation logic supporting decision-making (Savidis and Stephanidis, 2004b).

A Unified User Interface comprises a single (unified) interface specification that exhibits the following properties:

1. It embeds representation schemes for user- and usage-context- parameters and accesses user- and usage-context- information resources (e.g., repositories, servers), to extract or update such information.
2. It is equipped with alternative implemented dialogue patterns (i.e., implemented dialogue artifacts) appropriately associated with different combinations of values for user- and usage-context- related parameters. The need for such alternative dialogue patterns is identified during the design process when, given a particular design context for differing user- and usage-context- attribute values, alternative design artifacts are deemed as necessary to accomplish optimal interaction.
3. It embeds design logic and decision making capabilities that support activating, at run-time, the most appropriate dialogue patterns according to particular instances of user- and usage-context- parameters, and is capable of interaction monitoring to detect changes in parameters.

As a consequence, a unified interface realises:

• User-adapted behaviour (user awareness), i.e., the interface is capable of automatically selecting interaction patterns appropriate to the particular user.
• Usage-context adapted behaviour (usage context awareness), i.e., the interface is capable of automatically selecting interaction patterns appropriate to the particular physical and technological environment.

At run-time, adaptations may be of two types:

1. adaptations driven by initial user- and context- information known prior to the initiation of interaction, and
2. adaptations driven by information acquired through interaction monitoring analysis.

The former behaviour is referred to as adaptability (i.e., initial automatic adaptation) reflecting the interface's capability to automatically tailor itself initially to each individual end-user in a particular context. The latter behaviour is referred to as adaptivity (i.e., continuous automatic adaptation), and characterises the interface's capability to cope with the dynamically changing or evolving user and context characteristics. Adaptability is crucial to ensure accessibility, since it is essential to provide, before initiation of interaction, a fully accessible interface instance to each individual end-user (Stephanidis, 2001b). Furthermore, adaptivity can be applied only on accessible running interface instances (i.e., ones with which the user is capable of performing interaction), since interaction monitoring is required for the identification of changing / emerging decision parameters that may drive dynamic interface enhancements.

A particularly important aspect of developing unified user interfaces concerns their design. The following section describes the Unified User Interface design method, which has been elaborated as a part of the overall methodology to provide a process-oriented support framework for the design of Unified User Interfaces (Savidis et al., 2001, Savidis and Stephanidis, 2004a).

2. The Unified User Interface Design Method

2.1 Problem Being Addressed

Under a Universal Access perspective, interaction design increasingly becomes a knowledge-intensive endeavour. In this context, designers should be prepared to cope with large design spaces to accommodate design constraints posed by diversity in the target user population and the emerging contexts of use in the Information Society.

The main objective in such a context is to ensure that each end-user is provided with the most appropriate interactive experience at run-time. Producing and enumerating distinct interface designs through the conduct of multiple design processes would be an impractical solution, since the overall cost for managing in parallel such a large number of independent design processes, and for separately implementing each interface version, would be unacceptable (Savidis and Stephanidis, 2004a). Instead, a design process is required capable of leading to a single design outcome that appropriately structures multiple designs and their underlying user and context related parameters, facilitating the mapping of design to a target software system implementation. In this context, user interface adaptation is likely to predominate as a technique for addressing the compelling requirements for customisation, accessibility and high quality of interaction (Stephanidis, 2001a). Thus, it must be carefully planned, designed and accommodated into the life-cycle of an interactive system, from the early design phases, through to evaluation, implementation and deployment. In particular, the design of universally accessible applications and services is characterised by a wide range of design parameters, and related values. As a consequence, the need arises to adopt a design process which is capable of managing diversity.

The Unified Interface Design Method is a hybrid process-oriented design method enabling the organisation of diversity-based design decisions around a single hierarchical structure, purposefully developed to support the design of Unified User Interfaces (Savidis et al., 2001; Savidis and Stephanidis, 2004a). It proposes a specific design process to cater for the management of an evolving design space, in which alternative design artifacts can be associated to variations of the design problem parameters. The process of designing Unified User Interfaces does not lead to a single design outcome, but to a structured design space. It collects and appropriately represents alternative designs, along with the conditions under which each design should be made available at run-time (i.e., an adaptation-oriented design rationale). The Unified User Interface Design method is intended to be general, focusing on capturing and rationalising diversity in design, and encompasses a variety of techniques such as task analysis, abstract design, design polymorphism and design rationale.

2.2 Device / Technique(s) Used

The basic representation adopted in Unified User Interface design is called polymorphic task hierarchy, and combines: (a) hierarchical task analysis; (b) design polymorphism, i.e., the possibility of assigning alternative decompositions to the same (sub)task if required based on (combinations of) design parameters; and (c) user-task oriented operators.

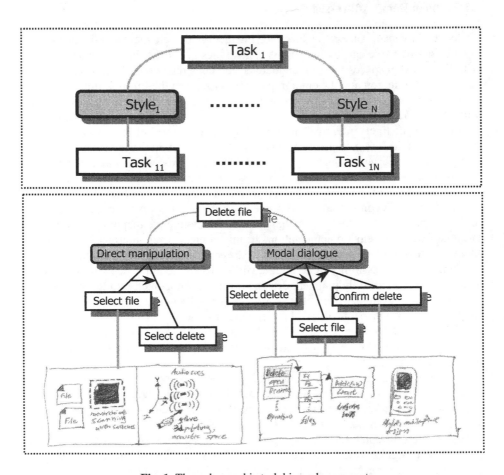

Fig. 1. The polymorphic task hierarchy concept

Figure 1 (from Savidis and Stephanidis, 2004a) depicts an example of polymorphic task hierarchy, illustrating how two alternative dialogue styles for a "delete file" task may be designed. Alternative decomposition "styles" are depicted in the upper part of the figure, and an exemplary polymorphic decomposition, which includes physical design annotation, appears in the lower part.

The hierarchical decomposition adopts the original properties of hierarchical task analysis (Kirwan and Ainsworth, 1992), enriched, through polymorphism, with the capability to differentiate and represent design alternatives for the same task according to varying design parameters. Task operators are based on the powerful Communicating Sequential Processes (CSP) language for describing the behaviour of reactive systems (Hoare, 1978), and enable the expression of dialogue control flow formulae for task accomplishment. Additional (or alternative) operators may be used as necessary. Additionally, the designer is not constrained to use CSP operators for describing user actions for device-level interaction (e.g., drawing, drag-and-drop, concurrent input). Alternatively, an event-based representation may be preferred (e.g., UAN, Hartson et al., 1990).

In a polymorphic task hierarchy, the root represents design abstractions, while leaf nodes represent concrete interaction components. Polymorphic decomposition leads from abstract design patterns to concrete artifacts. Three categories of design artifacts may be subject to polymorphism on the basis of user- and usage-context- parameter values, namely:

User tasks, relating to what the user has to do; user tasks are the centre of the polymorphic task decomposition process.

System tasks, representing what the system has to do, or how it responds to particular user actions (e.g., feedback); in the polymorphic task decomposition process, they are treated in the same manner as user tasks.

Physical designs, which concern the interface components on which user actions are to be performed; physical interface structure may also be subject to polymorphism.

Table 1 (from Savidis and Stephanidis, 2004a) summarises the basic task operators, which include sequencing, parallelism, logical exclusion and repetition.

In a polymorphic task hierarchy, the root represents design abstractions, while leaf nodes represent concrete interaction components. Polymorphic decomposition leads from abstract design patterns to concrete artifacts. Three categories of design artifacts may be subject to polymorphism on the basis of user- and usage-context- parameter values, namely:

- User tasks, relating to what the user has to do; user tasks are the centre of the polymorphic task decomposition process.
- System tasks, representing what the system has to do, or how it responds to particular user actions (e.g., feedback); in the polymorphic task decomposition process, they are treated in the same manner as user tasks.
- Physical designs, which concern the interface components on which user actions are to be performed; physical interface structure may also be subject to polymorphism.

Table 1. Basic task operators in the Unified User Interface design method

Operator	Explanation	Representation
before	*Task sequencing, documenting that task A must be performed before task B.*	*A B*
or	*Task parallelism, documenting that task A may be performed before, after or in parallel to task B.*	*A B*
xor	*Task exclusive completion, documenting that either A or B must be performed, but not both.*	*A B*
*	*Task simple repetition, documenting that A may be performed zero or more times.*	*A **
+	*Task absolute repetition, documenting that A must be performed at least one time.*	*A+*

User tasks, and in certain cases, system tasks, are not necessarily related to physical interaction, but may represent abstraction of either user- or system- actions. System tasks and user tasks may be freely combined within task "formulas", defining how sequences of user-initiated actions and system-driven actions interrelate. The physical design, providing the interaction context, is associated with a particular user task, and provides the physical dialogue pattern associated to a task-structure definition. Hence, it plays the role of annotating the task hierarchy with physical design information.

Each alternative polymorphic decomposition is called a decomposition style, or simply a style, and is attributed a unique name. Alternative task sub-hierarchies are attached to their respective styles. Polymorphism constitutes a technique for potentially increasing the number of alternative interface instances represented by a typical hierarchical task model. However, the Unified User Interface design method does not require the designer to follow the polymorphic task decomposition all the way down the user-task hierarchy, until primitive actions are met. A non-polymorphic task can be specialised at any level, following any design method chosen by the interface designer. When polymorphism is applied at the level of top or main tasks (e.g., edit a document, send an e-mail, perform spell-checking, construct graphic illustrations, etc), the designed interface instances are likely to be affected by structural differences, resulting in alternative versions of the same interactive environment, such as in the case of multiplatform interfaces (i.e., effect seems global).

Polymorphism on middle hierarchy levels (e.g., dialogue boxes for setting parameters, executing selected operations, editing retrieved items, etc.) introduces the effect of overall similarities with localised differences in interactive components and intermediate sub-dialogues. Finally, polymorphism at the lowest levels of the hierarchy, concerning primitive interactive actions supported by physical artifacts (e.g., pressing a button, moving a slider, defining a stroke with the mouse, etc.) causes differences on device-level input syntax and / or on the type of interaction objects in some interface components. If polymorphism is not applied, a task model represents a single interface design instance, on which no run-time adaptation is applied. There is therefore a fundamental link between adaptation capability and polymorphism.

2.3 Procedure for Using the Device

The key elements of the unified user interface design process are (Savidis and Stephanidis, 2004a):

- Hierarchical design discipline building upon the notion of task analysis, empowered by the introduction of task-level polymorphism.
- Iterative design process model, emphasising abstract task analysis with incremental polymorphic physical specialisation.
- Formalisation of run-time relationships among the alternative design artifacts associated with the same design context.
- Documentation recording the consolidated design rationale of each alternative design artefact.

2.3.1 The Space of User- and Context-Related Design Parameters

An essential prerequisite for conducting Unified User Interface Design is the conceptual categorisation of diversity aspects in all relevant dimensions (users, context of use, access terminal / platform), and the identification of the target design parameters for each design case (Savidis at al., 2001). This is based on the consideration that the degree to which a comprehensive taxonomy (or ontology) of design parameters can be achieved based on the current knowledge and wisdom of designing for diversity cannot be determined. Besides, not all parameters in such a taxonomy would be relevant for different design cases. For example, according to the targeted final user groups, different sets of design guidelines may need to be taken into account during design. Therefore, designers should be free to use case-specific design parameters, to experiment with different sets of them, and to create their own (partial) taxonomies according to the type of design cases they address and the target user population. Accumulated experience in designing for diversity is expected to progressively lead to the identification of more commonly valid classifications of design parameters. For example, human abilities relevant for determining alternative choices in a design case are likely to affect similar design cases. Some examples of attribute classes that designers may consider in Unified User Interface design are general computer-use expertise, domain-specific knowledge, role in an organisational context, motor abilities, sensory abilities, mental abilities, etc.

There is no predefined or fixed set of attribute categories or values which are chosen as part of the design process (e.g., by interface designers, or Human Factors experts). Values do not need be finite sets. The broader the set of values, the higher the potential for polymorphism (i.e., for alternative designs). For instance, commercial systems realising a single design for an "average" user have no differentiation capability at all.

It is the responsibility of interface designers to choose appropriate attributes and corresponding value ranges, as well as to define appropriate design alternatives when necessary. For simplicity, designers may choose to elicit only those attributes from which differentiated design decisions are likely to emerge. The construction of context and platform attributes may follow the same representation approach as users' characteristics. Examples of potential context attributes are acoustic noise and light sources, while examples of potential relevant platform attributes are processor speed, memory, secondary storage, peripheral equipment, resolution, screen physical size and graphics capabilities.

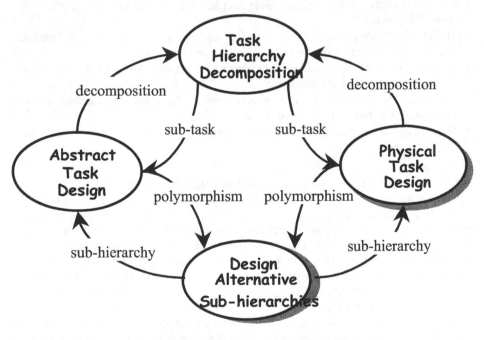

Fig. 2. The polymorphic task decomposition process

2.3.2 The Polymorphic Task Decomposition Process
The Unified User Interface design process realises an exhaustive hierarchical decomposition of tasks, starting from the abstract level, by incrementally specialising in a polymorphic fashion towards the physical level of interaction. In this process, different designs are likely to be associated with different (combinations of) user- and usage-context- attribute values.

The polymorphic decomposition process is depicted in Figure 2 (adapted from Savidis and Stephanidis, 2004a).

It starts from abstract- or physical- task design, depending on whether top-level user tasks can be defined as being abstract or not.

An abstract task can be decomposed either in a polymorphic fashion, if user- and usage-context- attribute values require different dialogue patterns, or following a unimorphic decomposition scheme. In the latter case, the transition is realised via a decomposition action, leading to the task hierarchy decomposition state. Polymorphic decomposition, on the other hand, leads to the design alternative sub-hierarchies state.

Reaching this state means that the required alternative dialogue styles have been identified, each initiating a distinct sub-hierarchy decomposition process. Hence, each such sub-hierarchy initiates its own instance of polymorphic task decomposition process. While initiating each distinct process, the designer may either start from the abstract task design state, or from the physical task design state. The former is pursued if the top-level task of the particular sub-hierarchy is an abstract one, while the second occurs in the case that the top-level task involves physical interaction.

From this state, the sub-tasks identified need to be further decomposed. For each sub-task at the abstract level, there is a sub-task transition to the abstract task design state. Otherwise, if the sub-task involves physical interaction means, a sub-task transition is performed to the physical task design state.

Physical tasks may be further decomposed either in a unimorphic fashion, or in a polymorphic fashion. These two alternative design possibilities are indicated by the "decomposition" and "polymorphism" transitions respectively.

In summary, the rules to be applied in polymorphic task decomposition are:

- If a given task does not involve physical interaction, start from abstract task design and:
- apply polymorphism, if decision parameters impose the need for alternative styles on user- / system- tasks and / or physical structure;
- apply decomposition, when alternative designs are needed for the same style.
- If a given task involves physical interaction, start from physical task design, and:
- apply polymorphism, if decision parameters impose the need for alternative styles on user- / system- tasks and / or physical structure;
- apply decomposition, when an alternative design is needed to realise the same style.

In Unified User Interface design, one of the key issues is to decide in which cases the diversity in design parameters leads to different concrete interface artifacts. Designers should take care that every decomposition step satisfies all constraints imposed by the combination of target user- and usage-context- attribute values. Polymorphic decomposition is required when different styles are appropriate for different execution contexts, based on the designer's decision. Differentiation decisions can be based on consolidated design knowledge, if available (e.g., design guidelines for specific target user groups, target platforms, etc), on the results of surveys or evaluation experiments, etc. There is no automatism in deciding when and how adaptation should be applied in the final interface.

2.3.3 Adaptation-Oriented Design Rationale

In the depicted process, the following primary decisions need to be taken:

- at which points of a task hierarchy polymorphism should be applied, based on the considered (combinations of) user- and usage-context- attributes; and
- how different styles behave at run-time. This is performed by assigning to pair(s) of style (groups) design relationships.

These decisions need to be documented in a design rationale recorded by capturing, for each sub-task in a polymorphic hierarchy, the underlying design logic, which directly associates user- / usage-context- parameter values with the designed artifacts.

Such a rationale should document (as a minimum requirement) the following (Savidis and Stephanidis, 2004b):

- related task
- supported execution context (i.e., design parameters)
- style properties
- design relationships with competing styles.

In Table 2 (from Savidis and Stephanidis, 2004a), an instance of such documentation record is depicted, adopting a tabular notation.

Table 2. An instance of design rationale documentation

Task: Delete File	
Style: Direct Manipulation	Style: Modal Dialogue
Users & Contexts: Expert, Frequent, Average	Users & Contexts: Casual, Naïve.
Targets: Speed, naturalness, flexibility	Targets: Safety, guided steps
Properties: Object first, function next	Properties: Function first, object next
Relationships: Exclusion (with all)	Relationships: Exclusion (with all)

Styles can be evaluated and compared with respect to any design parameter (e.g., Performance measures, Heuristics, User satisfaction, etc). Evaluation or comparison results can form part of the design rationale as annotations.

Four fundamental relationships among alternative styles (concerning the same polymorphic artefact) have been identified, reflecting the way in which artifacts may be employed during interaction for an individual user in a particular context (see Table 3, adapted from Savidis and Stephanidis, 2004a). These relationships in fact express the adaptation run-time behaviour of the designed interface, reflecting real-world design scenarios, and are motivated by the observation that different styles are not always mutually exclusive, even if they correspond to different (combinations of) design parameters values, since there are cases in which it is meaningful to make artifacts belonging to alternative styles concurrently available in a single adapted interface instance. These relationships also constitute the adaptation logic of the designed unified interface, i.e., they specify the conditions (parameters) under which alternative styles are activated at run-time.

Table 3. Design relationships among styles

Exclusion	Only one of the alternative styles may be present at run-time.
Compatibility	Any of the alternative styles may be present at run-time.
Substitution	When the second style is activated at run-time, the first should be deactivated.
Augmentation	In the presence of a style at run-time, a second style may also be activated.

This important aspect of the design process is likely to require in-depth experience on the part of designers, who will need to provide the designed unified interfaces with a complete adaptation logic, suitable for run-time execution.

2.4 Outcomes

In summary, the outcomes of the Unified User Interface Design method include:
1. the polymorphic task hierarchy
2. the design space populated by the produced physical designs
3. for each polymorphic artefact in the task hierarchy, a design rationale recording its run-time adaptation logic based on user- and context-related parameters.

The Unified User Interface Design method, being general and non prescriptive, does not require any specific format or notation for delivering the above outcomes, and designers are free to use any convenient encoding on a case basis or according to their personal preferences. In practice, the representation of end-user characteristics is best developed in terms of attribute-value pairs, using any suitable formalism, in order to allow the straightforward encoding of the relevant parameters into attribute-value-based user profiles at run-time. Concerning the polymorphic task hierarchy itself, it obviously needs to be hierarchically encoded with appropriate reference to the properties of each node in the hierarchy (i.e., sub-task or style). Physical design can also be conducted and delivered using any suitable device, such as textual design specifications, or, in the case of graphical interfaces, mock-ups and prototypes.

However, there is a requirement for the design outcomes to include an adaptation logic represented in a format directly supporting implementation. Such a format can be informal (e.g., design rationale tables), or a directly computable run-time decision logic (such as the Decision Making Specification Language, DMSL, Savidis and Stephanidis, 2004b) but, clearly, the designed logic must be sound and correctly based on the design parameters selected for each case.

Combined together, the outcomes of the Unified user interface Design process are meant to:
- Facilitate design re-use and incremental design. This is made possible by the linking of physical design artifacts to their respective tasks and execution contexts, and by the systematic organisation and documentation of all design artifacts,

facilitating the updating and extension of design cases. Potential changes or modifications can be applied on either polymorphic or unimorphic artifacts. Since the unified design method requires explicit annotation of the key design parameters, all updates are incorporated in a straightforward manner within their respective locations (according to the design parameters) in the unified design documentation structure. Additionally, the method emphasises capturing of the more abstract structures and patterns inherent in the interface design, enabling hierarchical incremental specialisation towards the lower physical-level of interaction, and making therefore possible to introduce design alternatives as close as possible to physical design. This makes it easier to update and extend the design space, since modifications due to the consideration of additional values of design parameters (e.g., considering new user- and usage-context- attribute values) can be applied locally to the lower-levels of the design, without affecting the rest of the design space.

- Facilitate the implementation of self-adapting interfaces through the provision of all the necessary knowledge for run-time decision making concerning alternative design artifacts. The method's outcomes constitute a starting point in order to potentially implement the captured interface instances as different facets of a unique run-time interactive system. All the knowledge required for run-time decision making concerning the alternative appearance and interactive behaviour of the interface need to be systematically integrated in the design outcomes. Specifically, the required knowledge includes the designed alternative styles along with their recorded design rationale. This is an important contribution of the method to HCI design, since it potentially bridges the gap between design and implementation, which has traditionally challenged user interface engineering.

2.5 Assumptions

The Unified User Interface Design method is targeted towards providing conceptual support for structuring and organising the design process of unified interfaces, rather than support for automating such a process, or supporting each step involved in detail. In this respect, polymorphic task decomposition is a prescriptive guide to what is to be attained, rather than how it is to be attained, and thus it is orthogonal to many existing design instruments (Savidis and Stephanidis, 2001d). This is considered as a particularly important feature in a Universal Access perspective, since user- and context-parameters diversity requires a logical structuring and rationalisation of the design space, but at the same time, different lower level design techniques may be required according to the specifics of each distinct design case. The process in Unified User Interface design is of incremental specification from abstract to concrete, i.e., it is a process of creatively mapping abstract tasks to a design space of multiple interaction artifacts interlinked through an adaptation logic.

The method is also open-ended, i.e., it does not impose any particular "ontology" or taxonomy or design parameters, and designers need to specify their own classification of attributes and related values sets for each design case, according to the specific target user population, type of application being designed, objectives of the development, etc. Therefore, one of the key issues in conducting Unified User Interface Design is the identification and conceptual categorisation, during the design process, of relevant design parameters, which need to be captured at an appropriate level of detail for enabling the rationalisation of design polymorphism. This important aspect of the design process is likely to require in-depth experience on the part of designers. Differentiation decisions can be based on consolidated design knowledge, if available (e.g., design guidelines for specific target user groups, target platforms, etc), of the results of surveys or evaluation experiments, etc. The open-world view fostered by Unified User Interface design also holds for interaction platforms, languages and artifacts.

Unified User Interface Design can be used in combination with any method deemed as appropriate for gathering and analysing design requirements and for evaluating designs. For example, it can be combined with the Universal Access Assessment Workshop method (see Chapter 11 of this book).

The above characteristics are believed to make Unified user Interface Design uniquely suited for its intended purposes. However, it is recognised that Unified User Interface design requires a higher initial effort and investment than traditional HCI design approaches (Savidis and Stephanidis, 2001d), as current design practices do not usually involve the identification of relevant design parameters, the design of alternative interface instances, the rationalisation of a complex design space and the final delivery of a complete interface adaptation logic. Towards assisting designers in the conduct of the Unified User Interface Design Process, the MENTOR tool has been developed, that aims at: (i) facilitating the conduct of Unified User Interface design by providing an appropriate interaction environment and editing facilities for all the phases involved in Unified User Interface design, as well as automated verification mechanisms for the adaptation logic embedded in design cases (Stephanidis et al., 2005, in print). The next section of this Chapter presents a validation case study of the Unified User Interface Design method conducted using MENTOR.

3. Case Study: The MediBridge C-Care Scenario

The Unified User Interface Design method focuses on capturing and rationalising diversity in design. Therefore, the first step of the validation case study reported here was to refine the C-Care application scenario (see Chapter 10 of this book) to introduce elements of diversity in design parameters related to users, contexts of use and platforms. Subsequently, the process of Unified User Interface design was conducted for the revised scenario using MENTOR, involving the following steps:

- The design parameters considered relevant for the design exercise were extracted and encoded.
- Polymorphic task decomposition was conducted based on selected tasks extracted from the revised scenario. The need for introducing polymorphic decomposition steps, dictated by divergence of design parameters and leading to different design styles, was detected at several points during this process and reported in the polymorphic task hierarchy, along with the associated design parameters (adaptation rationale).
- On the basis of the produced polymorphic task hierarchy, alternative physical designs were produced in the form of mock-ups.

- Using the related facilities of MENTOR, a design report has been generated documenting the above, including a complete adaptation logic for the designed interface in the DMSL language.

3.1 Developing and Refining the Scenario

The C-Care project focuses on personalised access to medical data anytime and from anywhere, through the provision of a centralised, continuously updated web-based repository of Electronic Health Records. In the context of the project, access to patient health data is envisaged for a variety of purposes in different situations, such as emergencies and medical visits, by users with different roles, and consequently different access rights to the system, and through a variety of platforms, such as the desk-top PC and the WAP phone. Therefore, C-Care constitutes a particularly interesting validation context for the Unified User Interface Design method, as it naturally lends itself to investigating diversity in design parameters, and envisaging alternative designs.

On the basis of the above considerations, it was decided to extend the original C-Care scenario to cater for the following cases:

- Doctors can have access to the C-Care system through a PC, a PDA or a mobile phone, viewing all types of data for any patient.
- Ambulance paramedic staff is equipped with a PDA or a mobile phone to perform specific tasks and view patient health data which are critical in emergency situations, and for emergency care (e.g., allergies, vaccinations).
- Nurses in the hospital can have access to patient administrative and medication data through a PC or a PDA.
- Patients themselves can have access to their data through a PC, a PDA or a mobile phone, and can opt to access all data or only the most recent (e.g., last week's blood test results).
- Users in all roles can easily send urgent notifications, including data from the EHR, to other users that may need to be informed (e.g., particular allergy data sent from the ambulance to a doctor in the hospital to obtain advice for emergency treatment, abnormal test results sent from the doctor to the patient or vice versa).

3.2 Conducting Unified User Interface Design

3.2.1 Definition of Design Parameters

The first phase of application of the Unified User Interface design method to the C-Care revised scenario was to define the user, and context-platform design parameters likely to affect interaction design for the design case highlighted above, and to cause design differentiations, i.e., polymorphism. These parameters are related to the users' role, the context of use and the selected access platform. Figure 3 and Figure 4 depict the MENTOR Design Parameters Editor with the user and context- platform design parameters defined for the case study. Three types of design parameters values are allowed in MENTOR, according to the specifications of the DMSL language: (i) enumerated, i.e., values belonging to a list of (more than two) strings specified by the designer; (ii) boolean, i.e., values True or False; and (iii) integer, which are specified by supplying the minimum and maximum bounds of the integer range allowed as a value. Value ranges define the space of legal values for a given attribute. All attributes defined in the C-Care design case have enumerated values.

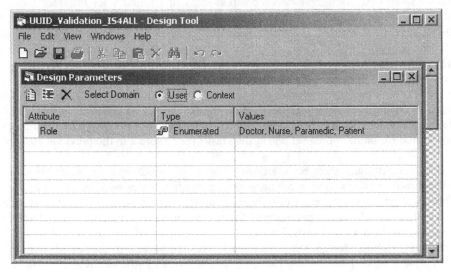

Fig. 3. Definition of user related design parameters in MENTOR

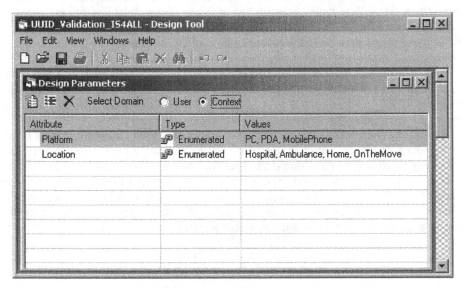

Fig. 4. Definition of platform and context related parameters in MENTOR

3.2.2 Polymorphic Task Decomposition and Adaptation Rationale Encoding

Once the design parameters to be used in the design case were defined, polymorphic task decomposition was performed using the Task Hierarchy Editor of MENTOR, which guides the decomposition process by contextualising the available decomposition actions according to the category of design artifact selected in the hierarchy and the admissible decomposition steps of Unified User Interface Design, as presented in Figure 2. Table 4 summarises the categories of design artifacts distinguished in Unified User Interface design, their icon representation in the MENTOR Polymorphic Task Hierarchy Editor, and the admissible decomposition steps for each category.

Table 4 also lists the properties that MENTOR allows to set for each design artifact category, using the Property Editor. For all categories, the artifact's name needs to be defined, and an informal description can also be encoded. Subtasks relationships can be defined for unimorphic user and system tasks (see Table 2 in the previous section).

Physical designs can be assigned images of mock-ups or prototypes. For polymorphic artifacts, design relations among children styles need to be defined (see Table 4 in previous section), while styles are assigned adaptation conditions, based on currently defined design parameters, for the purposes of encoding the adaptation rationale of the designed unified interface. These conditions are formulated, using the previously defined design parameters and the related values, in the DMLS language. Assigned design relations and style conditions are used by MENTOR to automatically derive the entire interface adaptation logic in DMSL. MENTOR also provides facilities for checking the consistency and hierarchical subsumption of assigned conditions, as well as their compatibility with the design relations linking them to other styles of the same polymorphic artifact (Stephanidis et al., 2005, in print). Examples of the above will be provided later on in this section.

Figure 5 depicts the high level decomposition of the overall task into two main sequential tasks, namely the unimorphic user task *Login* and the polymorphic user task *View EHR*.

The further decomposition of the *Login* task is presented in Figure 6. The *Login* task is decomposed into three unimorphic user tasks, namely Input User Name, Input User Password and Login Command. The availability of three different interaction platforms (PC, PDA and mobile phone) requires the adoption of different interaction styles for each of these tasks as well as for the overall *Login* dialogue. Therefore, the related physical designs are polymorphic, and further decompose to three unimorphic physical design styles, one for each available platform.

Table 4. Categories of design artifacts, and related icons, admissible decompositions and properties

Icon and Design Artefact Category	Admissible decompositions	Properties
Unimorphic User Task / Unimorphic System Task	• Unimorphic user task • Unimorphic system task • Polymorphic user task • Polymorphic system task • Unimorphic / Polymorphic physical design (only one)	• Name • Description • Subtask Relations
Unimorphic physical design	• Unimorphic physical design • Polymorphic physical design	• Name • Description • Image(s)
Polymorphic user task / Polymorphic system task	• Unimorphic user / system style • Polymorphic user / sytem style	• Name • Description • Design Relations
Polymorphic physical design	• Unimorphic physical design style • Polymorphic physical design style	• Name • Description • Design Relations
Unimorphic User Style / Unimorphic System Style	• Unimorphic user task • Unimorphic system task • Polymorphic user task • Polymorphic system task • Unimorphic / Polymorphic physical design (only one)	• Name • Description • Subtask Relations • Condition
Unimorphic physical design Style	• Unimorphic physical design • Polymorphic physical design	• Name • Description • Image(s) • Condition
Polymorphic User Style / Polymorphic System Style	• Unimorphic user / system style • Polymorphic user / system style	• Name • Description • Design Relations • Condition
Polymorphic physical design style	• Unimorphic physical design style • Polymorphic physical design style	• Name • Description • Design Relations • Condition

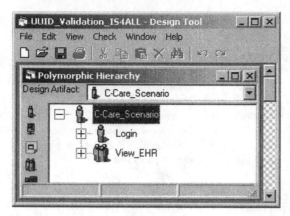

Fig. 5. High level tasks of the C-Care design case in the MENTOR Polymorphic Task Hierarchy Editor

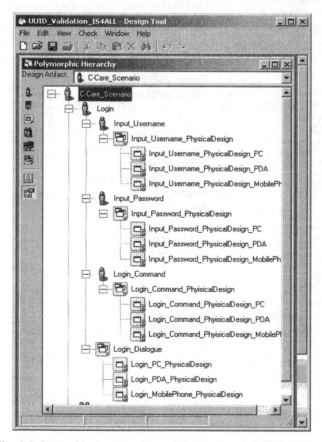

Fig. 6. Polymorphic decomposition of the Login task in MENTOR

Figure 7 shows the defined properties for the polymorphic physical design of the *Login* dialogue (Figure 7(A)), as well as for each of its three styles: PC (Figure 7(B)), PDA (Figure 7(C)) and mobile phone (Figure 7(D)). In Figure 7(A), the design relations assigned to three styles are evident. All styles are defined as mutually incompatible, as they are to be accessed by users through different platforms, and therefore cannot be provided simultaneously. In Figure 7(B), Figure 7(C), and Figure 7(D), the platform related conditions determining style selection at run-time appear, specifying the interaction platform for each style. The physical designs attached to each style are depicted in Figure 8.

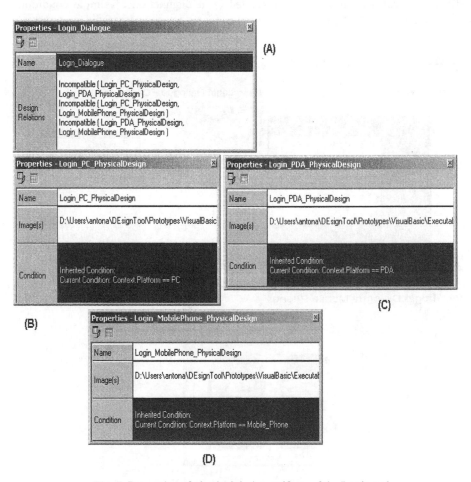

Fig. 7. Properties of physical design artifacts of the Login task

The *View EHR* task exhibits different characteristics form the *Login* task. First, it is a polymorphic user task, i.e., it is decomposed into two different styles according to the user role in the C-Care system. In this case, polymorphism does not concern the physical design of the task, but its sub-task decomposition: professional users (i.e., doctors, paramedic and nurses) need to select a patient for viewing the related EHR, while patient themselves directly access their personal data after login. As a consequence, the *View EHR* task is decomposed as depicted in Figure 9. Both styles defined for the View EHR polymorphic task are abstract, i.e., they are not associated with a physical design. Instead, they are further decomposed into user and system unimorphic tasks. Figure 10 shows the properties defined for the task (Figure 10(A)) and its styles (Figure 10(B) and Figure 10(C)). The two styles are defined as incompatible, as they are intended for users with different roles and access rights. The condition assigned to the style designed for patients (Figure 10 (C)) straightforwardly reflects the specific user role (patient), while the condition assigned to the style defined for professional users is constituted by a disjunction of simple conditions expressing user roles: the user in this case is either a doctor, a paramedic, or a nurse.

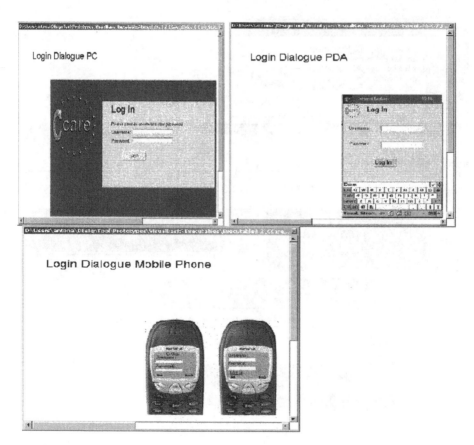

Fig. 8. The physical designs of the Login dialogue for the PC, the PDA and the mobile phone platforms in MENTOR

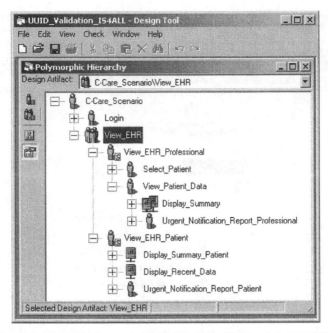

Fig. 9. Polymorphic decomposition of the View EHR task in MENTOR

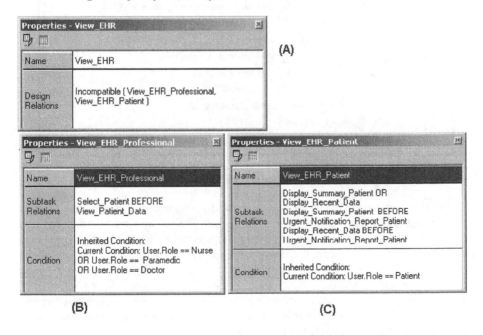

Fig. 10. Properties of the View EHR polymorphic user task and of its two decomposition styles

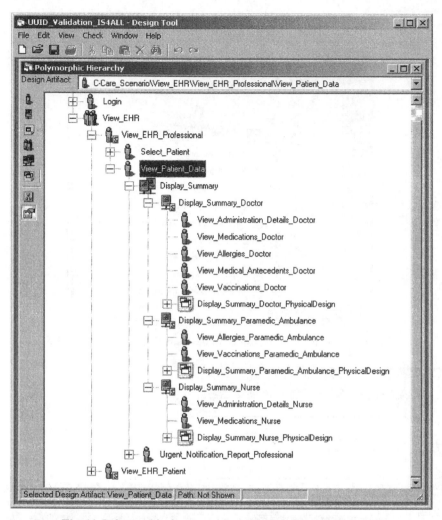

Fig. 11. Polymorphic decomposition of the Display Summary task

Another interesting example of polymorphic decomposition concerns the *Display Summary* subtask of the *View Patient Data* task. Polymorphism, in this case, is dictated by the need to present professional users with the type of patient data appropriate for their role and for the specific context in which the data are to be accessed. For example, doctors can view all patient data, nurses can view administrative and medication data, while paramedic personnel during ambulance emergency care can view data concerning allergies and vaccinations. Therefore the polymorphic system style Display Summary is decomposed into the three corresponding styles, as depicted in Figure 11.

The properties of the *Display Summary* task and of its styles appear in Figure 12. In Figure12(A), note the incompatibility design relation assigned to all style combinations, as each style is to be presented to users with different roles. In Figure

12(B), (C) and (D), note the conditions assigned to each style according to the specific user role.

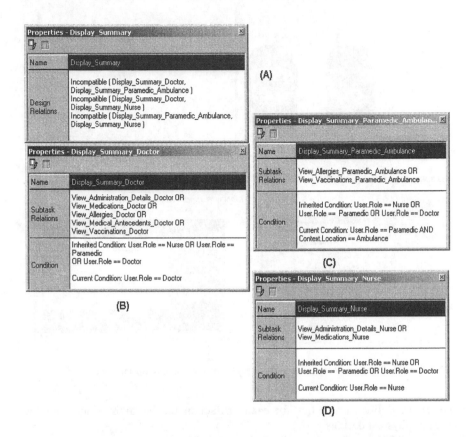

Fig. 12. Properties of the Display Summary polymorphic task and of its styles

In their turn, these styles have polymorphic physical designs, with styles appropriate for different platforms according to the type of access support provided by the system to the different user roles, i.e., PC, PDA and mobile phone for doctors, PDA and mobile phone for paramedic personnel during emergency care, and PC and PDA for nurses. Examples of these physical designs are depicted in Figure 13.

3.2.3 Outcomes

After encoding the Polymorphic Task Hierarchy and the properties of its design artifacts into the respective MENTOR editors, the design report for the C-Care case was automatically generated by the tool, including:

- the set of defined design parameters and allowed values
- a textual representation of the Polymorphic Task Hierarchy

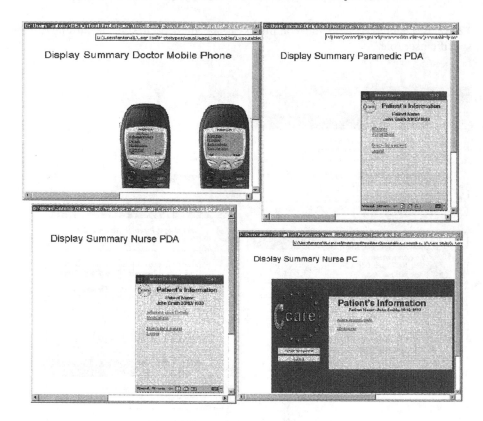

Fig. 13. Physical designs for various styles of the Display Summary task

- a list of the defined properties for each artifact in the hierarchy, including the images of physical designs
- the entire unified interface adaptation logic in DMSL.

Such a design report therefore constitutes the overall outcome of the application of the Unified User Interface Design method to the C-Care design case.

Figure 14 depicts a part of the generated adaptation logic.

4. Discussion and Lessons Learnt

In the validation experiment reported in the previous section, the Unified User interface Design method has been applied, in the context of the C-Care reference scenario, to a design case involving a small set of relevant design parameters, and exhibiting characteristics of system access through different platforms and in different contexts, as well by users with different roles and access rights.

The application of the method has led to the design of different interface instances that are adapted to: (i) different user roles and access rights; (i) different platforms and contexts of use. These instances constitute potential re-designs of the existing C-

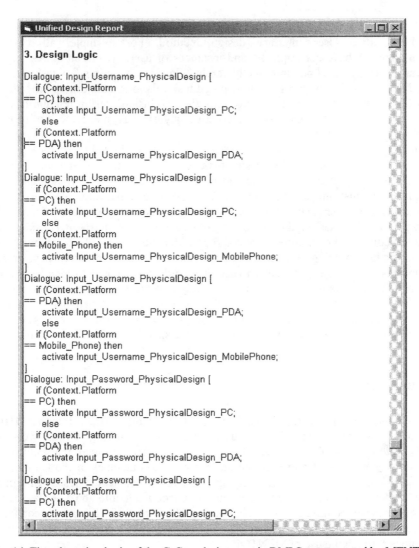

Fig. 14. The adaptation logic of the C-Care design case in DMLS, as generated by MENTOR

Care web prototype to cater for the diversity requirements likely to emerge when considering the issues of access and use of EHRs in a Universal Access perspective. The resulting design allows a unified implementation of the C-Care interface, and its run-time adaptation according to the occurrence of specified design parameters. The presented outcomes have been achieved through a series of steps, namely: (i) the selection of design parameters deemed relevant for the specific case; (ii) the identification of abstract application tasks and task structure; (iii) the identification of the necessary design alternatives according to the selected design parameters; and (iv) the physical design of the two envisaged interface instances. These steps are facilitated by MENTOR, which also supports the automatic derivation of the complete interface adaptation logic in DMSL.

The validation case study has involved many, albeit not all, the 'conceptual tools' of the Unified User Interface design method. For example, all types of decompositions have been applied, and instances of user, system and physical tasks appear in the produced polymorphic hierarchy. Conversely, only a few task operators have been necessary to represent the required task relations, and, due to the option of considering different access platforms, only the 'exclusion' design relation has been used, as none of the identified alternative styles was meant to be provided concurrently to the same user.

The application of the method in the validation case study, although limited for the sake of clarity to a simple set of design parameters, shows that the method is general enough for systematically capturing and rationalising diversity in design, and offers an appropriate instrument for proceeding from the conceptualisation of diversity at an abstract level to concrete physical designs reflecting the identified diversification. The design case addressed in this Chapter could easily be extended to consider other potential contexts. For example, one could consider the case in which somebody who has no medical training is involved in providing first aid in an emergency, or other similar cases. To extend the design case, it would be sufficient to identify the new relevant design parameters and add to the polymorphic task hierarchy the required new tasks and alternative styles. Therefore, it can be concluded that the method facilitates incremental design, allowing for progressively catering for emerging needs and requirements in the field of application (in the specific case, Health Telematics).

5. Summary

This Chapter has presented an application of the Unified User Interface Design method to a selected application scenario, namely the MediBridge C-Care web-based EHR system. Towards this end, the Chapter has first outlined the fundamental objectives, conceptual framework, design process and outcomes of the Unified User Interface design method. Subsequently, the Chapter has presented selected fragments of an experimental case study based on: (i) introducing into the C-Care scenario elements of user, context of use and interaction platform diversity, and (ii) conducting the Unified User Interface design process for such a scenario and delivering its outcomes through the use of MENTOR.

Acknowledgments

The authors would like to thank Mr. Antonis Natsis of the HCI Laboratory of ICS-FORTH for contributing to the realisation of the interface mock-ups for the case study presented in this Chapter.

Chapter 13
Using Non-functional Requirements as
Design Drivers for Universal Access

Demosthenes Akoumianakis[1] and Constantine Stephanidis[1,2]

[1]Foundation for Research and Technology – Hellas (FORTH)
Institute of Computer Science
Heraklion, Crete, GR-70013, Greece
cs@ics.forth.gr
[2]University of Crete
Department of Computer Science, Greece

Abstract. This Chapter elaborates on a technique aiming to provide early insight into the identification of universal access software quality attributes. The technique, referred to as Non-Functional Requirements Analysis (NfRA), constitutes a preliminary step in a scenario-based inquiry motivated by an explicit focus on non-functional requirements (NfRs) as drivers for scenario retooling (Erskine et al., 1997). This Chapter will illustrate the method by focusing on four main NfRs that are critical for universal access, namely adaptability, scalability, platform independence and user tolerance or individualisation. These are general NfRs applicable to a broad range of interactive software, irrespective of their functional scope, interaction platform or intended use.

1. Introduction

The present work is motivated by recent advances in software engineering aiming to make non-functional requirements an explicit goal in the process of software design. A representative effort in this direction is the work reported in Chung et al. (1999), where the authors elaborate a pragmatic approach to building quality into software systems. Systems must exhibit software quality attributes, such as accuracy, performance, security and modifiability. However, such non-functional requirements (NfRs) are difficult to address in many projects, even though there are many techniques to meet functional requirements in order to provide desired functionality. To perplex matters, the NfRs for each system typically interact with each other, have a broad impact on the system and may be subjective. In the present work, we are interested in NfRs relevant to universal access.

Functional requirements denote what a software system is expected to do in terms of functions or services for supporting user goals, tasks or activities. Non-functional requirements (NfRs) specify global quality constraints that must be satisfied by the software. These constraints, also known as *software global attributes*, typically

C. Stephanidis (Ed.): Universal Access Code of Practice in Health Telematics, LNCS 3041, pp. 141-155, 2005.
© Springer-Verlag Berlin Heidelberg 2005

include performance, fault-tolerance, availability, security and so on. Closely related to NfRs, transactional requirements state the demand for a consistent, transparent and individual execution of transactions by the system. The well-known ACID properties (Atomicity, Consistency, Isolation and Durability), summarise these transactional requirements.

During the software development process, functional requirements are usually incorporated into the software artefacts step by step. At the end of the process, all functional requirements must have been implemented in such way that the developed system satisfies the requirements defined at the early design stages. NfRs, however, are not implemented in the same way as functional requirements. To be more realistic, NfRs are hardly considered when software is built. This is due to several reasons. First of all, NfRs are more complex to deal with. Second, they are usually very abstract and stated only informally, and rarely supported by tools, methodologies or languages. Third, it is not a trivial matter to verify whether a specific NfR is satisfied by the final product or not. Fourth, very often NfRs conflict with each other, i.e., availability and performance, making a step-by-step implementation of NfRs impossible. Finally, NfRs commonly concern environment builders rather than application programmers.

Kotonya and Sommerville (1998) classify non-functional requirements into three main categories, namely product requirements, process requirements and external requirements. Product requirements specify the desired characteristics that a system or subsystem must possess. Process requirements put constraints on the development process of the system. External requirements are constraints applied to both the product and the process and are derived from the environment where the system is developed. An alternative classification for NfRs distinguishes between the executing (final) system and the work products (e.g., architecture, design and code) that are generated throughout the development process. In the first category, the relevant NfRs include *usability* (ease-of-use, learnability, memorability, efficiency, etc), *configurability, reliability, availability, security, scalability*, etc. On the other hand, qualities relevant to the work products generated in the process of creating the system include reusability, modifiability (i.e., ability to add properties), evolvability, etc.

In the recent literature, the above have been identified as increasingly critical NfRs, and there have been various studies aiming to provide metrics for some of them (cf., metrics of software adaptability). However, none of these studies have emphasised their role as design drivers in the context of HCI design or their relevance to the cause of universal access engineering. On the other hand, it becomes increasingly evident that many of the quality targets assumed by universal access are explicitly related and positively correlated to the level of consideration given to certain non-functional quality attributes. Consequently, it is of paramount important for software design teams concerned with universal access to be able to identify relevant NfRs, gain insight into how they are intertwined and accordingly plan their design and development efforts.

In the following sections, we present a version of non-functional requirements analysis (NfRA), with the intention to describe how developers can systematically deal with a system's universal access-specific NfRs, and the way in which this approach influences the process and outcomes of HCI design. The rest of the Chapter is structured as follows. The following section describes NfRA in terms of problem being addressed, devices used, process for using the device, outcomes and assumptions. Then, we elaborate the validation of NfRA in the context of a case study revealing how NfRA can be used to set design drivers for universal access. The Chapter concludes with a discussion and conclusions.

2. The NfRA Method

2.1 Problem Being Addressed

NfRs have been used to address a variety of problems in the software engineering literature, including software requirements specifications, software architectural components, evaluation metrics, etc. In the context of the present work, however, they serve a slightly different purpose. In particular they serve as drivers for interaction design providing the means for unfolding design options and building interaction design spaces. Specifically, although design space analysis is a well-known and established practice in HCI, the drivers leading designers to populate design spaces are not always clear and concise. In the past, advocates of design space analysis have based their techniques on notions such as design questions as in Question, Options and Criteria (McLean, et al., 1991) and psychological claims as in claims analysis (Carroll et al., 1992), without however specifying a concise method for devising appropriate questions or claims, other than tentative guidelines (Bellotti et al., 1991). NfRA serves precisely this purpose in the context of universal access engineering.

2.2 Devices Used

In IEEE/ANSI 830 (1993), IEEE Recommended Practice for Software Requirements Specifications, defines thirteen non-functional requirements that must be included in the software requirements document, namely performance, interface, operational, resource, verifications, acceptance, documentation, security, portability, quality, reliability, maintainability and safety. Table 1 provides informal definitions for some of these requirements.

In the context of universal access, the above and perhaps other NfRs constitute the prime design drivers or criteria motivating the need for generating alternatives and building a design space. In other words, each one (out of the range chosen) is embodied in a reference scenario and then articulated by means of growth scenarios. This is depicted in the diagram of Figure 1.

Table 1. Non-functional requirements

NfR	Definition
Availability	Rate of hardware and software component failure (mean time between failures)
Cost of ownership	Overall operating costs to the organisation after the system is in production
Maintainability	Ability of the support programming staff to keep the system in steady running state, including enhancement
Data integrity	Tolerance for loss, corruption, or duplication of data
Development cost	Overall cost of development
Extensibility	Ability to accommodate increased functionality
Flexibility	Ability to handle requirement changes
Functionality	Number, variety, and breadth of user-oriented features
Leveragability/Reuse	Ability to leverage common components across multiple products
Operability	Ease of everyday operation; level of support requirements
Performance	Ability to meet real-time constraints in batch and online
Portability	Ability to move application to different platforms or operating systems
Quality	Reduced number of severe defects
Robustness	Ability to handle error and boundary conditions while running
Scalability	Ability to handle a wide variety of system configuration sizes
Installability	Ease of system installation on all necessary platforms

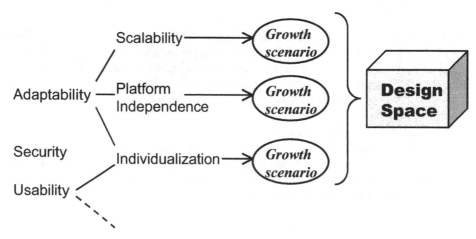

Fig. 1. Role of non-functional requirements in design space analysis

2.3 Procedure for Using the Device

NfRA requires a reference scenario, which may be a description of an existing system and the corresponding use practices or a hypothetical account of a system to be designed. Once the scenario is available, subsequent stages should aim at identifying user tasks documented on the scenario, identifying NfRs and studying how they are intertwined, and finally populating the design space through growth scenarios and iterative prototyping (see Figure 2). It should be noted that the concept of growth scenarios links Non-functional Requirements analysis with the Universal Access Assessment Workshop (UA^{2}W) method (see Chapter 11 of this book), which could provide a context for some of the stages of NfRA.

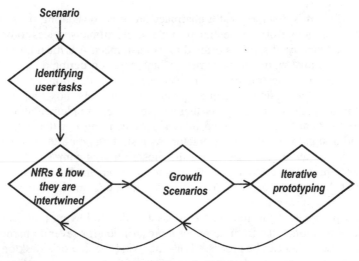

Fig. 2. Steps in NfRA

2.4 Outcomes

The prime outcomes of the NfRA, irrespective of how it is conducted (e.g., individually or in a group) should include two primary outcomes, namely, the NfRs hierarchy with clear indication of the specific NfRs considered and how they are intertwined, and a rich NfR-populated design space with mock-ups and low-fidelity prototypes accompanied by design rationale linking the various options to the NfRs hierarchy.

2.5 Assumptions

A key characteristic of the approach is that it provides a systematic way to produce a *design space* rather than a single artefact. The alternatives compiled and documented in the design space need only be prototypes of some sort (e.g., paper sketches, or computer mock-ups). In terms of skills, NfRA assumes that the team understands non-functional requirements and their implications on software design.

3. A Reference Scenario

To illustrate the technique, we will make use of a scenario-based approach to illustrate two main goals, namely:
- How scenario-based design can be applied to facilitate the development of a new system, from initial concept to design and prototype.
- How the scenario-based perspective can be improved and enhanced by means of integrating in the analysis a systematic account of non-functional requirements for universal access.

To this effect, it is assumed that a pharmacy store is considering the transition of some of its operations from conventional mode to electronic services to broaden the type, range and quality of services offered to its customers. A critical business area is related to on-line prescription management, which entails ordering drugs and clearing financial transactions electronically. The service is intended for a wide audience, including medical professionals such as general practitioners, hospitals, and citizens either in the hospital or at home. As there is no current implementation of such a system, the pharmacy has outsourced the tasks of carrying out the initial stages of analysis and design to an external contractor. As a starting point, the two parties have agreed to concentrate on the case where the prescription is compiled by the general practitioner to provide a reference use case, and to incrementally extend the scope of the use case by introducing new requirements detailing alternative strategies for service delivery and user access.

Thus, for purposes of illustration, let us assume that following a patient's visit to the General Practitioner, the latter compiles a prescription for several pharmaceuticals items. The prescription can be processed on-line using the doctor's desktop terminal, which can access the on-line pharmacy store. One of the tasks to be performed entails the on-line pharmacy store's request for specifying payment details for processing the transaction. In the longer term, the pharmacy is interested in widening the scope of use of the services by means of making it available for citizens at home or the pharmacy's own personnel moving around and visiting customers at their own sites.

4. Application of NfRA

Having briefly described the high-level scenario and the requirements of the pharmacy, let us now consider a possible set of activities to be carried out by the external analyst towards the development of prototypes. To address the task, the analyst considers that a conventional approach to system design, whereby key target users are identified and requirements are collected through interviews, questionnaires or other means, may not be the optimal choice for the task at hand. This is because the analyst realises that in effect the service to be offered by the pharmacy store is intended for a wider audience including all authorised citizens, medical professionals, and personnel of the pharmacy store, etc. Aiming to investigate the specific requirements of each of those target user categories could be an endless task. Instead, an alternative approach is considered appropriate, whereby key tasks envisioned in the target system are conceptualised in terms of non-functional requirements, and subsequently refined to become tailored to specific use cases, target users or contexts of use. According to this approach, the steps to be followed include:

- Identification of user tasks to be supported
- Analysis of key non-functional requirements relevant to the system envisioned
- Iterative design and prototyping to suit alternative design options.

The actual tasks carried out by the analysts in each one of those steps are briefly described below.

4.1 Identifying Core User Tasks and Deriving a Tentative Design

For purposes of illustration, this section focuses on a particular task, and namely the design of the dialogue to be used to enter information about the customers' credit card number. Very quickly the analyst compiles a list of user tasks. These include entering information about:

- Type of card, chosen from a range of cards such as MASTERCARD, VISA, AMERICAN EXPRESS, etc.
- Card number, typically a numeric entry
- Expiry date of card, indication of day, month and year
- User's name as printed on the card
- Billing address information

Moreover, the analyst builds a table designating each of the above user tasks to a primitive interaction task, which could be used as a building block of the dialogue components.

Table 2 depicts the derived designations.

Table 2. User tasks versus primitive interaction tasks

User task	Candidate (primitive) interaction task
Enter type of card	Selection
Enter card number	Text entry
Enter expiry date of card	Selection or text entry
Enter user's name as printed on the card	Text entry
Enter billing address information	Selection or text entry

Following this step, the analyst starts to compile design representations translating the above into design issues to be addressed. An extract of the design representation is depicted in the upper part of Figure 3, in the form of enumerated design issues. Working with this representation, the analyst develops paper mock-ups of possible design options (see lower part of Figure 3 that can be used to provide an interactive manifestation for the above tasks. The above have been used as reference material to derive an early computer mock-up, as shown in Figure 3.

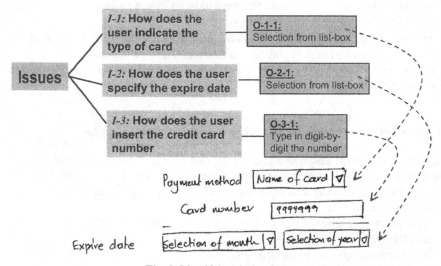

Fig. 3. Identifying design issues

Payment method: | MasterCard |

Credit card number: | |

Expiration date: | 01 (January) | | 2001 |

Cardholder's name: | |
(as it appears on the card)

continue

Fig. 4. Early computer-based mock up for some of the user tasks

4.2 Identifying Relevant Non-functional Requirements

Having developed a preliminary computer-based mock up to be used for consultations with the pharmacy store and target users, the analyst pauses the design tasks to consider some of the critical NfRs that the system should meet, how they are intertwined ,and the way in which they influence subsequent design phases. From the pharmacy store's statement of objectives, the analyst identifies various critical NfRs, including *security of transactions, performance, usability, adaptability*, etc. Following, a review of these NfRs with the pharmacy store management team, it is decided that indeed all identified NfRs are valid and important but the analyst should explicitly concentrate on the system's adaptability, as this is considered a vital differentiating factor of the service. Moreover, adaptability is to be considered in all its possible dimensions, including system adaptability to scale of operations, system adaptability to interaction partners (i.e., end users) and system adaptability to platforms of use (i.e., interaction platforms and terminals). In order to gain a deeper insight of adaptability as a NfR, the analyst consults the relevant literature to obtain an understanding of what adaptability is and how it is intertwined with other system quality attributes. The results of this activity are summarised below.

4.2.1 Adaptability

According to ISO 9126 (1991) adaptability is defined as "...attributes of software that bear on the opportunity for its adaptation to different specified environments without applying other actions or means than those provided for this purpose for the software considered". (ISO 9126: 1991, A.2.6.1). An alternative formulation is that adaptability refers to the capability of an interactive system to tolerate changes in its target execution context without external intervention. A system supporting adaptability is capable of undertaking context-sensitive processing to *recognise* the need for change, *determine* the plausible alternatives that satisfy the change and *effect* the optimal option in order to generate new behaviour (Akoumianakis, Savidis and Stephanidis, 2000).

From the review of the relevant literature and past experiences, the analyst concludes that the criticalness of adaptability is twofold. First of all, a commitment to support this NfR frequently imposes decisions, which do not only undermine the entire lifecycle of an interactive system, but are also hard to revise at later stages. For example, adaptability has implications on the architectural abstraction of the system, while commitment to an architecture that does not support adaptability may render some of the requirements of the on-line pharmacy store impossible to achieve or very resource demanding and consuming. For example, as the on-line pharmacy service is to be accessible from multiple access terminals or target user groups, including elderly people and people with disabilities, a commitment to a rigid architecture that does not support adaptation will be a binding constraint for subsequent developments. Second, adaptability correlates with, or assumes, other (first-order) NfRs such as scalability, user tolerance, platform interoperability and individualisation, all of which are very important for universal access.

In what follows, we provide a brief account of each NfR, emphasising their intertwining with adaptability and pointing out in each case the scope of the desirable adaptable behaviour that a software system should exhibit in order to support the NfR.

4.2.2 Scalability

A scalable system is one that can undertake the required context-sensitive processing to cope with changes of scale in the system's target execution context. Changes of scale in the execution context of the on-line pharmacy, necessitating adaptation, may result from increases in the number of inputs to the software (for example, from 10 inputs per second to 1000 inputs per second (scale up)), or from variations in the modality of the input (for example, from multimedia input steams to textual strings (scale down)). Scalability is also relevant to the system's outputs and, in particular, to the way in which they are manifested to the user. Thus, for instance, a system may have to scale upwards to present a piece of multimedia information (e.g., Web content) on a powerful desktop terminal, or scale downwards to present the same (Web) content on a portable device such as a PDA or a uni-modal terminal (e.g., a kiosk) located in a public space. Scaling up or down as needed will allow the on-line pharmacy to accommodate such changes in the course of designing the required adaptable behaviour. It is therefore claimed that, in the context of universal access, an adaptable system needs to be scalable to cope with (certain types of) changes in its execution context.

4.2.3 User Tolerance and Individualisation

Another source of change in the execution context of an interactive system may result from the target (or current) users. Specifically, users differ with regards to levels of expertise, interests, requirements, preferences, roles assumed, etc. ISO 9241 - Part 10 identifies individualisation as an important principle (or software ergonomic criterion) for dialogue design, pointing out explicitly that dialogue systems should be designed to support suitability for individualisation, by exhibiting the capability to adapt to the user's needs and skills for a given task. Accordingly, an adaptable system could foresee such variations and modify its behaviour accordingly.

For example, the lack of the required resources on behalf of the current user to interact with the software may force interaction to take place through an alternative channel or communication medium (e.g., non-visual). This is the case not only with novice users, elderly, people with disabilities, but also users in circumstances that cause a situational loss of certain abilities. Thus, an adaptable system should be capable of identifying and responding to situations where the user is motor-impaired, not possessing certain abilities sufficiently (e.g., fine spatial control, finger isolation) · to operate an input device such as the mouse; or the user is vision-impaired or his/her visual channel is pre-occupied (e.g., driver), thus not being able to intuitively articulate information presented in a visual modality. It can therefore be concluded that, in the context of universal access, an adaptable system should also exhibit user tolerance and individualisation.

4.2.4 Platform Independence

Platform independence, as a NfR of a software system in the context of universal access, refers to the degree of tightness of the system or of units of the system, but mainly of its interactive elements, to a particular class of target environments (or platforms). Platform independence can be realised either as a sort of portability, which is typically programmed, or as a result of compiling a more abstract specification. In the software engineering literature, portability constitutes a NfR indicating the easiness of porting a software system across a class of target environments. Though important, this type of system adaptability (regarding the target platforms) does not suffice for the purposes of universal access, since current implementations maintain a tight link with the run-time environments of the target platforms.

In previous work (Savidis et al., 1997, Savidis et al., 2001a, Savidis et al., 2001b), it has been demonstrated that the later approach (e.g., compiling specifications to realise this sort of adaptability), though more demanding, is more appropriate and relevant for universal access. This is due to the facilitation of the automatic selection of designated platform-specific artefacts (from a repository of implemented artefacts and dialogue patterns registered to various target platforms), while avoiding direct "calls" to the platform. In this manner, the specification can be updated (with regards to target platforms) and re-compiled to utilise new interaction facilities.

The specifications approach has been shown to be demanding in terms of underlying tool support and corresponding engineering practices. Nevertheless, it remains the only comprehensive proposal adequately addressing the development challenges posed by universal access. Thus, it is claimed that, in the context of universal access, an adaptable system should also exhibit platform independence.

4.3 Intertwining of NfRS

From the above brief analysis of NfRs, it becomes evident that the designated NfRs are positively correlated. The resulting correlation is depicted in Table 3.

Table 3. Intertwining of NfRs

	Adaptability	Scalability	Individualisation	Platform indep/ce
Adaptability		+	+	+
Scalability	+		+	+
Individualisation	+	+		+
Platform independence	+	+	+	

The positive signs in the table convey the impact of the each NfR on the others. Thus, for example, an increased level of scalability in the target system results in an increase in the degree of the system's adaptability, and vice versa. The main conclusion that the analysts draws from the above is that the target system should be designed in such a way so as to provide alternative manifestations for user tasks depending on situational aspects such as who the current user is, what terminal is being used, from where the system is accessed, etc. In other words, subsequent design phases should not aim to develop one design proposal, but several which are to be initiated under specific conditions or circumstances.

4.4 Iterative Design and Prototyping

The design targets set following the NfRs analysis point to several properties to be exhibited by the on-line pharmacy. These are summarised as follows:
- The on-line pharmacy should be adaptable to different users, including general practitioners, and the citizens consuming pharmaceutical products, their relatives making orders on their behalf, etc.

- The online pharmacy should be accessible by, and scalable to, various terminals such as PCs, PDAs, and other network attachable devices.
- The on-line pharmacy store should be accessible across contexts of use, including the office, the residential environment of a consumer, and while moving from one place to another.

Clearly, the current prototype, as depicted in Figure 4, does not suffice to facilitate all (or some of) the above. This is because it has been formulated on the basis of certain implicit assumptions. Specifically, the design presented in Figure 4 is based on the assumption that, in order to complete the task, the user will have to fill in a form through a Graphical User Interface, providing information such as type of card, card number, expiry data, user's name as printed on the card, billing address information, etc.

Such a scenario designates a particular execution context for the task that implicitly assumes at least the following:

- The target user is a professional with access to a personal computer, and in possession of all necessary human capabilities to operate the designated dialogue
- The underlying technology platform offers the needed resources, in terms of software libraries, input / output devices, etc, to realise the graphical dialogue
- The task is to be executed from a residential or business context of use.

Such assumptions can be made explicit by considering the requirements of each interaction object and the compound dialogue as a whole. Examples of the implicit assumptions characterising the artefact of Figure 4 are presented in Figure 5.

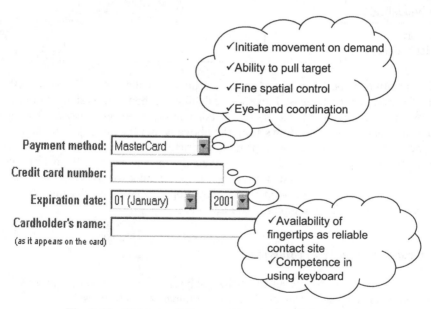

Fig. 5. Identifying implicit assumptions in the original prototype

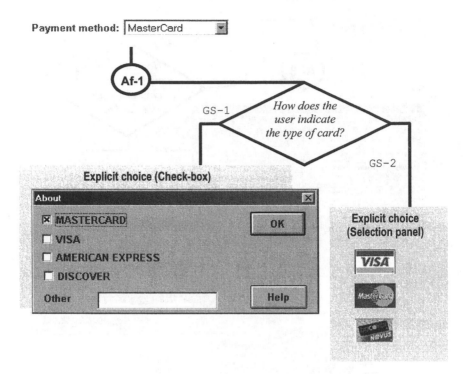

Fig. 6. From concrete to abstract design

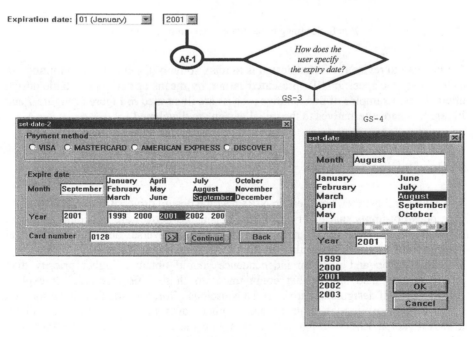

Fig. 7. Alternatives for entering expiry date

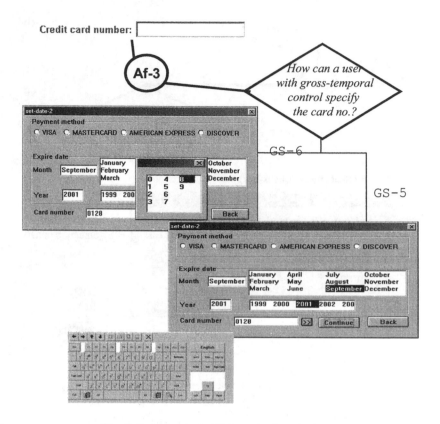

Fig. 8. Scanning to facilitate motor-impaired access

One way to revise the initial design is to relax some of the implicit assumptions so as to satisfy the specific NfRs presented earlier, by means of deriving suitable design alternatives. Examples of this iterative process are illustrated in Figure 6, Figure 7 and Figure 8, where alternatives to the initial design are developed.

5. Concluding Remarks

This Chapter illustrated how certain NfRs become design drivers for universal access. This does not imply that other NfRs (not considered above) are not important for a software system, but simply points out that when universal access is the critical design goal for a system, then certain NfRs such as adaptability, scalability, individualisation and platform independence should obtain a higher priority than others. It was also shown that commitment to these NfRs requires an explicit consideration of design alternatives and a conscious effort towards their incorporation (or encapsulation) into the target system. In other words, the focus should be not only to investigate and build design alternatives with the intention to compare them and select an optimal option, but also to facilitate their co-existence in the final implementation so as to provide the resources for realising the required level of adaptability. It can therefore be concluded that such a process of incrementally revising and extending the scope of the system by introducing new artefacts to suit emerging requirements is an inherent property of a universal access design life cycle.

Chapter 14
Screening Models and Growth Scenarios

Demosthenes Akoumianakis[1] and Constantine Stephanidis[1,2]

[1]Foundation for Research and Technology – Hellas (FORTH)
Institute of Computer Science
Heraklion, Crete, GR-70013, Greece
cs@ics.forth.gr
[2]University of Crete
Department of Computer Science, Greece

Abstract. This Chapter describes screening, a well-known technique widely used in a variety of disciplines, such as industrial design, urban planning, engineering design disciplines, assistive technology, etc., and the social sciences (e.g., economics and product innovation). A variety of screening models (both formal and semi-formal) are available to facilitate product assessment at various stages of development. We will briefly review the technique and then describe its application in the context of Universal Access.

1. Introduction

In Chapter 11, we described the Universal Access Assessment Workshop (UA[2]W) which makes explicit reference to the concept of screening a scenario to identify barriers in use, usability problems etc. Here, we will provide additional details on a general technique referred to as *screening artefacts*, targeted to facilitate early insight into Universal Access. Screening an artefact may be as simple as a checklist of criteria in the form of questions that fall into a small number of categories (e.g., "must-meet", "should-meet", "meets"). Typically, "must-meet" criteria are questions used to determine the viability of the artefact (i.e., required features or qualities). In most cases, these criteria are structured as closed-ended questions and are designed to provide go/no-go decision points. On the other hand, "should-meet" criteria are often more specific and depict recommended or desirable features or product qualities.

However, screening may also be a more complex activity entailing formal or semi-formal models and quantification before it can bring about useful results. Four general categories of screening models have been identified in literature, namely:
- *Ranking* models that compare one product idea against others on some specified evaluation criteria – the highest ranked product is selected.
- *Scoring* models that use criteria considered critical to a products' performance – product exceeding a minimum acceptable score (when summed up across all evaluative criteria) are selected.
- *Economic* models that are based on deterministic or probabilistic payoffs, profits, etc. – the product meeting some desired level is selected.

C. Stephanidis (Ed.): Universal Access Code of Practice in Health Telematics, LNCS 3041, pp. 156-174, 2005.
© Springer-Verlag Berlin Heidelberg 2005

- *Optimisation* models that involve some mathematical function – products that maximise this function are selected.

Depending on the choice of model and its parameters, quantification may be simple or complex. For example, in case of a multi-parameter model, it may be appropriate to devise a weighted scoring system to evaluate each parameter, which may have different weighting value, and subsequently compute the aggregate score. In all cases, screening should be a structured and well-targeted activity, which is carried out either by an individual or a group of people. In what follows, we tailor the general concept of screening to suit the aims and objectives of a Universal Access inquiry.

2. The Screening Method

2.1 Problem Being Addressed

The method is intended to facilitate an approach to Universal Access that is based on structured argumentation about a tentative design based on designated quality attributes, heuristics and criteria. Screening seeks to identify at an early stage desirable features of a software system, which if supported, would avoid potential barriers to use and to develop design proposals to support their implementation. It may be used on its own or as part of the UA^2W method.

2.2 Device / Technique(s) Used

The prime technique used when screening a tentative design is filtering through designated filters. For the purpose of Universal Access, such filters may take several forms. The most popular is that of questions which seek to provide insight into alternative execution contexts for a task. In terms of theoretical background, they can be considered as similar to "issues" in IBIS (Rittel, 1972), or "questions" in QOC (McLean et al., 1996) or "claims" in Claims Analysis (Carroll, 1995), or even as usability heuristics in discount usability (Nielsen, 1992). In the following section, some examples of filters are provided, which could be of potential value to a Universal Access inquiry.

2.2.1 Categories of Filters

In the context of Universal Access, we have identified three main categories of screening filters, namely user-, context- and terminal or platform-specific, corresponding to the sources of change in the tasks execution context, i.e., change due to user variation, change due to context variation, and change due to platform variation.

User-specific filters are formulated from the study of permanent or situational user characteristics and abilities. Some indicative examples of user-specific filters are the following:

- How is the task performed by a user who possesses alternative reliable control acts, such as movement of one / both hands, directed eye-gaze, head movement, movement of lower limbs, vocalisation.
- How is the task performed by a user who cannot push and pull targets or cannot isolate finger movement or cannot initiate movement on demand or does not have fine spatial control.

User specific filters such as the above may be extracted by consulting assessment manuals or human performance criteria.

Terminal-specific filters are formulated on the basis of characteristics of terminals or interaction platforms. Filters under this category may fall under several clusters, which may be used to characterise, amongst other things, the following aspects of a terminal:

- External features, labels and instructions
- Location and access to the terminal
- Card systems and Keypads
- Typefaces and legibility
- Touch screens
- Screens and instructions
- Operating instructions
- Training materials, etc.

In addition, under this category there may be filters, which relate explicitly to the user interface software, i.e., architectural properties and corresponding interactive behaviour.

Context-specific filters depict physical and social conditions in the environment in which a task is executed. Examples of context-specific filters include:

- Locating and accessing the terminal
- The terminal's location signs are easy to read
- The terminal's lighting levels are adequate
- The terminal's queuing arrangements are adequate
- The path to the terminal is wheelchair accessible
- The terminal is equipped with a location system for blind users.
- Usage pattern
- Informative feedback on task progress
- Responsiveness to monitored interactions
- Responsiveness to external stimuli
- Awareness of non-users
- The system "observes" usage and accordingly modifies its behaviour
- The system detects changes in the usage pattern and accordingly modifies its behaviour.
- Ubiquity
- The system's design does not presuppose a particular context of use
- The system can be used from different geographic locations
- The system can be accessed through different terminals
- The system detects changes in the context of use and accordingly modifies its behaviour
- The level of security is adequate.

The above may also be combined to provide a structured and general-purpose instrument for screening particular types of products. An example of this is depicted in Figure 1, where a screening form is presented to assess subjectively a product's adherence to Universal Access principles. It should be noted that the subjective nature of the form assumes that people recording their opinion have had previous exposure to the product.

Sample Screening Form			
Screening interactive software to assess universal access compliance			
This form collects the opinions and observations of end users and / or experts who screen interactive software to determine its adherence to universal access principles. This form can be adapted for use with multiple types of interactive software as well as multiple types of end users and / or experts.			

Date: _____

Product (Name, brand, company): _____

Title / position of user: _____

Occupation & speciality: _____

	User-specific considerations	Does not meet expectations	Meets expectations	Exceeds expectations
1	The system implements mechanisms to elicit information about the user.			
2	The system keeps track of my personal preferences.			
3	The system provides sufficient guidance and support for the user, as needed.			
4	The system takes reasonable time to became aware of my personal preferences.			
5	The system makes the right assumptions about myself.			
6	The system's user model is sufficiently visible.			
7	The system's user model can be inspected.			
8	The system's user model is sufficiently transparent.			
9	The system prohibits unauthorised access to the user model.			
10	The system consults the user to confirm some of its assumptions.			
11	I can inform the system about misuse of assumptions.			
12	The system asks my approval before it updates the user model.			

Fig. 1. An example screening form

2.3 Procedure for Using the Device

Screening or filtering is ideally carried out as a group activity, although this need not be the case. There are four steps involved in using the filtering technique, irrespective of whether it is used by an individual analyst, a group of analysts (e.g., collaborative workshop) or in the course of a participatory design inquiry.

2.3.1 Defining the Filters

First, the design team defines the filters to be used. The filters should be clustered into groups seeking to assess specific qualities in the reference system (i.e., availability of user model, hardware configuration, architectural qualities, user interface software attributes, etc). Filter clusters should reveal how an artefact is currently used, as well as what features of the artefact prohibit access by different categories of users, in different contexts of use and through alternative interaction platforms.

2.3.2 The Screening Phase

Screening should aim to address a two-fold purpose: on the one hand it should characterise the current execution context of a task, and on the other hand, it should lead to envisioning new execution contexts by reflecting changes in the target user groups, the context of use and the access terminal or platform on which the product is to be executed. The screening phase should be carried out by at least one, but preferably more, participants or experts. It is important to note that this is an expert activity since it entails an understanding of the designated filters and interpretation of the case in hand.

2.3.3 Identification of Break Downs

In this stage, the group consolidates problems in the reference system and summarises intended uses of the system that are not supported by the current implementation. For example, the system could fail criteria such as:

- Accessibility (i.e., the system is not accessible by certain target user groups)
- Platform independence (i.e., the system can only be accessed in a specific environment such as Windows and it is not available as WWW or WAP application or service)
- Scalability (i.e., the content of the system does not scale up or down to meet platform or access terminal requirements or capabilities)
- Ubiquity (i.e., the system or service does not support anyone, anywhere and anytime access)
- User-adaptable behaviour (i.e., the system cannot be customised either automatically or manually to diverse requirements)
- User-adaptive behaviour (i.e., when in operation the system does not monitor user's interaction behaviour to adjust aspects of interaction)
- Use-adaptable and adaptive behaviour (i.e., the system takes no account of the context of use to accordingly modify its interactive behaviour)
- Localisation (i.e., the system cannot be localised)

2.3.4 Concept Formation and New Artefacts

Finally, new artefacts are devised as paper mock-ups or low-fidelity prototypes to depict improvements resulting from the identified breakdowns.

2.3.5 Some Techniques to Facilitate Filtering

The filtering process, which is schematically depicted in Figure 2, may be informal, i.e., based on intuition or (semi-) formal, i.e., informed by empirical evidence or analytical insight. Unfortunately, the empirical ground available for Universal Access is still limited and narrow. The research community is just beginning to undertake efforts in this direction, but these will take time to yield consolidated results in the form of design criteria, recommendations or rules. Thus, many of the techniques to be reviewed in this section are based either on the designer's intuition or on techniques which have been developed in other fields of inquiry such as HCI design, and which can provide a methodological basis for analytical assessment of Universal Access.

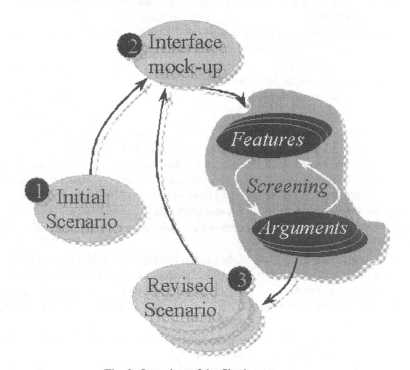

Fig. 2. Overview of the filtering process

Feature inspection
This technique involves the inspection of task related features of a mock-up by experts. Typical features to be inspected include:

- Availability of a user model
- Transparency, modifiability and capability to inspect the system's model of the user

- Appropriateness of the user interface for completing a task
- Availability of certain functions (i.e., help, undo, redo, etc)
- The ability to be self explanatory
- Error tolerance and other usability aspects.

Heuristics

This is a well-known technique popular amongst HCI design and usability engineering practitioners. It involves the assessment of a tentative mock-up or low-fidelity prototype against a set of general or domain-specific heuristics. In a heuristic evaluation, domain specialists judge whether each element of a user interface follows a list of established heuristics. Typically, two or three experts evaluate the system with reference to established guidelines, note usability problems, and rank them in order of severity.

An example of heuristics, which according to Katz (see http://www.acm.org/sigchi/web/chi97testing/katz.htm) promote Universal Access and usability of web sites, is the following:

- Enable all essential information to be accessed using alternative modalities
- Use explicit labelling of content and structural elements
- Minimise Visual Strain
- Enable the user to locate information quickly
- Minimise the users' memory load

Design criteria and principles (i.e., Universal design principles)

Design criteria may be extracted from standards or best practice examples. For instance, the seven universal design principles constitute an example of general guidelines intended to ensure that the proposed design is inclusive and respects diversity in human abilities. The seven principles are as follows (Story, 1998):

- *Equitable use* - the design is useful and marketable to any group of users.
- *Flexibility in use* - the design accommodates a wide range of individual preferences and abilities.
- *Simple and intuitive use* - use of the design is easy to understand, regardless of the user's experience, knowledge, language skills or current concentration level.
- *Perceptible information* - the design communicates necessary information effectively to the user, regardless of ambient conditions or the user's sensory abilities.
- *Tolerance for error* - the design minimises hazards and the adverse consequences of accidental or unintended actions.
- *Low physical effort* - the design can be used efficiently and comfortably and with a minimum of fatigue.
- *Size and space provided* - for approach, reach, manipulation, and use regardless of user's body size, posture or mobility.

2.4 Outcomes

Screening delivers three main types of results:

- A list of designated Universal Access Filters (input to filtering grid)
- Universal Access problem descriptions (or breakdowns) and corresponding mock-ups of new artefacts which remedy the problems (input to filtering grid)
- Argumentative rationale for new artefacts and accompanying design logic.

The above may be optionally documented in a filtering grid (see Figure 3). Each column in the grid represents a typical task in the use of the product (i.e., searching for, reviewing, updating and Electronic Patient Record, etc). Rows in the grid list the agreed designated filters or screening criteria. In each cell, designers may denote the relative performance of each task against the respective criterion or screening heuristic.

It is important to note that in this type of screening, the objective is not merely to identify a particular system or system specification to be selected out of a range of plausible ones. Instead, the aim is to identify how the same system (or its tasks) performs against the screening heuristics and to reveal failures. The greater the number of failures identified, the richer the insight gained in the system's global execution context.

		User tasks								
		Task 1	*Task 2*	*Task 3*	*Task 4*	*Task 5*	*Task 6*	*Task 7*	...	*Task v*
Designated Universal Access Filters	*Filter 1*									
	Filter 2									
	Filter 3									
	Filter 4									
	Filter 5									
	Filter 6									
	...									
	Filter v									

Fig. 3. The filtering grid

2.5 Assumptions

It is important to note that Universal Access Filters do not provide answers. Rather, they motivate designers to think about a problem or certain aspects of the problem.

Another shortcoming is the fact that Universal Access Filters are not of general-purpose; usually they are category-, platform-, domain- or context-specific. This means that when there are several categories of users or several contexts of use to be considered, Universal Access Filters within one category may conflict with those of another category, thus increasing both the complexity of design and the range of issues to be addressed.

3. Application of the Method

3.1 Reference Scenario

The target reference scenario comes from HYGEIAnet, which is the Virtual Health Telematics Network of the Region of Crete, Greece (Tsiknakis et al., 1997; see also Acknowledgement). An extract of our reference scenario is depicted in Exhibit 1.

> **Exhibit 1**
>
> *Following last night's notification by the Local Service Center, Dr Fred logs on to HYGEIAnet Electronic Patient Records service from his office in the University Hospital of Heraklion. Dr Fred asks the system to present demographic data about the patient N. Stathiakis, who was admitted last night into the hospital. The doctor wishes to have an overview of the patient's demographic data and health condition before visiting him in the clinic. The system responds to the request and presents two screens in sequence (see Figure 4a and Figure 4b) regarding demographics. From last night's briefing Dr Fred was informed that the patient suffers from asthma and this was the cause of his recent admission to the hospital. To obtain an insight into the patient's past treatment, Dr Fred requests to review the patient's previous drug treatment for asthma. The system responds with the screen of Figure 4c. Having obtained a sufficient insight about the patient's history, past treatment and current conditions, Dr Fred decides to visit the patient in the clinic.*

3.2 Screening

The objective of the conducted exercise was to make use of the screening method in order to gain insight into new execution contexts for the tasks mentioned in the narrative of Exhibit 1. The exercise was conducted in the context of a UA^{2}W session. Participants invited to attend included one analyst (responsible for the conduct of the UA^{2}W sessions), one representative of the HYGEIAnet development team and one independent designer with no prior exposure either to the notion of UA^{2}W or the HYGEIAnet electronic patient record system. All participants were informed by the analyst through email about what was to be done in the course of the two UA^{2}W sessions, the design materials to be used (i.e., scenario narrative, mock-ups, etc) and the expected outcomes.

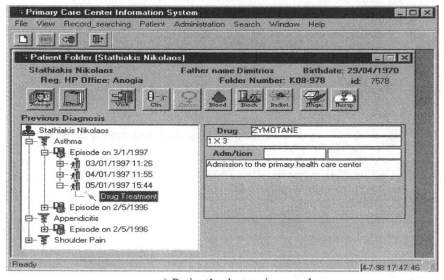

(a) Patient's demographic data

(b) Patient's condition of residence

c) Patient's electronic record

Fig. 4. Examples of designated tasks in the current implementation

Screening entailed the engagement of participants in an argumentative phase, whereby implicit assumptions embodied in the original scenario and the corresponding artefacts were identified and subsequently formulated as filters. Participants were informed that we are interested primarily in three categories of implicit claims, relating to the underlying implementation platform, the target users and the context of use. By inspection of the initial scenario, participants identified the tasks involved (e.g., presentation of the patient's demographics record) and made a variety of comments regarding the implicit assumptions embedded in the scenario. Some of them are depicted as implicit or explicit claims in the left-hand column of Table 1.

Table 1. Record of assumptions identified and corresponding access filters

Platform	"The user interface follows the desktop-based, windows-style of interaction"	How can the following tasks be manifested in a non-windows / non-desktop based style of interaction?	
		✓ WAP phone	GS1
		✓ Portable device such as iPAQ	GS2
		✓ Kiosk located at a specified area	GS3
		✓ WWW	GS4
User	"The user interface is designed for professional users, typically doctors of medicine"	Should and how could the task be carried out by:	
		✓ other medical professionals, such as nurses or paramedics?	GS5
		✓ patients	GS6
	"System users are in possession of fine spatial control, fine eye-hand coordination, ability to pull and push targets, ability to initiate movement on demand", etc.	How can the task be carried out by patients who possess: Gross temporal (as opposed to final spatial) control Upper-limbs as the reliable contact act and fist as primary contact site Ability to produce movements in timed patterns	GS7
Context of use	"Users (e.g., doctors) access the system using PCs located in their offices in the hospital"	How can the task be carried out when:	
		✓ User is moving around in the ward	GS8
		✓ User is at the patient's bed	GS9
		✓ User is at home	GS1 0
		✓ User is in a public area of the clinic (e.g., coffee bar)	GS1 1

The other two columns of Table 1 capture the essence and outcomes of scenario screening. Notably, the second column in the table depicts normative filtering statements intended to generate thinking and design deliberations towards the conceptualisation of new execution contexts. Specifically, filters such as those listed in the middle column of the table depict abstract characterisations of envisioned task execution contexts designated by corresponding growth scenarios (right hand column in Table 1). It is worth pointing out that some of the envisioned growth scenarios can have relationshisp such as those reported in Alspaugh and Anton, (2001). For our purposes additional relations between scenarios X and Y are considered (see Table 2), which are useful constructs in deciding the exact number and scope of the growth scenarios to be selected and elaborated.

Table 2. Relationships between growth scenarios

Expression of relation	Interpretation
X assumes Y	Y is required before X can be realised
X complements Y	X and Y are complementary- either one can be active but not both concurrently
X augments Y	Y adds specific features to X to make it more adaptable; as an example consider the use of scanning in a WWW style
X parallel_to Y	X can be active in parallel to (or concurrently with) Y

For example, GS7 is a special case of GS6, thus when detailing the latter, one needs to accommodate the former. Similarly, GS1 presents an alternative to GS2, GS3 and GS4, thus when detailing any of them, one needs to accommodate the other two. Identifying such relationships between alternative growth scenarios helps in specifying interrelated execution contexts that should be reflected in the Universal Access implementation. Specifically, such interrelationships define the scope of adaptation (both adaptability and adaptivity, according to Stephanidis 2001) that the Universal Access implementation should exhibit. Adaptability can be used to implement scenarios related either through the relationships *assumes*, *complements* and *augments*, while adaptivity should be the prime technique to implement scenarios which are related with the relationship *parallel_to*.

Concluding the screening phase, and following the above design deliberations, the design team agrees upon and formulates a set of relevant Universal Access requirements, for each of the designated tasks, and for the system globally. Once agreed by participants, these requirements are documented in the UA²F (upper parts in Figure 5) for each of the tasks respectively.

Task/artifact	Context of use
Present the patient demographics	Doctor's hospital office
Style	
Windowing-based, form-like interaction style	

	Objective
Screening phase	Doctors should be able to review the patient demographics while moving around (e.g., outside the office, in the ward of the hospital, etc)
	HYGEIAnet should be able to present the patients demographics using a variety of presentation styles suitable to different devices (e.g., WAP phone, iPAQ)
	Parts of the HYGEIAnet electronic patient record system should be also accessible by patients at home or on the move.
	The parts of the HYGEIAnet electronic patient record system which is accessible by patients at home or on the move should also be accessible to people with disabilities and specifically motor-impaired patients from their residence environment

	Growth scenarios	**Priority**	**Constraint**
Growth scenarios	Scalability to a WAP platform to present demographic information on a WAP phone (GS1)	High	WAP page
	Scalability to present the patient's medical history on the iPAQ (GS 2)	High	Small screen device Stylus
	Adaptability to motor-impaired users (GS 3)	High	Scanning Gross temporal control (switches)

Fig. 5. Extract from the UA2F

3.3 Compiling Growth Scenarios

Relaxing some of the assumptions depicted in Table 1 facilitates insight into novel execution contexts. Articulating concrete proposals for these novel execution contexts is the essence of growth scenario compilation. To this effect, the potentially large number of plausible growth scenarios implied from the screening phase (see Table 1) should eventually be consolidated to a concise subset intended to address the specific Universal Access requirements as agreed by the team (see Figure 5), taking into account the interrelationships between scenarios, thus arriving at aggregate formulations of a small number of designated growth scenarios. For the purposes of our example, three separate and complementary growth scenarios have been developed, depicting the new execution contexts introduced in the lower part of the UA^{2}F of Figure 5.

Exhibit 2 summarises each of the three growth scenarios and their intended purpose. The three growth scenarios seek to expand the execution context of the designated tasks beyond their desktop embodiment, by introducing alternative interactive styles, suitable for WAP phones, the iPAQ and WWW access.

Exhibit 2

GS 1	→	*Dr Fred issues a search query to the HYGEIAnet service and receives the patient's demographic information and condition of residence as WAP pages on the mobile phone (see Figure 6)*
GS 2	→	*Dr Fred has now arrived by the bedside of the next patient. He makes use of his iPAQ to obtain information on the patient's medical history (Figure 7)*
GS3 (GS 4 ∧ GS6)	→	*Assumes an augmented WWW style for searching the electronic patient record using scanning (for users with motor impairments) – see Figure 8*

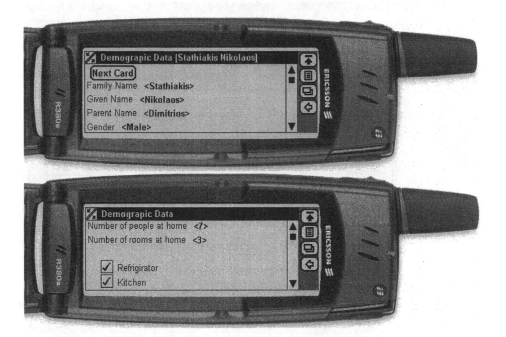

Fig. 6. WAP pages for presenting the patient's demographics

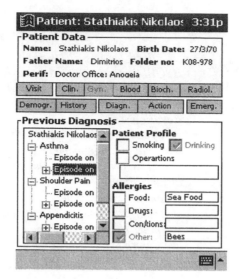

Fig. 7. iPAQ interface for reviewing the patient's medical record

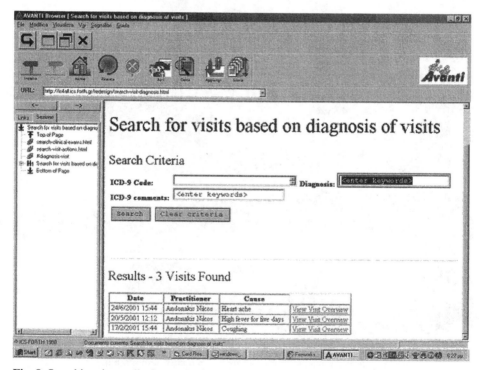

Fig. 8. Searching the medical record using an augmented WWW-style and a scanning interface

Furthermore, the WWW style is augmented so as to allow motor-impaired users to execute the designated task. Finally, some sort of prototyping technique or tool is considered appropriate for visualising early design ideas embedded in the growth scenarios.

It should be noted that the final quality attribute detailing the relationships between the various growth scenarios also defines the scale and scope of adaptable and adaptive behaviour to be exhibited by the Universal Access implementation of these growth scenarios. Thus, it provides developers with a concrete statement of the systems adaptability requirements, which, in turn, allows informative decisions to be made about critical aspects of the system, such as, for example, its architectural abstraction, the choice of interaction techniques, and the conditions under which alternative styles of interaction are to be initiated.

Table 3 depicts some of the rationale for the designated growth scenarios and the reasoning behind the computer mock-ups introduced earlier. As shown, the quality attributes elaborated for each scenario include: initiator (user-adaptability), context of use, flow of events, exceptions, pre- and post-conditions and relationship with other growth scenarios.

4. Discussion

It is important to clarify that the examples presented above are only indicative of the type of work and corresponding outcomes of screening and compiling growth scenarios. Nevertheless, they demonstrate clearly that the UA^{2}W is essentially a creative process involving elements of both analysis and synthesis.

Analysis is the main objective in the course of building an initial reference scenario and subsequently when screening the scenario to identify implicit or explicit assumptions about the designated users, the tasks they carry out and the way in which these tasks are computationally embodied and manifested. On the other hand, compiling growth scenarios is effectively the creative stage, which nevertheless is tightly linked with the analysis carried out. The type and scope of the screening is only bound by the specific Universal Access requirements relevant to the system at hand. In other words, the assumptions identified may highlight a broad range of new execution contexts for the designated task, shaped by variations in the user and context of use characteristics relevant for such a task. Accordingly, several growth scenarios may be needed to describe exactly the scope of Universal Access envisaged for the designated task(s). In this effort, the design team should mind the relationships governing these growth scenarios and how these relationships are to be implemented, which in turn will determine non-functional qualities of the system such as portability from one platform to another, adaptability to users or contexts of use, adaptive features, etc. As illustrated in our GS 3, the WWW style developed is the same for both able- bodied users and motor impaired users. The only difference is at the level of the user interface and the underlying interaction techniques. Thus, it can be argued that in realising GS3 the system needs to be designed in such a away so as to support adaptability in the form of user-adapted interaction facilities.

Table 3. Elaboration of growth scenarios

	Growth Scenario 1 (WAP phone)		Growth Scenario 2 (PDA)		Growth Scenario 3 (WWW & scanning)	
Initiator	Professional user (Dr Fred)		Professional user (Dr Fred)		Patient at home	
Context of use	The user (Dr Fred) outside the office		The user (Dr Fred) is moving around in the ward and has arrived by the bed of the patient		The user (with motor-impairments) is at home and wishes to review his medical record	
	User	*System*	*User*	*System*	*User*	*System*
Flow of events	▪ The user connects to the HYGEIAnet server and logs-in ▪ The user specifies service by typing in a numerical value ▪ The user types in the name of the patient	▪ The system responds to notify user's login and asks the user to select a service ▪ The system notifies the user that service is available ▪ The system asks for the name of patient ▪ The system retrieves the patient's medical record and posts the results	▪ The user connects to the HYGEIAnet server and logs-in ▪ The user selects an application ▪ The user makes a selection from the list of patients	▪ The system responds to notify user's login and presents set of application options on PDA ▪ The system list of patients in the ward ▪ The system presents parts of the medical record o\n PDA	▪ The user connects to the HYGEIAnet server and logs-in ▪ The user selects an application ▪ The user makes a selection from the list of patients	▪ The system responds to notify user's login and presents set of application options on PDA ▪ The system list of patients in the ward ▪ The system presents parts of the medical record o\n PDA
Exceptions	▪ Network problems ▪ Error in login procedure		▪ Network problems		▪ Network problems	
Pre-conditions	▪ User is authorised ▪ HYGEIAnet offers the service		▪ User is authorised ▪ HYGEIAnet offers the service		▪ User is authorised ▪ User is familiar with scanning	
Post-conditions	▪ System has inferred the task's execution context ▪ WAP style automatically initiated		▪ System has inferred the task's execution context ▪ PDA style automatically initiated		▪ System has inferred the task's execution context ▪ WWW style automatically initiated	
Relationships	▪ Parallel to GS 2 and GS 3		▪ Parallel to GS 1 and GS 3		▪ Parallel to GS 1 and GS 2 ▪ Augments the basic WWW growth scenario	

Regarding the design outcomes compiled in the course of UA^2W sessions, it is important to note that the UA^2F is intended to capture formative design deliberations and decisions and to provide a record of design rational. The UAQM should be seen as a summative artefact. More importantly, however, both these provide a mechanism for capturing the team's history of encounters in the course of the UA^2W sessions, thus offering a "living memory" of the team's cooperative exchanges. In other words, the analyst should make every effort to record the collective wisdom, agreed rationale and the consensus reached in the course of the UA^2W sessions, thus maintaining a tacit record of intensive collaboration, argumentation and negotiation between group members.

5. Concluding Remarks

Our experience with the screening and growth scenarios method in the context of HYGEIAnet has revealed several recommendations for best practices related to the method. It turns out that a critical factor of success in applying such a technique is the analyst's preparation and commitment throughout the various stages in the method's application. The specific demands placed upon the analysts relate to, amongst other concerns, the choice of reference scenario, the choice of participants, the management practices followed in the course of scenario screening and compilation of growth scenarios, etc. In the planning stage, and independently of the method used to generate the scenario, the analyst should ensure certain quality attributes in the reference scenario. First of all, the scenario should be relevant to Universal Access, in the sense that it should not lead to growth scenarios which are unrealistic or impractical, given the scope of the system or the business objectives. Second, the scenario should be meaningful and comprehensive, while formulated in a manner that depicts actual use rather than intended use of a system. Third, the scenario should have the agreement of the relevant stakeholders with regards to the tasks described and to the designated goals of these tasks. Provided that these conditions are met, the method can be very rich in its design outcomes and very satisfying for all parties concerned, inheriting all the positive consequences of cooperative design inquiries.

Another important consideration relates to the composition of the design team (to be invited by the analyst) and the measures taken to make the agreed scenario part of the group's deliberations. Specifically, since the method heavily relies on analysing artefacts and generating proposals for new execution contexts for these artefacts, the results are likely to be correlated with the design deliberations made in the course of conducting the method. In other words, the results will be of higher quality and value if participants fully understand the scope of the exercise and engage actively in scenario screening and compiling growth scenarios. To this end, the analyst should take all appropriate measures to invite participants who are willing to become involved and competent to contribute.

Finally, it is important to highlight that at the heart of the work described in this Chapter is an implied focus on proactively accounting for Universal Access in the course of early design and development activities. The basic argumentation instruments of scenario screening and compilation of growth scenarios serve precisely such a proactive cause, irrespective of whether a prototype system exists or not, or of the fidelity of the prototype. Specifically, although validation case studies thus far have involved prototypes of existing systems, the method does not pre-suppose their availability. In fact, in cases where a system is not available, the reference scenario can be solely based on statements of functional requirements, while prototypes may depict envisioned tasks using low-fidelity mock-ups (e.g., paper-based).

Acknowledgement

The authors would also like to explicitly acknowledge the co-operation with the Centre for Medical Informatics & Health Telematics applications (CMI-HTA) of the Institute of Computer Science, Foundation for Research and Technology – Hellas. The CMI-HTA Laboratory is the developer of HYGEIAnet.

Chapter 15
W3C-WAI Content Accessibility Auditing

Pier Luigi Emiliani and Laura Burzagli

Consiglio Nazionale delle Ricerche
Istituto di Fisica Applicata "Nello Carrara"
Via Panciatichi, 64
Firenze 50127, Italy
{p.l.emiliani, L.Burzagli}@ifac.cnr.it

Abstract. This Chapter describes W3C-WAI Accessibility Auditing as a technique aiming to improve accessibility of web-based information systems. We consider the role of WAI Content Accessibility Guidelines (WCAG) in two complementary phases, namely the summative phase where WCAG can be used to identify accessibility problems and the formative stage where WCAG provide a means for proactive design inherently accessible.

1. Introduction

The World Wide Web Accessibility Initiative (WAI, http://www.w3.org/wai) has formulated three sets of guidelines for Web sites, Web authoring tools, and browsers, in an effort to consolidate previous experience on accessibility and to provide design recommendations that can improve the accessibility of WWW for people with disabilities. Specifically, people with different kinds of disabilities can experience difficulty using the Web due to a combination of barriers in the information on Web pages, and barriers in the "user agents" (browsers, multimedia players, or assistive technologies such as screen readers or voice recognition).

The W3C-WAI guidelines are written for a variety of audiences, including people who design Web sites, people who check existing Web sites for accessibility, organisations that wish to request a given level of accessibility for their Web sites; and others who are interested in ensuring that people with disabilities can access information on the Web. For sites that follow the guidelines, logos are available which can be placed on web pages to show conformance. Also, partially automated checkers have been developed to help in assessing compliance of Web sites to designated W3C-WAI guidelines.

C. Stephanidis (Ed.): Universal Access Code of Practice in Health Telematics, LNCS 3041, pp. 175-196, 2005.
© Springer-Verlag Berlin Heidelberg 2005

2. Problem Being Addressed

2.1 Web Content Accessibility Guidelines

The Web Content Accessibility Guidelines constitute a specification providing guidance on accessibility of Web sites for people with disabilities. This document is based upon two main principles:
- Ensuring Graceful Transformation
- Making Content Understandable and Navigable

The specification contains fourteen guidelines or general principles of accessible design, which focus explicitly on barriers related to Web pages.

2.2 Authoring Tool Accessibility Guidelines

The Authoring Tool Accessibility Guidelines (ATAG) Working Group (AUWG) develops guidelines and techniques to assist authoring tool software developers to make their tools, and the content that their tools generate, more accessible to people with disabilities. The guidelines address both the accessibility of Web content produced by authoring tools and the accessibility of authoring tool interfaces.

2.3 User Agent Guidelines

The user agent guidelines provide guidance for designing user agents that lower barriers to Web accessibility for people with disabilities (visual, hearing, physical, cognitive, and neurological). User agents include HTML browsers and other types of software that retrieve and render Web content. A user agent that conforms to these guidelines promotes accessibility through its own user interface and through other internal facilities, including its ability to communicate with other technologies (especially assistive technologies). Furthermore, all users, not just users with disabilities, are expected to find conforming user agents more usable.

In the remaining of the present report we provide a generic account of the use of W3C-WAI guidelines irrespective of their type and focus.

3. Device / Techniques Used

3.1 Guidelines, Checkpoints, Priority Levels

W3C-WAI guidelines are formulated as generic statements of design principles and good practice. Each guideline is associated with one or more checkpoints describing how a particular guideline applies in a typical reference scenario. In other words, checkpoints associated with a particular Web Content Development guideline describes how the guideline applies in a specific content development scenario.

Each checkpoint is assigned one of three priority levels. Priority one is for checkpoints that a developer must satisfy, otherwise some groups of people will be unable to access information on a site; priority two characterises checkpoints that a developer should satisfy or else it will be very difficult to access information; priority three characterises checkpoints that a developer may satisfy, otherwise some people will find it difficult to access information.

The specification defines three "conformance levels" to facilitate reference by other organisations. Conformance level "Single-A" (A) includes priority one checkpoints, "Double-A" (AA) includes priority one and two, and "Triple-A" (AAA) includes priority one, two and three.

3.2 Design Input

There are two (complementary) pathways towards making use of the W3C-WAI guidelines. First, the guidelines may be used as a formative design technique to inform concept formation and early design decisions. Second, the guidelines may be used to facilitate experts tasked to carry out assessment and compliance audits once a prototype of the system is available.

3.2.1 Formative

As a technique for formative design, W3C-WAI guidelines may inform designer's efforts to shape and arrive at preliminary design concepts for the target system. These concepts may be prototyped, refined and extended in the course of iterations and given user feedback. For such a task to be effective, designers need to possess a detailed and in depth understanding of the guidelines and their relevance to the target application domain. The typical outcomes of using the guidelines as a formative design method are depicted in the various prototypes of the system (i.e., choice of components used in a Web document, attributes of the components, etc).

3.2.2 Summative

The guidelines may also be used to assess compliance of a high fidelity prototype or an existing system to principles embedded in the guidelines. In this case, the technique is used to facilitate summative evaluation of the system and can be conducted as an inspection-based inquiry or audit. The relevant literature reports several efforts providing details of how the technique may be used in this context. Moreover, there have been tools developed which can partially automate this task and generate reports depicting segments of a Web document which violate checkpoints of specific guidelines. These tools may also indicate the level of compliance asserted, namely Single-A, Double-A and Triple AAA compliance. As an example of these tools to assess a web site, we can consider Bobby (http://bobby.watchfire.com/ bobby/html/en/index.jsp).

Bobby was developed by CAST to enable authors to determine if their sites are accessible and now Watchfire Corporation, a provider of Website Management software and services, has acquired it. Bobby does this through automatic checks as well as manual checks. It also analyses Web pages for compatibility with various browsers. Bobby may be downloaded and executed locally, or alternatively it may be used through a Web interface on Watchfire's site. A downloadable version is written in Java and takes advantage of the accessibility support in Java.

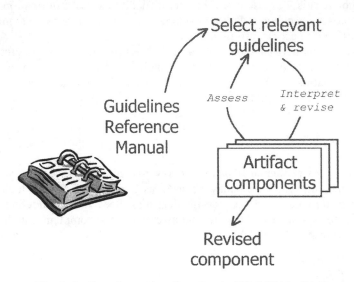

Fig. 1. Outline of procedure for using the W3C-WAI guidelines

4. Procedure for Using the Device / Technique

4.1 Process Outline

The general procedure for using the W3C-WAI guidelines, either for formative or summative design input is as follows (see Figure 1).

- Step 1: Select the level of accessibility suitable for the specific application, (A, AA, AAA).
- Step 2: Choose in the document the guidelines, relative to the web pages under analysis.
- Step 3: Verify (given a prototype or an existing system) all the checkpoints relative to the selected guidelines necessary for the selected priority level.

  Automatic applications (see previous section) exist and can be used for the validation, as Bobby (http://bobby.watchfire.com/bobby/html/en/index.jsp) but only as the first step of the procedure, and cannot entirely substitute human judgment.

4.2 Recommendations Regarding the Conduct of the Process and Problems That May Occur

Designers should be aware of some of the problems associated with all kinds of software ergonomics and human factors guidelines, including those published by

W3C-WAI. In this section, we provide a brief account of these problems in an effort to inform designers of potential shortcomings when adopting guidelines and in particular the W3C-WAI guidelines for design purposes, and to identify means of potential improvement.

First, W3C-WAI accessibility guidelines, in the majority of cases, are expressed as general recommendations independent from context. In other words, the guidelines do not take account of the specificities of a particular application domain, such as EPRs. This raises a compelling need for contextual interpretation of the relevant guidelines; this task is both interaction and collaboration intensive. Moreover, any interpretation effort is bound by the capability, experience and breadth of knowledge of the designer (or the specialist involved) regarding alternative access solutions, technical characteristics, etc.

Second, W3C-WAI accessibility guidelines are not experimentally validated. The currently available experimental work is generally considered as rather limited, and does not cover the broad range of alternative solutions. Moreover, due to radical changes that occur in the mainstream Information Technology industry, some of the past experimental results rapidly become invalid or out of context. This is further complicated by the general lack of comprehensive evaluation methodologies and experimentation frameworks that may be necessary particularly in the context of people with disabilities.

Third, they are difficult to communicate to developers. Recommendations derived from guidelines are not always comprehensible or easily appropriated by the development team. This is not only due to the typically demanding task of implementing these recommendations, but also due to the doubts that are frequently expressed regarding the validity of a particular recommendation in a given design case.

Fourth, guidelines are difficult to implement, as they require substantial programming-intensive efforts. As the industry lacks high-level tools for developing accessible user interfaces, the implementation task required to account for accessibility recommendations is complex. It typically requires substantial programming-intensive efforts, which in general, cannot be reused across design cases. As a result, the cost of developing and maintaining the interface is high, and it increases dramatically with the number of different target user groups.

Finally, accessibility guidelines make use of special vocabulary. The special vocabulary used by some of the available guideline manuals introduces an additional problem. This arises from the language used in these documents, which is not always comprehensible by the designers or the developers of user interfaces. As a consequence, additional training is usually required before the development team could effectively and efficiently use a guideline manual and implement the relevant recommendations.

5. Outcomes

The primary outcomes include:
- Identification of accessibility/usability problems
- Indication of corrective actions

Depending on the outcome of a W3C-WAI compliance audit, a web site may be registered as one of the following options:

- Single A conformance with a particular set of guidelines indicates that the site has met a minimum standard of accessibility by satisfying all applicable Priority 1 checkpoints.
- Double A conformance indicates satisfaction of all Priority 1 and Priority 2 checkpoints.
- Triple A conformance indicates satisfaction of all applicable checkpoints irrespective of priority level.

6. Underlying Assumptions

The technique assumes:
- Competence in the use and interpretation of the guidelines
- Availability of a tentative design mock-up or a prototype.

7. An Example from the IFC Electronic Patient Record

IS4ALL has validated the method in the context of one case study. The case study comes from IFC, the Clinic Physiology Institute of the Italian National Research Council in Pisa.

IFC have provided a scenario in a Health Telematics context, starting with a doctor visit at the home of the patient, her admission to the hospital and, after an operation, the discharge (see Chapter 5). The scenario includes many important elements about the realisation and the use of a clinical record. This scenario consists of 7 steps, namely, General practitioner visit, Cardiology ward admission, Surgery consultant, Massa Hospital, Anesthesiological and Surgical procedures, ICU (Intensive Care Unit) and Patient discharge and follow-up.

At every stage there is an updating of the information in the electronic clinical record. This information can be represented in different formats, such as text, image or table. These components, requiring different physical and sensory abilities, could introduce some accessibility problems for disabled people, who, for example, can't use a visual output and must use an audio or tactile output. The W3C WAI guidelines give explanations about the accessibility barriers and suggestions for the building of accessible web documents, without specific references to any application field.

In this Chapter, we discuss the application of the W3C-WAI Guidelines to the specific field of the clinical record. The Chapter is not a complete validation process of the IFC scenario web pages compared with W3C-WAI 1.0, but a discussion about the application of some guidelines in the EPR field.

7.1 Guidelines Application Procedure

This Chapter aims to discuss some examples of possible barriers. Since not all the possible information elements considered in the WCAG are present in clinical documents (EPR), only the guidelines relevant to the elements present in the scenario will be analysed. The general procedure is depicted in Figure 2.

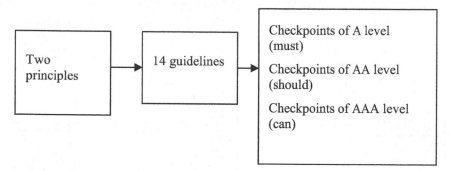

Fig. 2. Auditing procedure

During the realisation of a web document, the author can introduce several different components, such as different media, (i.e., text or image), but also different structures for the presentation (rendering) of the information (i.e., tables or lists). For any of these elements the author must be able to adapt his/her work to the accessibility guidelines listed by W3C-WAI.

In this work we have selected the components present in the IFC scenario, namely text, image and table. For every element we consider the guideline/s concerning this element with the relevant checkpoints and then we describe the application of this/these rules to clinical data. The WCAG have generic characteristics. So when these rules are applied to a specific application domain, such as medical records, some aspects can assume a special meaning. In some cases their application results easier than in the general case, while in other cases problems can become more severe.

It is very important to identify the components of the web document that can introduce barriers for disabled people. In the IFC scenario, the clinical records contain several types of information and several structures for the presentation. We can find, for example, text, images and tables. In the following, these elements will be considered and compared with WAI Guidelines. The steps to be followed include identification of the web presentation element, selection of the guideline/s and the checkpoint of reference, general application to the clinical record, and specific application to the clinical record.

7.2 The Element: TEXT

First of all, the text present in the clinical record is examined. In the IFC scenario, the surgeon report or the discharge letter can be considered (see Figure 3).

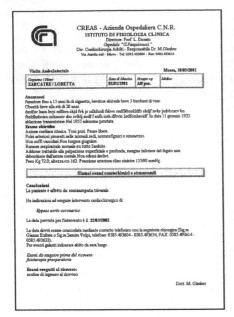 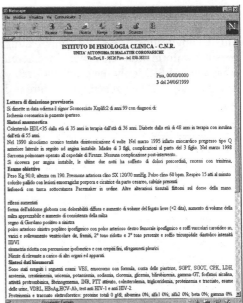

Fig. 3. Surgeon report and discharge letter

Both these web pages contain portions of text, for which WCAG designate several guidelines and associated checkpoints as illustrated below.

Guideline of reference n. 14: Ensure that documents are clear and simple
Checkpoints

14.1   Use the clearest and simplest language appropriate for a site's content. [Priority 1]

14.2   Supplement text with graphic or auditory presentations where they will facilitate comprehension of the page. [Priority 3]

14.3   Create a style of presentation that is consistent across pages. [Priority 3]

Guideline of reference n. 2: Don't rely on colour alone
Checkpoints

2.1   Ensure that all information conveyed with colour is also available without colour, for example from context or markup. [Priority 1]

2.2   Ensure that foreground and background colour combinations provide sufficient contrast when viewed by someone having colour deficits or when viewed on a black and white screen. [Priority 2 for images, Priority 3 for text].

7.2.1 A General Application to EPR

Assessment of compliance with the three assumptions related to the guideline no. 14, (at priority 1 and priority 2 level) is not automatic. Checkpoint 14.1 is critical, because in a clinical record it is necessary to introduce a particular language with specialised terms in order to describe the clinical situation. Checkpoint 14.2 is difficult to apply in a clinical record, because it is rather difficult to find graphical components to represent this type of information. The auditory component is not necessary because it can be obtained by means of an alternative device (e.g., screen reading software). For checkpoint 14.3, it is possible to create a style of presentation consistent across pages, (using the same structure to report different data). For example it is useful that important fields, such as the specific information of every web page, the navigation bar and the link to the navigations aids are always in the same position on the page. The user can read easily the clinical record, because, after an initial training, s/he always finds information in the same position. And it is also easy to evaluate the application of this checkpoint with an examination of different pages of the clinical record.

The application of the checkpoint 2.1 is of particular interest concerning the presentation of the numerical data. As shown later on, the colour red marks the values out of range. The checkpoint states that the web page's author cannot rely only on colour to distinguish the data in the right range from the data out of range. The adoption of a different colour can be only used as redundant information. The primary rendering method must be able to present the difference without the use of colour, for example with a textual comment. In the following sections we will illustrate practical examples of the application of the above. Finally, it should be noted that the application of the checkpoint 2.2 does not imply particular considerations for an EPR.

7.2.2 Practical Applications

The EPR language usually involves technical terms that can make it inaccessible for non-professionals and patients. Various techniques are available to reduce the accessibility problems introduced by incorrect use or complex language. An easy solution can be implemented with the introduction of a little glossary (in the form of a list of terms) to clarify some specific medical terms. By linking each complex term to an element of this list, it is possible to clarify the difficult terms (see Figure 4). Moreover, it is possible to consider alternative renderings of the glossary page. First of all, the glossary can be placed at the end of the referent page (see Figure 5). This option would not bring radical changes in the referent page, other than the introduction of the list of terms for clarifications, if needed. In other words, a patient not familiar with medical terms would obtain useful information by consulting the glossary, while a professional such as a physician who may read the document, need not be disturbed by the presence of the glossary. Thus, improved accessibility and quality is brought to all potential users without having to create alternative versions of the page, which would add complexity from a technical point of view.

Alternatively, it is possible to insert the glossary in an alternative page, linking every element of the referent page, which requires an explanation, to an element of the second page. This solution allows the author to maintain the first page without changes, but of course, introduces the need for authoring an additional page. Another solution is to provide an alternative page written in a different and more simplified language. In this case, the introduction of a link at the beginning of the first document would be necessary to direct a user to the alternative or simplified page. The result can also be very good, but the complexity of the document increases, because of the need to author two separate documents and establish a link between them.

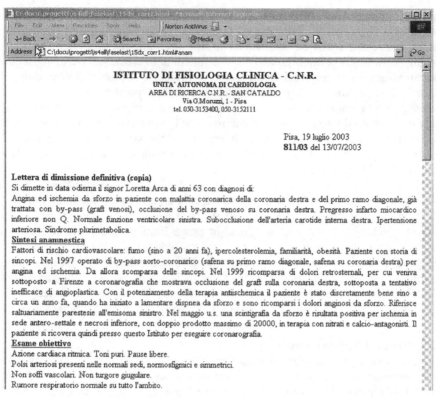

Fig. 4. Every difficult term is linked to an element of the glossary

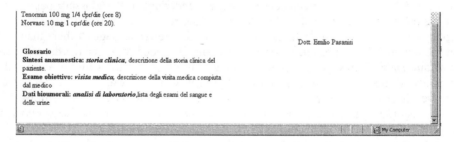

Fig. 5. At the end of the page a short glossary is inserted for the patient

7.3 The Element: IMAGE

Several examples of this component can be found in EPR. They come from radiological analysis.

Guideline of reference n. 1: Provide equivalent alternatives to auditory and visual content.

Checkpoints

1.1   Provide a text equivalent for every non-text element (e.g., via "alt", "longdesc", or in element content). [Priority 1]

1.2   Provide redundant text links for each active region of a server-side image map. [Priority 1]

1.3   <u>Until user agents</u> can automatically read aloud the text equivalent of a visual track, provide an auditory description of the important information of the visual track of a multimedia presentation. [Priority 1]

1.4   For any time-based multimedia presentation (e.g., a movie or animation), synchronise equivalent alternatives (e.g., captions or auditory descriptions of the visual track) with the presentation. [Priority 1]

1.5   <u>Until user agents</u> render text equivalents for client-side image map links, provide redundant text links for each active region of a client-side image map. [Priority 3]

7.3.1   A General Application to Clinical Record

In the clinical records, several images are present coming, for example, from the radiological analysis. Figure 6 contains an example of a frame of a coronography and an example of Web view of echocardiography results.

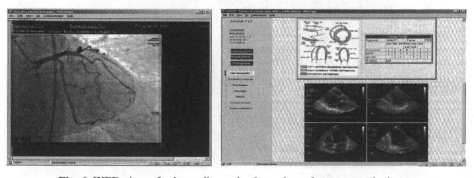

Fig. 6. WEB view of echocardiography & results and coronography image

The application of the checkpoint 2.2 implies that a text must be added to every image. This text can be, for example, the radiological report. But it can be also the description of the function of the image, for example "ECG results". It depends on the user of the EPR. These alternative renderings are not sufficient in all situations, for example for the surgeon, who needs the image. However, these texts can give useful information when a visual rendering is not possible, for example when a user is blind or when only an auditory output is available. Additionally, texts can provide an alternative rendering for results of many clinical examinations, usually realised as images in the web pages. However, these translations may appear quite difficult for the peculiarity of graphic information. Checkpoints from 1.2 to 1.5 are not relevant to our examples, because they refer to image maps or to multimedia presentations. Multimedia presentations are not present in the available clinical records.

7.3.2 Practical Applications

For this kind of information we can consider the results coming from the coronography. The first result of a coronography is a movie, from which the most significant frames are extracted (see Figure 7). Depending on the intended use, the movie, the images or the text can be considered. Generally, when an image is considered, the accessibility of the documents in electronic format requires an alternative, for example a text. In this case the report of each frame, which normally exists, can be used as "alternative text" (see Figure 8).

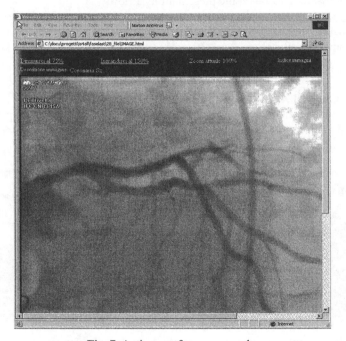

Fig. 7. An image of a coronography

The "alternative text" ("Coronaria Sx, 15.5 CRA, 21.4 LAO: Tronco Comune: presenta irregolarità, una stenosi subcritica minore del 50%. L'arteria discendente anteriore è normale per calibro e profilo. L'arteria circonflessa e' normale per calibro e profilo.") is not visible in the normal presentation. This text will be read in an audio presentation.

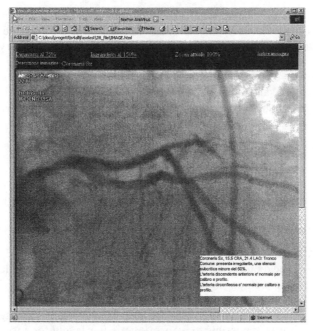

Fig. 8. The previous image with the alternative text

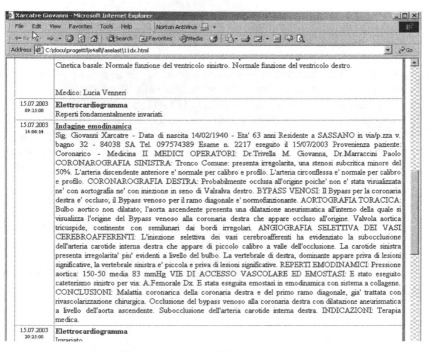

Fig. 9. The report of the coronography

It is not possible to completely substitute the images of the coronography with the report, but in certain circumstances it could be sufficient, for example for a General Practitioner who is interested in obtaining an overview or a summary of the result rather than a complete analysis.

We can also have a textual report for the entire coronography, for example in the list of instrumental examinations (see Figure 9) where it is possible to insert a link for the graphical presentation. On the other hand, the movie, if required, will be available for the surgeon.

7.4 The Element: TABLE

A common example of this element is the presentation of the blood examination results.

Guideline 5. Create tables that transform gracefully.

The list of WAI checkpoints establishes a difference between the two different uses of the tables within the web pages. We can use tables to structure data, and this is the most common use and interpretation of the tables. Nevertheless, there is another common use of the tables in the web: for the structuring of the page. Before the creation of CSS it was impossible to realise a particular layout for a web page without the aid of the tables, but at present the layout can be realised with this technique (Checkpoints 5.3, 5.4).

Checkpoints

5.1   For data tables, identify row and column headers. [Priority 1]
      For example, in HTML, use TD to identify data cells and TH to identify headers.

5.2   For data tables that have two or more logical levels of row or column headers, use markup to associate data cells and header cells. [Priority 1]
      For example, in HTML, use THEAD, TFOOT, and TBODY to group rows, COL and COLGROUP to group columns, and the "axis", "scope", and "headers" attributes, to describe more complex relationships among data.

5.3   Do not use tables for layout unless the table makes sense when linearised. Otherwise, if the table does not make sense, provide an alternative equivalent (which may be a linearised version). [Priority 2]

5.4   If a table is used for layout, do not use any structural markup for the purpose of visual formatting. [Priority 2]
      For example, in HTML do not use the TH element to cause the content of a (non-table header) cell to be displayed centred and in bold.

5.5   Provide summaries for tables. [Priority 3]
      For example, in HTML, use the "summary" attribute of the TABLE element.

5.6   Provide abbreviations for header labels. [Priority 3]
      For example, in HTML, use the "abbr" attribute on the TH element.

7.4.1 A General Application

The table (for an example see Figure 10) is an important element of a clinical record. This element is used for the presentation of results, such as blood examination. Every cell can have different meanings depending on the meaning of the corresponding row and column. In Figure 10 every cell contains the value of a blood parameter (row) at a particular time of the day (column). But many other different data presentations exist, depending on the value of the row and of the column.

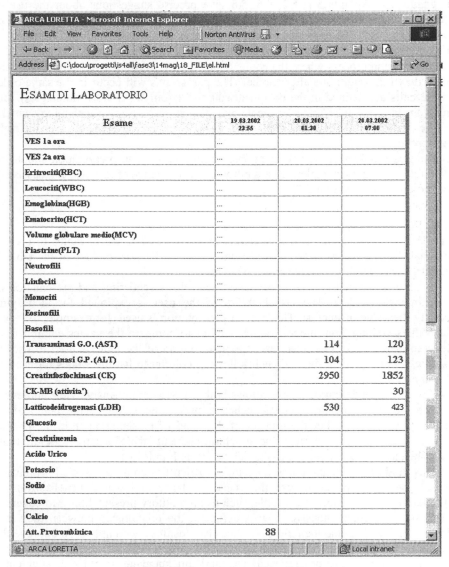

Fig. 10. Presentation with a table

The use of the table is difficult, because a table is essentially a visual presentation of the data and the interpretation of the content with a different rendering can introduce misunderstandings. When a user (i.e., the patient, for example) uses a non-visual device for the output (and this is necessary for some users), he must be sure about the position of the data, because an uncorrected position suggests an uncorrected interpretation of the data themselves. And this is a situation to avoid.

The WAI guideline suggests several tricks to override the problems concerning this special format through the use of particular elements and attributes of the mark-up language. Checkpoints 5.1, 5.2, 5.5, 5.6 give precise suggestions about the use of elements and attributes that can be interpreted by assistive technology devices. For example the use of the row and column headers is considered. With this information the user agent and the assistive technology are able to create a linearised version. "A table rendering process where the contents of the cells become a series of paragraphs (e.g., down the page) one after another. The paragraphs will occur in the same order as the cells are defined in the document source." (from W3C-WAI Guidelines). But there are several different user agents and devices for assistive technology on the market, making it difficult to be sure that every combination gives the user the right interpretation.

For this problem in crucial situations, an alternative data presentation should be available to ensure a complete accessibility to a larger range of terminals and assistive technologies (Checkpoint 5.3).

7.4.2 Practical Applications

The IFC scenario, as implemented today, makes extensive use of tables to present medical data on the web. Moreover, in the majority of cases the use of the table is such that accessibility requirements are not met.

A table is a visual type of presentation that allows rendering and presentation of two-dimensional data. The visual ability of the user is exploited for identifying exactly the value of interest. This type of presentation is used, for example, to report the values coming from blood examinations or to compare the values coming from different samples. In the latter case, the first column of the table is used to list the sample's name or identifier and each following column to list the values for each of the samples.

The visual rendering of a table allows both a first comprehensive view and every subsequent check of the correspondence between the value in the cell and its reference parameters. For the transfer of this kind of presentation from the printed format to the electronic format, the structural element "table" seems to be the most suitable and commonly used one (see, for example, Figure 10).

This kind of presentation presents a lot of difficulties both for disabled people and for all people who cannot use the visual modality and would benefit from an alternative manifestation of the table, such as an auditory presentation. Moreover, in cases where a comprehensive view is deficient, the relationship between the value under consideration and the reference values can result very complex. To improve the accessibility of information presented through tables, web designers have several options, such as using properties of the mark up language in order to augment a particular design or introducing alternatives styles as needed.

7.5 Making Use of Mark Up Language Properties

A first option is to make use of the properties offered by the use of mark up language. When the author gives a structure to the document using a mark up language, he can insert all the options required by the assistive technology and provided as mark up properties. As a result, elements such as column or row headers or the attribute "summary" and the element "caption" may be introduced.

The example depicted in Figure 11 illustrates the use of the "caption" element "Risultati analisi del sangue" and the "summary" attribute "Esami del sangue del 19.03.2002 ore 23:55, del 20.03.2002 ore 01:30, del 20.03.2003 ore 7.00." This second component is manifested only in a non- visual presentation. Moreover, the example implements all the necessary headers, according to Guideline n. 5 of the WCAG, which designates the steps to create tables that transform gracefully.

It is important to note that the introduction of these components does not completely change the presentation of the page in the standard version, but now the page contains structural information for correct implementation of alternative renderings, such as an audio presentation with the use of a screen reader.

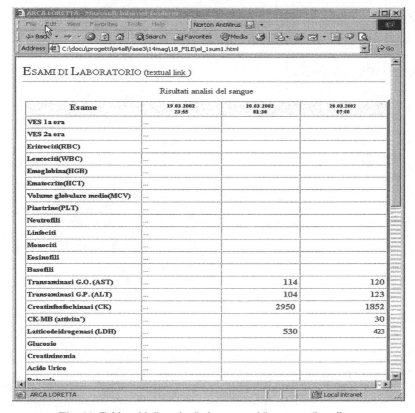

Fig. 11. Table with "caption" element and "summary" attribute

7.6 Introducing Alternative Styles: Articulating a List Element

An alternative to using mark up language properties to assure accessibility is the introduction of new (or alternatives styles). This option is frequently necessitated because of the limited capability of (some) assistive technologies and devices / software applications to correctly interpret all mark up language codes. Thus, even when all the needed accessibility options have been introduced in the document, accessibility may still be sub-optimal due to the limitations of the assistive technologies to interpret designated mark up language codes.

In such cases, different presentations of the information can be introduced, which turn out to be more useful for a non-visual rendering. For example, let us consider a list where elements of the list represent the name of an examination. If the date of the sample and the relevant value are added (see Figure 12), even with a sequential access, for example in audio format, the results will be clear.

This page can be reached starting from the previous page, with the selection of the link at the beginning of the page. At the end of the browsing, the user can go back to the previous page.

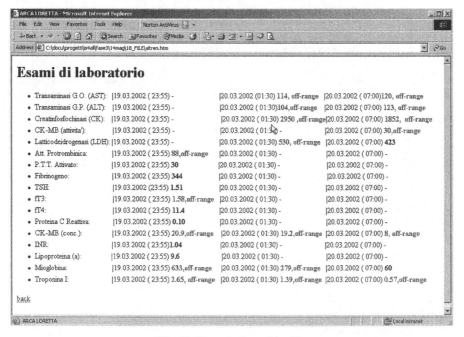

Fig. 12. Presentation with a list

This type of presentation also involves the problem of the different needs coming from users with different degrees of experience, in particular between a "beginner" and an "expert" user. For a "beginner", this kind of presentation is clear and does not create doubts. On the contrary, for an "expert" this presentation is boring and repetitive, especially when, after a lot of reading, the user will have learnt the mental pattern of the reference values.

It would be useful to implement a presentation with two different levels of navigation, so that the user can alternate the two different styles. Technically speaking, this can be implemented by means of the introduction of a kind of navigation via TAB key. It is possible to identify some elements within the document and mark them, and it is possible to jump from one to another, skipping all the information between them (see Figure 13). In our case it is possible, for example, to avoid the repetition of the examination date and list only to the values. The implementation of the list can also be made automatically, eliminating all exams that are not available on that date. This operation is important, because with a visual presentation the user can easily skip the rows without values, while with an audio presentation all rows would be read, with a very inefficient result.

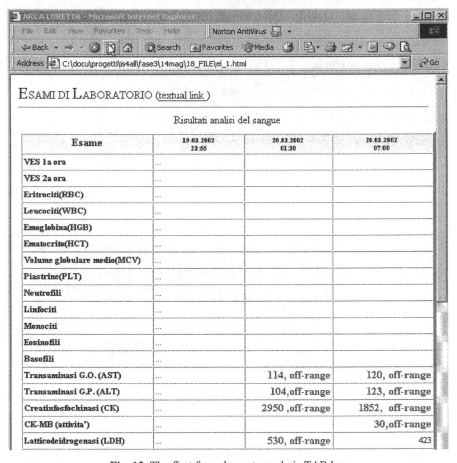

Fig. 13. The first four elements read via TAB key

7.7 Information Conveyed by Colour

In the same example of the table, there is another issue posing potential accessibility problems, namely the incorrect use of colour. It is not possible to distinguish by using colour alone the values within and outside a specific range. A possible solution to this problem is to associate every wrong value with expression like "off-range" or even a character like "*", with a footnote for its explanation. This solution (see Figure 14 and Figure 15 for examples) would be more appropriate even for an audio rendering and would satisfy the WCAG guideline n.2, which states, "Do not rely on colour alone to convey information".

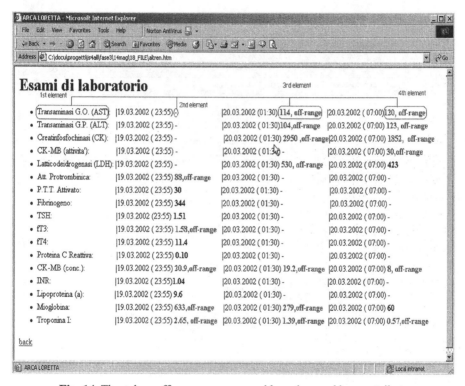

Fig. 14. The values off-range are conveyed by colour and by an attribute

8. Conclusions

This Chapter has reviewed the problem of accessibility of EPR, the WAI guidelines and some typical examples of Web accessibility problems found in an EPR application. We have then discussed potential solutions and improvements with the intention to remedy the accessibility problem and at the same time improve the quality of the application.

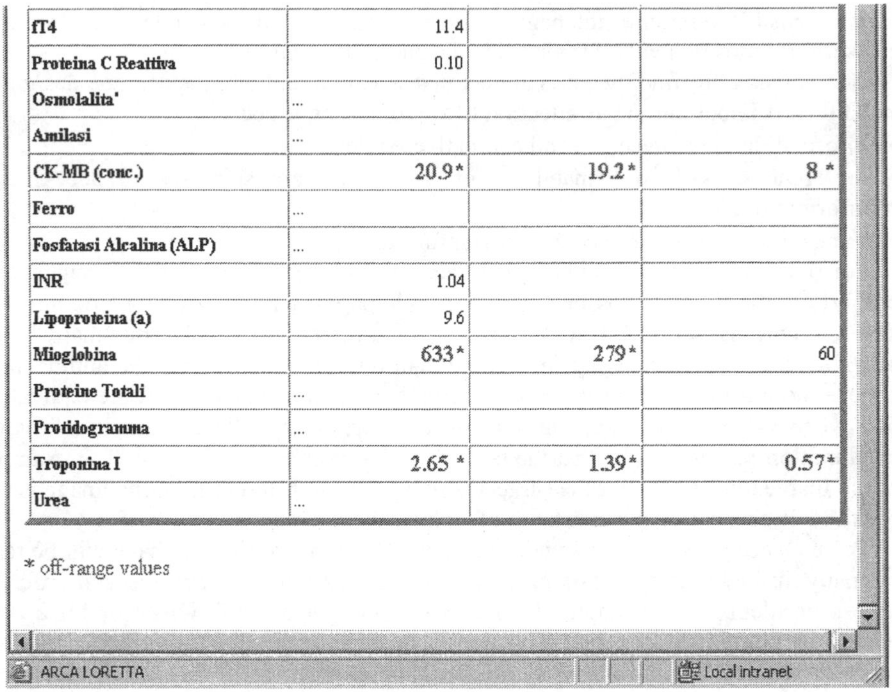

fT4	11.4		
Proteina C Reattiva	0.10		
Osmolalita'	...		
Amilasi	...		
CK-MB (conc.)	20.9*	19.2*	8 *
Ferro	...		
Fosfatasi Alcalina (ALP)	...		
INR	1.04		
Lipoproteina (a)	9.6		
Mioglobina	633*	279*	60
Proteine Totali	...		
Protidogramma	...		
Troponina I	2.65 *	1.39*	0.57*
Urea	...		

* off-range values

ARCA LORETTA   Local intranet

Fig. 15. Off-range values conveyed by colour and an "*" char to refer to the footnote

In our analysis we have considered the accessibility of the presentation and the interaction e.g., adding alternative text to an image or introducing a short text to information conveyed only with colour. This is the first aspect of the problem, and can be handled by the author mainly through technical solutions, which assume knowledge of the possibilities offered by the mark up languages. The author can add elements or attributes of the specific mark up language and create pages that have a different rendering on different terminal configurations. This approach illustrates that it is not always necessary to create several different pages, (such as "alternative version" or "text version") for each type of disability, but it is often sufficient to insert some particular language options, (for example rows headers or summary for the tables), as suggested by W3C-WCAG 1.0, to have different presentations. During this phase the author must also keep in mind that a particular piece of information can be manifested with different presentations. For example, blood examination results could be presented by means of a table, similar to the printed version, but also through a list, which is more appropriate for an auditory presentation. However, this first level, which relates to the presentation and interaction, is not sufficient to solve all accessibility problems, because one may also have to consider content accessibility as, for example, when the language of a discharge letter is complex or inappropriate for the patient. In this case, even though the information can be perceivable, it is not understandable by the patient. To address content accessibility problems, the author will typically need the help of the medical staff to introduce redundancy of information in the system, in such a way that every category of user can access a comprehensible version of the page. In such cases, a useful technique to explore is a glossary of terms typically introduced at the end of the page.

Generalising our findings, it is argued that when an author considers the design of an EPR, it is important to pay attention to the following aspects:

- Information to be presented and alternatives styles,
- Preferences, skills or capabilities of users who are supposed to access this information,
- Types of devices to be used to access information.

For the first aspect, the author must keep in mind that if the mark up language is properly utilised, it is possible to write web pages with different renderings on different terminal settings. However, it is also important to remember that many kinds of information could be assigned to more than one presentation and the author must choose the most suitable or introduce alternatives. Some presentations are equivalent for every category of user, but this is not always true. The example of blood examination results tells us that the table can be substituted with a list. The example of the image tells us that for the surgeon a presentation different from the image is not possible. In this phase, the assistance of a physician is essential.

For the second aspect, the author must keep in mind that the web page will be read by many different categories of users, who can have different disabilities and different access problems. For example, the access barriers for a blind person or for a deaf person are completely different. This remark does not mean that the author can ignore other differences among the users, such as the experience in the use of electronic systems or the level of medical knowledge, because these aspects can imply the need or the preference for different presentations. Every solution taking in account these elements has to be considered more comprehensive. Regarding the device used to present information, it is important to keep in mind that EPR data information is likely to be accessed through several different devices with distinct capabilities and characteristics for both input and output. For every target device, for example a PC, a notebook or a PDA, the author must take into account the constraints or capabilities of the device and provide a proper presentation.

At the end of this analysis phase, the author(s) can choose the desirable level of accessibility of the EPR system and a strategy for its implementation. The author(s) can also choose a solution that is not complete, for example, that is only effective for a PC presentation or for blind people, but he should know the limits of the implementation. Different technical solutions are always possible, for example with dynamic or static pages, with one or more versions of the same page and with different user identification systems. Finally, the choice also depends on the authoring tool features.

Acknowledgement

The authors would like to thank Mr Stefano Dalmiani (CNR-IFC, Pisa, Italy) for his assistance with regards to EPR data.

Chapter 16
Usability Inspection of the WardInHand Prototype

Panagiotis Karampelas[1], Demosthenes Akoumianakis[1]
and Constantine Stephanidis[1,2]

[1] Foundation for Research and Technology – Hellas (FORTH)
Institute of Computer Science
Heraklion, Crete, GR-70013, Greece
cs@ics.forth.gr
[2] University of Crete
Department of Computer Science, Greece

Abstract. This Chapter describes the process and outcomes of the evaluation of a user interface prototype running on a Personal Digital Assistant (PDA). The prototype was developed in the context of the IST-funded project WardInHand and implements a PDA version of a ward information system. The evaluation was based on a usage scenario comprising mock-ups and textual descriptions of the typical tasks of the system. Although the evaluation revealed a broad range of usability problems, in this Chapter we consider only those which feature prominently in the vast majority of PDA-based applications, such as adaptability, individualisation, user profiling, alternative dialogue styles, localisation, etc., and propose design solutions of general purpose, as a basis for improved design practice.

1. Introduction

Personal Digital Assistant (PDA) devices have become increasingly popular for a wide variety of tasks, ranging from simple tasks such as storing information (e.g., phone numbers or documents), maintaining to-do lists, to more advanced activities such as searching databases (e.g., Dunlop & Davidson, 2000) and web browsing (e.g., Buchanan and Jones, 2000; Buyukkokten et al., 2000). From these developments, it becomes evident that PDAs are not just about organising personal data, but, more importantly about access to information. Text editors and pocket-sized database programs can let the user take a wealth of information everywhere. More recently, there has been a strong push towards applications-oriented developments making use of PDAs. An example is in the3 domain of Health Telematics, where PDAs are used to carry out a broad range of professional activities, from accessing and ordering pharmaceuticals to data collection in clinical settings and workflow management.

This Chapter pertains to the usability of the user interfaces of mobile devices and in particular user interfaces running on palmtop information appliances, such as PDAs. Our normative perspective is to investigate the application of screening (based on popular HCI guidelines and heuristics) in situations where palmtop devices are

C. Stephanidis (Ed.): Universal Access Code of Practice in Health Telematics, LNCS 3041, pp. 197-208, 2005.

used to carry out domain-specific tasks, other than mere information handling. We approach this target by considering a reference scenario from the domain of Health Telematics and making use of well-known user interface principles to gain insight to the design of the user experience with such devices. It is claimed that PDAs have their origin in information centric devices such as desktop computers and as a result their interfaces are based on models such as the Graphical User Interface (GUI). Thus, principles of GUI design could be used to inform user interface design for PDAs.

Our reference scenario is based on WardInHand (Chapter 8, see also Virtuoso and Dodeerob, 2001). The WardInHand system aims to support the day-by-day activities of healthcare professional (i.e., doctors, nurses) within a hospital ward by providing a tool for workgroup collaboration and wireless access to the patient's clinical records. Such a system should respond accurately, reliably, effectively and efficiently under the challenging situation of a hospital ward, where the user should devote his attention to the patient and not on how the device is operated. The demands on mental workload should be minimal, while instant access and fast response times are required for robust system operation. Furthermore, special design constraints are imposed by specific properties of the target device. Limited screen resolution, absence of keyboard, pen-based manipulation of the widgets, point and click as primary interaction technique, are some of the design constraints that should be taken into account when designing user interfaces for PDAs.

The rest of the Chapter is structured as follows. The next section describes the evaluation procedure and the methods used. Then we present the results of the evaluation by means of discussing usability problems encountered and proposals for design improvements. The emphasis is not to exhaustively list all usability faults of the system, but rather to point out typical problems encountered with PDAs and corresponding design solutions of general applicability. Finally, the Chapter concludes with a list of general guidelines and recommendations for designing user interfaces for PDAs.

2. Usability Evaluation Method

For the purposes of evaluation, the WardInHand reference scenario comprised mock-ups and textual descriptions of the typical tasks and user experience with a high fidelity prototype of the system. The resulting scenario formed the basis for usability evaluation using a mix of heuristic techniques. In this section, we report the procedure, which was followed as well as the methods used to carry out the evaluation.

2.1 Procedure

The evaluation case study was realised on the premises of Human - Computer Interaction Laboratory of the Institute of Computer Science, Foundation for Research and Technology - Hellas, Crete, Greece. The evaluation procedure was initiated by a presentation of the prototype by the project coordinator of the WardInHand consortium. The presentation provided a thorough review of all functions and computer-mediated tasks supported by the device. Following this presentation, a tentative scenario was drafted and sent back to the WardInHand project coordinator for comments. Following iterative exchanges, aspects of the scenario were refined and a final version was compiled for future reference. Subsequent evaluation phases made use of this final version of the scenario. Finally, in terms of the procedures used, it should be noted that experts taking part in the evaluation had not been previously exposed to the prototype, while the only reference materials at their disposal were the final version of the scenario and a WardInHand conference paper outlining the aims and objectives of the system.

2.2 Instruments

The evaluation methodology used is screening system mock-ups based on three different methods, which are briefly described below.

2.2.1 Cognitive Walkthrough

A cognitive walkthrough involves the inspection of the effectiveness of the user interface by analysing how easily a user can learn to interact with the interface and comprehend the functionality of the interface. In our case, the materials inspected were paper screenshots as documented in the scenario. Two expert evaluators performed a thorough and detailed examination of how easily a user can learn to interact with the user interface, identifying at the same time potential problems of conception that the user may encounter. The profile of the target users, namely doctors and nurses, was analysed and useful conclusions were formulated regarding their potential attitude towards the system. It turned out that doctors and nurses usually exhibit high reluctance to divert from traditional techniques of completing tasks, low motivation to use sophisticated technology and devices, and low willingness to spend time learning to interact with new devices.

2.2.2 Feature Inspection

This technique involves the inspection of task related features of the user interface by examining the appropriateness of the user interface for completing a task, the availability of required functions, the ability of being self explanatory and other usability aspects. For example, a common task for doctors using the interface could be the reviewing of blood pressure measurements. Features of the specific task e.g., how easily the user can access the respective screen, or how much memory load is required to comprehend the visual output of the screen, were examined and tentative suggestions and comments were produced.

One usability expert who focused on specific features of the user interface carried out feature inspection. The most important features analysed were the alternative navigation dialogues, the interaction alternatives, the consistent presentation of the interface elements, the self-explanatory interface components, the accessibility of the user interface elements, and the adaptability of the user interface according to user requirements.

2.2.3 Heuristic Evaluation

Heuristic evaluation entails inspection of several characteristics of the user interface against a set of guidelines or general principles by examining the visibility of system status, the user control and freedom, the consistency of the system, the error prevention, and further usability aspects. In our case, three different usability experts examined individually the WardInHand user interface. The typical list of heuristics was used to generate the systematic comments on the usability aspects of the user interface. As a result, inadequate presentation of information, lack of user guidance, inconsistent design, difficulties in data manipulation were some of the problems encountered.

3. Results

In this section we summarise the results of the usability evaluation and develop design solutions that could eliminate some of the problems encountered. Many of the proposed solutions are general enough to be applicable to other design cases involving the use of PDAs to carry out domain-specific activities.

3.1 Navigation Concepts and Styles

Navigation in user interface design is one of the key issues for the success and acceptability of the entire system. Robust, self-explanatory navigation helps the user to understand the structure of the application, to access faster the requested task, and to use effectively and efficiently the application. Several guidelines have been developed concerning navigation in traditional GUI applications and websites. PDAs design constraints such as limited screen size, absence of keyboard etc, impose a very careful design of the navigation functions. A set of guidelines that the designer should bear in mind when designing the navigation style include: consistent presentation, use of alternative navigation tools (adaptability), retaining major option accessibility, self-explanatory navigation. Following the above guidelines, WardInHand navigation, which is depicted in Figure 1, could be revised as shown in Figure 2.

The revised implementation combines a toolbar and a status bar in the upper part of the screen containing all the necessary navigation aids, like the Home icon which will always return the user to the main application screen (current screen), the Next and Back icons which will guide user in the other screens of application and the logout icon which will help users to quit the system immediately after completing a set of tasks. In addition, useful information is displayed on the left part of the bar, such as the name of the user logged in and the name of the patient whose electronic record is currently active. These features allow the user to carry out additional tasks, such as changing either his profile by tapping on his name or switching over into another's patient record by just tapping on the patient name and selecting from the combo box the name of the other patient. It must be noted that only the available options are enabled in the bar, while the unavailable options are visible for consistency purposes but greyed and inactive.

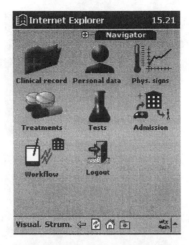

Fig. 1. The current prototype

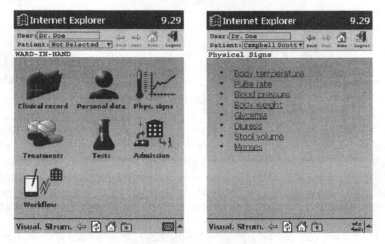

Fig. 2. Revised navigation

A parallel navigation method is also implemented for providing users with an alternative navigation style (see Figure 3). All navigation functions are available as nested menu options organised in logical groups. The unavailable options are inactive and greyed.

3.2 On-Screen Keyboard

The absence of a real keyboard enforces the implementation of a virtual one in the available space. The virtual keyboard currently implemented in the WardInHand application can be seen in Figure 4.

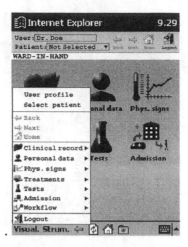

Fig. 3. Alternative navigation implementation by menu dialogue

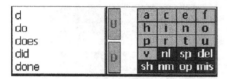
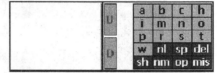

Fig. 4. Virtual Keyboard

If a first time user of the system came across this keyboard, it is more than likely that he/she would not be able to understand its operation. He would wonder where the rest of the characters are. Where are the numbers? What do these blue buttons stand for? What is the functionality of "U" and "D" button? Why are all these words starting with "d" presented in the text field where the user should type in his username? Why in the second screenshot has the keyboard changed? What is the criterion of displaying characters?

All these questions can be answered by the developers of the system, but there is no way for the user to understand any of those by just viewing the keyboard. On the contrary, the built-in virtual keyboard of the iPAQ implements the metaphor of a traditional 'qwerty' keyboard, which is familiar to the user. The built-in keyboard of the iPAQ is illustrated in Figure 5.

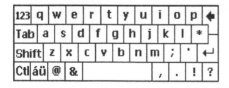
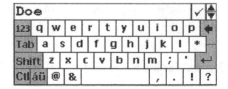

Fig. 5. Built in Virtual Keyboard   **Fig. 6.** A smart context sensitive keyboard

Using an application oriented virtual keyboard sometimes accomplishes the opposite of the expected results. Specifically, the user is familiar with the use of the built-in keyboard since he uses it for all the applications, therefore he could use it efficiently and effectively, while a new keyboard layout encountered for the first time could be confusing.

An alternative is to provide a virtual keyboard that is familiar to the user e.g., a 'qwerty'-like keyboard, enhanced with context-sensitive capabilities. For example, if the context of use of the keyboard is the login screen, then an enhanced keyboard could be presented, as shown in Figure 6. The functionality of this keyboard is easily understood. The user types the first letter of the username and the sensitive list presents the first username that starts with the character pressed. By tapping the tick (✓) the user inserts the selected word in the login name field. Using up (▲) and down (▼) buttons the user can view the previous and next words in the list. In the context of entering the name of a drug the list should display only the affiliated names of drugs. In free context of use where the user could type anything, the list would contain all the available words in the vocabulary. Figure 7 demonstrates how the context sensitive keyboard could behave in a complex data entry screen.

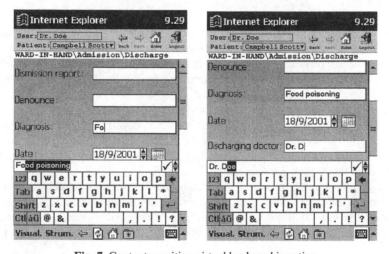

Fig. 7. Context sensitive virtual keyboard in action

In the picture on the left, the user (a doctor in the specific case) starts filling in the diagnosis text entry field using the context sensitive virtual keyboard. The keyboard binds its reference vocabulary to the set of diagnosis keywords. By tapping the 'f' character, the first entry related to diagnosis which starts with 'f' is displayed on the attached panel of the virtual keyboard. By tapping the second character 'o' the relative word is displayed, in this case is 'Food poisoning'. If this is the right diagnosis, the doctor has just to press the tick (✓) button in the attached panel of the keyboard in order to enter the diagnosis. From the example it becomes evident that the user completes the text entry task by tapping three times on the virtual keyboard, instead of tapping fourteen times, which is required to complete the phrase 'Food poisoning'. It is clear that context sensitivity greatly improves user performance and comfort, provided that the context-related vocabulary is sufficiently rich. Date and time field entries could be handled with another approach as presented in the following section.

The picture on the right introduces a more advanced feature for the implementation of the context sensitive virtual keyboard. When the keyboard is ready to accept input for the 'Discharging doctor' field, it automatically adds the title abbreviation 'Dr.', and then expects the doctor's name to be entered. The context associated with the entry field is the list of the doctor names, thus the user can select with minimal interaction the desired name. The field could also be automatically filled in by the doctor's name that is currently logged in. Additional intelligence could be incorporated in the context sensitive virtual keyboard, for instance when a field requires a person's name the first character could be capitalised automatically by the keyboard, without obliging the user to change to capital letters, tap the first letter, change to small letters and continue writing the name. Utilising such quick and easy procedures in the framework of a portable device can dramatically increase the usability of the device, even for the most unwilling users.

3.3 Data Entry

Due to constraints implied by the design of the PDA device, several considerations should be taken into account during the design phase of an application. The absence of keyboard (as a physical input device) forces the designers to attempt to reduce the necessity for data input. The main interaction method with the device is through point and click using the stylus. An alternative interaction method is by using the navigation buttons of the device which provide reduced functionality (four directions navigation). An approach to overcome these constraints entails a tolerable implementation of a virtual keyboard. Nevertheless it is not the cure for data entry. Hence the designers should design carefully the data entry dialogues, by reducing to the minimum the request for data entry.

Some general guidelines could help towards this direction, namely use of combo boxes with predefined values, use of numerical input fields with default values and provision of suitable functionality for the user to increase or decrease the value, use of a context sensitive virtual keyboard. Examples of these input methods are given in Figure 8.

3.4 Colour Coding

Colour coding is a favourite usability issue since the introduction of coloured monitors in the early phases of graphical interaction. For that reason many guidelines and conclusions have been formulated to regulate the use of colours in computer based applications. Some of the most important ones are: use colour sparingly, use colour consistently with user expectations, use colours that contrast well, don't use blue for text, don't use saturated colours, use colour redundantly, let users tailor colours. Standard conventions in real life such as red for stop, yellow for caution and green for go are also combinations that apply in computer applications.

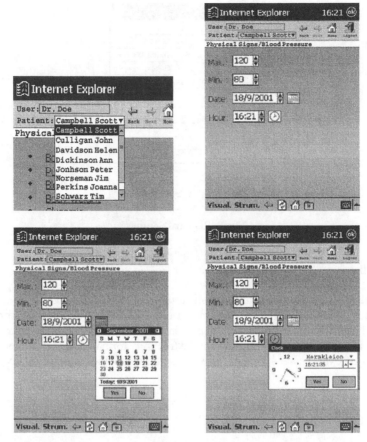

Fig. 8. Sample of input techniques for data entry

3.5 Date / Time Format

Use a global Date/time format usually from the default regional settings of the operating system as it is shown in Figure 9.

In date/time fields, indicate visually whether the user should enter only the date or the date and time. This will facilitate user's input and will save mistake-correcting time. It is also recommended that visual indication for the expected format of the date/time input is provided. For instance, if the user is supposed to enter the time in hour and minute format the design should provide a visual indication that the expected input is hours and minutes but not seconds. Date fields should also be filled automatically, for example, when a test is prescribed then the date of the test could be filled with the date of the next day, or of the current date if it is known that the implementation of this test is immediate. A pop up window with the calendar should also be available for selecting dates close to the current date.

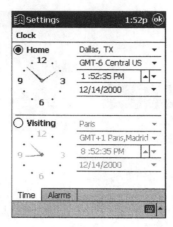

Fig. 9. Regional Settings

3.6 Localisation

If an application is multilingual, a priori design considerations should be taken into account for facing the difficulties that may be brought about by alternate formatting. The most important issues that the user interface designer should bear in mind include: use of regional settings for extracting format for date/time/currency, allocation of extra space allocated, use of standard graphics instead of text for task representation.

3.7 Help Functions

A help function is generally considered as necessary, especially for novice users. Help functionality like the one provided by the device could be offered as an option in the main menu, as it provided for the default applications (see Figure 10). The user consequently could use this help screen for acquiring information for the specific application functionality. Another important aspect of the specific help implementation is that it provides an overview of the application's functionality. When browsing the help screen the user can understand the task organisation of the system, since the help categorisation depicts the actual structure of the system, and helps exploring and learning its specific functions.

3.8 Use of Buttons

The general navigation method presented earlier should be adequate for interacting with the system. However advanced functionality requires additional manipulation, which could be accomplished by the use of buttons. The operating system implementation encourages the position of the confirmation button in the Title bar of the application. The same approach should be adopted for the dialogues that require only affirmative response. For generic situations, the use of buttons should follow the

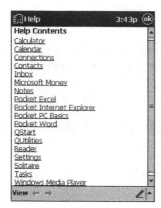 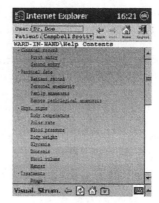

Fig. 10. System help vs. Application help

general guidelines for interactive windows graphical objects (widgets), namely: frequently used option should be available as buttons, size buttons should be relative to each other, buttons should be grouped into panes, buttons should be labelled carefully, industry/icon standards should be used for labels, greying out should be used to show button's unavailability, buttons should be placed in the centre of the screen or in the bottom right part of the screen for right-handed users.

4. Discussion and General Recommendations

User interface design, in general, is based not only on the aesthetics and visualisation of the information, but mainly on the logical flow of information and how the interface satisfies the task specifications and user expectations. Several constraints should be born in mind during the design, which are mainly affected by the physical characteristics of the PDA. A list of the most important guidelines that the user interface designer should have in mind when designing for a PDA could be summarised as follows:

- Keep user interaction minimal. Provided that a PDA is not a traditional computer, but just a personal digital assistant, the user would expect to complete the necessary tasks as fast as practically possible.
- Minimise data entry. The absence of a physical keyboard makes the data entry an awkward and time consuming task.
- Provide intelligent (context sensitive) data input where possible. Make extensive use of combo boxes where possible for entering text. For numerical values use default values and provide up and down sliders for correcting the exact value of an entry. Moreover, task-oriented vocabularies could help towards an increase in data entry completion times.
- Retain design consistency. Use the same look and feel throughout the application. Do not present and hide functionality in different screens. Use the same approach for completing a task in a uniform way.
- Provide self-explanatory navigation with alternatives. Make the navigation through the different screens as simple as possible. Provide visual clues to the user to direct

attention to the part of the application he/she is interacting with. Disable the unavailable options without hiding them.

- Use system format for date/time/currency fields. In order to avoid user's confusion, use consistently the system format from the regional settings information to present information about date, time and currency.
- Use standard graphics buttons instead of text buttons. For international applications, standard icons and graphics are recommended to avoid translation incompatibilities. The limited screen size can be a barrier to the appropriate translation of a text. By using a standard icon, there is no need for translating and localising the text of a button.
- Provide help functionality. Offer general hyperlink-based help to explain the functionality of the application.

Chapter 17
Multimodal Interfaces – A Generic Design Approach

Noëlle Carbonell

Université Henri Poincaré - Nancy 1
LORIA (CNRS, INRIA, Universités de Nancy)
Campus Scientifique, BP 239
Vandoeuvre-les-Nancy Cedex F-54506 France
Noelle.Carbonell@loria.fr

Abstract. Integrating new input-output modalities, such as speech, gaze, gestures, haptics, etc., in user interfaces is currently considered as a significant potential contribution to implementing the concept of Universal Access (UA) in the Information Society (see, for example, Oviatt, 2003). UA in this context means providing everybody, including disabled users, with easy human-computer interaction in any context of use, and especially in mobile contexts. However, the cost of developing an appropriate specific multimodal user interface for each interactive software is prohibitive. A generic design methodology, along with generic reusable components, are needed to master the complexity of the design and development of interfaces that allow flexible use of alternative modalities, in meaningful combinations, according to the constraints in the interaction environment or the user's motor and perceptual capabilities. We present a design approach meant to facilitate the development of generic multimodal user interfaces, based on best practice in software and user interface design and architecture.

1. Problem Being Addressed

At present, specific off the shelf components are available that can process and interpret data from a wide range of input devices reliably. However, these components are monomodal, in the sense that they are dedicated to a specific medium and modality. There is not yet, outside research laboratory prototypes, any software platform capable of interpreting multimodal input data.

Similarly, software on the market is available for the generation of monomodal output messages conveyed through various media, whereas the generation of multimodal presentations is not yet supported.

In the next section, we present a design approach that makes it possible to:

- Interpret users' multimodal commands or manipulations/actions using partial monomodal interpretations, each interpretation being elaborated by a dedicated component which processes the specific input data stream transmitted through one of the available media. This treatment may be viewed as a *fusion* process of events or data.

C. Stephanidis (Ed.): Universal Access Code of Practice in Health Telematics, LNCS 3041, pp. 209-223, 2005.
© Springer-Verlag Berlin Heidelberg 2005

- Match these global interpretations with appropriate functions in the current application software, or *translate* them into appropriate commands (i.e., execution calls of the appropriate functions in the kernel of the considered software).
- As regards system multimodal outputs, break up the information content of system messages into chunks, assign the resulting data chunks to appropriate modalities, and input each of them into the relevant monomodal generation/presentation component. This treatment is often viewed as a data *fission* process in contrast with multimodal input fusion.

In most current applications, stereotyped system messages only need to be implemented in order to achieve efficient interaction, so that simple techniques can be applied to generate appropriate multimodal system messages. Modality selection can be easily performed using available ergonomic criteria. As regards accessibility, the World Wide Web Consortium's (W3C) Web Access Initiative (WAI) has designed accessibility guidelines (http://www.w3.org/WAI/) which have been implemented in software tools such as Bobby[1]. Efficient generation software components also exist for many output modalities (except for haptics, a modality which still needs further research studies), namely, speech, sound, graphics and text.

The fusion of multimodal inputs and their global interpretation in terms of executable function calls are, on the other hand, much more complex, due mainly to the relative complexity of users' utterances and the limitations of current monomodal interpreters, especially concerning modalities such as speech, gestures and haptics.

The approach presented in the remainder of this Chapter is meant to help designers to overcome these difficulties in contexts of use where the semantics of the information exchanges between user and software amounts only to the expressive power of Direct Manipulation (Shneiderman, 1993).

As this Chapter is focused on software architecture issues, it does not include some of the sections that are present in the other Chapters, namely:

- The 'Procedures for using the device' section, since numerous software design methods exist, and most companies have evolved their own design and development methodology, practice and standards. In addition, software design issues have motivated the publication of numerous manuals and best practice case studies; see, for instance, (Bass et al., 1998) for design issues, and (Clements et al., 2001) for evaluation methods.
- 'Outcomes' or rather the advantages of the software architecture proposed for multimodal user interfaces are briefly discussed in the relevant section of this Chapter.
- The 'Assumptions' section is not relevant to this Chapter: as the proposed architecture framework aims at genericity, no restriction should be placed on its applicability.

---

[1] Bobby (http://bobby.watchfire.com/), a Watchfire Corporation product, is meant to help Web application designers to comply with these guidelines by exposing accessibility problems in Web pages and suggesting solutions to repair them.

2. Device / Technique(s) Used

After providing brief definitions of what we mean by "modality" and "multimodality", we shall present a generic overall software architecture for multimodal user interfaces. This generic architecture is based on a five-layer software model, each layer being designed according to component programming principles. Inter-component information exchanges implement the W3C SOAP message exchange paradigm[2]. It is meant to facilitate multimodal input and output processing. In particular, the interpretation of users' multimodal utterances simply consists of matching them with the appropriate functions in the considered specific application software, in order to achieve robust human-computer interaction while limiting development complexity and cost. As it is largely application-independent, generic interpreters and generators on the market can be used for processing monomodal inputs and outputs.

2.1 Definitions

Modality here refers to the use of a medium, or channel of communication, as a means to convey information (Maybury, 1993). In the context of remote information exchanges, the sender translates concepts (symbolic information) into physical events which are conveyed to the recipient through an appropriate channel or *medium*, and the recipient interprets the incoming signal in terms of abstract symbols.

More precisely, in the context of HCI, these processes involve the user's senses and motor skills and, symmetrically, the system input/output devices and software. According to the taxonomy presented in (Bernsen, 1994), several modalities may be supported by the same medium (e.g., text and graphics used as output modalities). In this context, '*media*' and '*modalities*' are often defined contrastingly; see (Coutaz and Caelen, 1991), (Maybury, 1993; 2001) and (Bernsen, 1994), among others. The first term is used for referring to the hardware and software channels through which information is conveyed, and the second one for designating the coupling of a medium with the interpretation processes required for transforming physical representations of information into meaningful symbols or messages.

To sum up:

'... by *media* we mean the carrier of information such as text, graphics, audio, or video. Broadly, we include any necessary physical interactive device (*e.g.*, keyboard, mouse, microphone, speaker, screen). In contrast, by *mode* or *modality* we refer to the human senses (more generally agent senses) employed to process incoming information, *e.g.*, vision, audition, and haptics.' (Maybury, 2001).

Multimodality refers to the simultaneous or alternate use of several modalities. According to the above definitions of medium and modality, multimodality is not synonymous with multimedia. For instance, outgoing multimodal messages are meaningful in addition to being multimedia (since they are conveyed via several media); the system uses a symbolic representation of their information content to

---

[2] See (W3C (b), 2003) for an overview of this message exchange framework.

process them. Such a representation is not required for manipulating multimedia documents.

Authors of the W3C document on multimodal interaction requirements[3] use *sequential* in place of "alternate" for designating modality switching.

They also refine the above classification by considering two subclasses of simultaneous usage of several modalities. They restrict the use of *simultaneous* to characterise multimodal messages whose monomodal components can be processed separately[4], while they use *composite* to characterise multimodal messages that have to be treated as single meaningful entities[5].

2.2 Overall Software Architecture

To our mind, a multimodal user interface will be considered as generic if:
1. Additional modalities (i.e., monomodal interpreters and/or generators) can easily be plugged in, and existing modalities unplugged;
2. It can be easily interfaced with the functional kernel of any standard application software.

To fulfil these requirements a multi-layer architecture is first needed. The five layer ARCH metamodel[6] appears as a better candidate than the three layer Seeheim architecture[7], due to its finer granularity, and hence, its greater flexibility.

A slightly modified version of the original ARCH model is represented in Figure 1. This new version is meant to answer the specific requirements for multimodal interactive software architecture. In particular, it takes into account the requirement in W3C (a), 2003, subsection 4.3, that advocates the "separation of data model, presentation layer and application logic".

We briefly describe the role of the five components in the following subsections.

2.2.1 Functional Core
This layer includes all functions in the application software that operate on objects in the application domain; it constitutes the kernel (somewhat like in Unix) of the application software.

---

[3] See (W3C (a), 2003).

[4] In other words, monomodal components of multimodal messages that convey unrelated chunks of information and can each be viewed as an autonomous message. For instance, the user may simultaneously dictate a letter using dedicated software that displays orthographic transcripts of her speech utterances in one window, and browse on the Web using direct manipulation in another window.

[5] For instance, see the multimodal (speech and pointing gestures) composite command in Bolt, 1980.

[6] See (UIMS Tool Developers Workshop, 1992), and, for an application of the slinky metamodel to object oriented design (Carrière, Kazman, 1997).

[7] cf. (Pfaff, Hagen, 1985).

2.2.2 Functional Core Adapter

The functional core adapter serves as an interface between the functional core and the dialogue controller. In particular, it is in charge of translating:

- abstract meaningful representations of the user's multimodal commands (coming from the dialogue controller) into appropriate executable requests to the functional core (see the descriptions of the multimodal and monomodal interpreters/generators below); and,
- results of the functional core activities into abstract representations intended for the dialogue controller.

These representations of the meaning of user inputs and system outputs are independent of the available input/output modalities[8]. In cases when the information to be conveyed cannot be appropriately expressed using the available modalities, the functional core adapter is in charge of generating information that captures the original data at the very best and can be expressed through the available modalities. For instance, if speech and haptics are the only output modalities available (e.g., the user interface is meant for blind users), this component will transform pictures into abstract representations appropriate for haptic and/or oral presentation, possibly using dedicated software for such transformations. The functional core adapter also sorts out conflicting interpretations of input (from several modalities) provided by the dialogue controller, using knowledge of the application functionalities and contextual information (on the current state of the interaction mainly). It may select one of them, and then notify the dialogue controller of its choice so that the latter can update the dialogue history appropriately and possibly inform the user accordingly. Or it may reject all of them, and then request the dialogue controller to initiate a clarification sub-dialogue with the user.

2.2.3 Dialogue Controller

The dialogue controller or manager is the key component in the interactive multi-thread system. It is responsible for task-level synchronisation and scheduling. In other words, it controls both the flow of commands and events from the user towards the functional core and, symmetrically, the flow of both results from the functional core and events from the application domain towards the user. It manipulates abstract representations of input and output information. For synchronising input, output and external events, it orders them relatively to each other from the time stamps attached to them, in accordance with the MMI-A17 requirement in W3C (a), 2003. For the management and control of the dialogue with the user (initiative of exchanges, clarification sub-dialogues, etc.), it may use information from the dialogue context (see the 'Context' subsection below). Typically, the dialogue between the user and the system may be user-driven or application-driven; mixed initiative may also be considered.

The dialogue controller uses the common abstract representation format for exchanging information with other components in the system, namely the functional core adapter and the multimodal interpreter-generator.

---

[8] In compliance with, and as a generalisation of, the recommendation in (W3C (a), 2003, section 2.6 'Semantics of input generated by UI components').

2.2.4 Mutimodal Interpreter and Generator

The multimodal interpreter performs the "fusion" of the partial interpretations produced by the various monomodal input components with a view to building valid commands, namely commands that the functional core will be able to carry out successfully. Fusion algorithms operate on time stamped monomodal inputs from the user. This component also orders the global interpretations of monomodal inputs (sequential multimodality) or of multimodal inputs (composite multimodality) according to the confidence scores computed by the monomodal interpreters. As for the multimodal generator, its main function is to split up the information content in a message generated by the functional core into chunks. These information chunks are processed by the appropriate monomodal generators which build the monomodal components of the multimodal presentation of the overall message. The assignment of information chunks to the available media follows general ergonomic and semantic criteria. The multimodal generator also defines the temporal and spatial layout/organisations of the message presentation to the user. Before passing the abstract representation of the information content of a message to the multimodal generator, the dialogue controller may modify and/or annotate it to take account of the current user profile and the current interaction context/environment (using the global context discussed further in the subsection 'Context'). In the case of sequential (alternate) multimodality, the fusion (or fission) processor is not activated. The abstract representation generated by the monomodal interpreter (or the dialogue controller) is simply forwarded to the dialogue controller (or the appropriate monomodal generator).

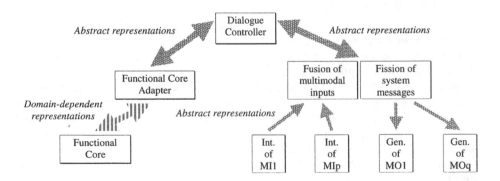

Fig. 1. The ARCH metamodel adapted for multimodal user interfaces.

– 'Fusion of...' and 'Fission of...': these components represent the multimodal interpreter and generator.
– 'Int.' and 'Gen.' designate interpreters and generators.
– 'MI1',..., 'MIp', 'MO1', ..., 'MOq' designate monomodal input/output data (p/q different modalities).

2.2.5 Monomodal Interpreters and Generators

These components include, for each modality, the software[9] necessary for:
- interpreting input events or signals from the user, and
- generating output from the information chunks delivered by the multimodal generator.

Any plug-in software on the market can be used as a monomodal component provided that it is encapsulated appropriately. In particular, interpreters should be capable of translating monomodal recognition results into "phrases" in the abstract representation language, while generators should have the necessary knowledge for translating abstract representations into appropriate internal specific representations.

Each generator should, in addition, include both a styling and a rendering module (according to W3C (c), 2003).

2.2.6 Communication Between Components

Information exchanges between components have been limited to pairs of components as shown in Figure 1, in order to simplify message management. They are implemented using message-passing techniques in order to facilitate the use/reuse of available components or plug-ins. Message content and structure are defined according to the XML SOAP framework proposed by the W3C (W3C (b), 2003), thus making distributed implementations of the proposed architecture over the Internet easier to develop.

SOAP provides a framework for the exchange of structured and typed application-specific information between peers in a decentralised distributed environment. It is a one-way message exchange protocol that can be used to create interaction patterns, for instance request-response. A SOAP message is an XML Infoset that includes a description of its information content. SOAP also provides the means to specify the actions to be taken by a SOAP node on reception of a message.

2.2.7 Context

For applications involving sophisticated interaction techniques such as dynamic adaptation or natural language interaction, it is possible to add a global context component to the architecture in Figure 1. This component, which is consulted and updated by the dialogue controller exclusively, may be viewed as a repository of dynamic knowledge on the overall context of the interaction between the user and the application. It may include a history of the interactions, the current user's profile, the current state of the application/display, the context of use (e.g., mobile device, PC), etc.

Some components may need specific contextual information. For instance, dynamic adaptation of speech recognition algorithms to the type and intensity of background noise results in a significant improvement of speech recognition accuracy.

The functional core adapter also needs a private context component in order to keep some trace of the semantics of the interaction between the user and the system. This history should at least include the last activated application function and the current state of the application. This information is needed, for instance, to process

---

[9] Especially monomodal device drivers and signal handlers (W3C (a), 2003).

conflicting interpretations and incomplete or non-existing commands (see subsection 'Functional core adapter' above).

It is possible to take such requirements into account by adding a specific context component to the architecture in Figure 1, and restricting access rights[10] (to the information stored in this repository) to the component that needs it.

However, as soon as a piece of contextual information may prove useful for several components it will be stored in the global context rather than in a private repository so as to retain the simple message management strategy that has been chosen by reason of its easy implementation within the ARCH architecture framework (see above the subsection 'Communication between components').

3. Outcomes

The proposed architecture is generic and can be applied to any application, provided that application-specific information is input into the components as initialisation parameters. This information should be specified in text form, using XML files with appropriate metadata and structures, in order to facilitate the implementation of components as plug-ins. Components will have to ensure its translation into proprietary internal formats, directly or through encapsulated software.

For any given application, this approach may be used to feed in specific static information to components in the user interface, for instance: input and output speech vocabularies to the speech processor, dialogue strategies (e.g., initiative of exchanges) to the dialogue controller, abstract representations of the possible commands in the application to the functional core adapter, etc.

4. Validation of the Approach: the Tele-Home Monitoring Scenario

To illustrate how the generic user interface architecture presented in the previous section can be tailored to meet the specific requirements and constraints of real applications in the area of TeleCare, a tentative overall functional architecture for the multimodal user interface to a tele-home monitoring application is described in this section.

This application, which is described in Chapter 9 of this volume, is meant to control a set of home monitoring devices connected to a distant medical centre. These devices are capable of transmitting measurement results to the medical centre, which stores them in the patients' EHR (Electronic Health Record). They have also some limited capability to interact with patients while they are carrying out measurement procedures.

As this case study implements the general design principles and recommendations underpinning the proposed generic architecture, it may contribute to validating them on top of the architecture.

---

[10] i.e., consultation and updating rights.

The scenario, as it is described in Chapter 9, offers only very limited opportunities for multimodal interaction, due to the limitations of the technology used for the home monitoring set-up. Before presenting a possible architecture for the multimodal user interface to this environment, we shall describe an extension of the scenario, which favours multimodal interaction.

4.1 Scenario Extension

As mentioned in the initial description of the scenario, "all industrial societies are aging" (Chapter 9). Then, patients suffering from ESRD (End Stage Renal Disease) may also suffer from the usual chronic pathologies associated with aging, most of these pathologies being liable to progressively reduce their mobility, nimbleness, visual and auditory acuity. Seniors are also often confronted with solitude.

Providing these patients with enhanced facilities for remote dialoguing with the medical staff (GPs and specialists) and flexible interaction with home monitoring devices is likely to improve their daily lives significantly.

One major step towards achieving this goal is the design and development of an adaptable multimodal user interface that provides patients at home with appropriate facilities for consulting the medical staff in charge of home care, accessing their EPHRs, and interacting with home monitoring devices.

The feasibility and availability of such a user interface clearly fall in with a short-term prospective outlook. The home monitoring equipment described in Chapter 9 needs only to be supplemented with a PC equipped with a small electronic remote control device.

This device might have the appearance (overall size and weight, size of screen, etc.) of present PDAs. However, the present functionalities of PDAs ought to be sensibly augmented through the addition of the following hardware components in order to enable easy and flexible multimodal interaction through current interaction modalities:

- a microphone and a loudspeaker for speech input and speech/sound output;
- a radio connection[11] with the PC; and,
- possibly, a keypad (with a restricted set of keys) or a set of control buttons.

Such a device would make it possible to develop a great variety of usable monomodal and multimodal user interfaces.

Patients would be able to interact with their telematic health care home environment using either one of the following input modalities or combinations of two or more of them:

- speech,
- direct manipulation (with a stylus or a keypad in place of the mouse),
- text entered using handwriting (with a stylus) or a multi-function keypad or a 12 key onscreen keyboard meant for PDAs (see Nesbat, 2003).

Regarding output modalities, the system responses could be conveyed to the user through speech synthesis, sound and the standard output modalities available on PDAs.

---

[11] supported, for instance, by a blue tooth type of device.

Accessibility requirements of patients suffering from a large variety of minor physical disabilities could be easily satisfied with such a device which would also meet the mobility requirements imposed by its usage at home in the course of everyday activities, thanks to its physical characteristics and its radio connexion to the PC, the home monitoring equipment[12] and the phone.

The technology does exist at present. Major remaining issues concern the deployment of this technology, in particular the design and development of a reliable multimodal interaction platform.

4.2 Multimodal User Interface Architecture

In this section, we propose and describe a possible functional architecture, which takes into account the specific application context and device set-up presented above. The augmented PDA remote control device is designated by the acronym APDA.

4.2.1 Tailoring the Generic Architecture Model to the Application Requirements
Several constraints on architecture choices can be inferred from the given application context.
1. A distributed architecture is clearly needed and should be considered.

   For instance, real time speech recognition requires storage and processing capabilities beyond those of the APDA; the speech input from the user should then be processed by the PC. Similarly, the PC rather than the APDA should take charge of the generation of the system natural language messages, as well as the text-to-speech and speech synthesis algorithms.

   For the same reason, The PC should also host the dialogue controller and its context. Consequently, it should also collect and process the output data yielded by the various monitoring devices with a view to defining the information content of the feedback to be delivered to the user and selecting the appropriate modalities for conveying this information according to the user's profile.

   These data include warnings and instructions on the operation of the monitoring devices (see the initial description of the scenario in Chapter 9) besides measurements which have to be transmitted to an ODBC database but also conveyed to the user in a form that he/she can understand easily considering his/her general and medical knowledge.

2. The information exchanges between the user and the application are standard in the sense that they can be expressed adequately using direct manipulation. The user needs only a simple command language to convey his/her requests for information. Implementing multimodal interaction in a context where it is a mere substitute for direct manipulation and does not enrich the scope or the throughput of information exchanges may seem superfluous.

---

[12] The description of the real scenario in Chapter 9 implies that such a connection is possible, since the monitoring devices are capable of sending their measurements to the "Home hub" which is a microcontroller communication link capable of transmitting data over conventional phone lines.

However, two major benefits (in comparison with direct manipulation) are to be expected from the integration of the modalities listed in the previous section into the user interface of the given application:
- greater accessibility, given the specific user community it is meant for (patients with various physical disabilities);
- easier and more efficient interaction, given the specific context of use (every day activities at home and home monitoring).

The first specific requirement implies the use of the SOAP framework for designing message exchanges between application components.

To meet the second specific requirement, the implementation of both *supplementary* and *complementary* multimodality is needed.

According to W3C (a), 2003:

"An application makes supplementary use of multimodality if it allows to carry every interaction (input or output) through to completion in each modality as if it was the only modality.",

whereas:

"an application makes complementary use of multimodality if interactions in one modality are used to complement interactions in another."

The architecture considered for the multimodal user interface of the given application is presented in the next subsection. It takes into account the specific constraints mentioned in the present subsection.

4.2.2 Multimodal User Interface Architecture – Application to the Tele-Home Monitoring Scenario
The overall architecture of the user interface is presented in Figure 2, and commented on in this subsection. Comments are focused on the specific features and components that have been added to adapt the generic architecture in Figure 1 to the home monitoring application context.

4.2.3 Global Context
For the given application, the global context component mainly includes the current user profile which the dialogue controller needs to be aware of in order to implement supplementary multimodality as a means for enhancing accessibility.

This profile may be established and updated by the user, possibly with the help of the system, or defined automatically by the system from the data in the patient's EPR[13] which the controller will obtain by sending a request to the application functional core via the functional core adapter.

In most cases, adaptivity is not needed. Adaptability will prove satisfactory for achieving accessibility, since the criteria for selecting an appropriate modality or combinations of modalities in this context amount to the physical perceptual and motor capabilities of the user, which are relatively stable in the course of time.

---

[13] Electronic Patient (Health) Record.

Adaptivity will prove useful for dynamically updating output modalities according to the user's current location and activity. However, identifying and tracing users' daily home activities accurately is still a research area (Yu and Balland, 2003; Oliver and Horvitz, 2003). Then, the implementation of adaptivity for the purpose of taking into account the user's mobility and activity is still to be viewed as prospective.

The global context may also include device profiles for specifying such features as media type, processing requirements, performances, location, etc. (W3C (c), 2003). This information may be of use to the dialogue controller both for selecting output modalities, and for advising users in their choices of input modalities while they define or update their user profiles, or in cases when the performances of the currently used modalities deteriorate due to external events or changes in the interaction environment.

4.2.4 Monomodal Interpreters and Generators

Some interpreters and generators may need specific contextual information which will be stored in a private context component.

For instance, in question/answer oral dialogues, participants tend to use the same words as their interlocutors, rather than synonyms. Therefore, a specific context component including a lexicon of the meaningful words employed by the user will sensibly improve the usability and effectiveness of natural language system messages. This context will be initialised and updated by the speech interpreter and consulted by the natural language generator.

Similarly, sophisticated speech recognisers that model background noise and use the resulting models to improve recognition accuracy need private context components (including captors) which will provide them with the necessary data.

Narrowing the interpretation scope by predicting the information content of the incoming written or spoken user message from available contextual information may improve the accuracy of handwriting and speech recognition.

Using the global context, the dialogue controller is capable of evolving such predictions which will be conveyed to the appropriate components via the multimodal interpreter.

4.2.5 Integration of Home Monitoring Devices as User Interface Components

The integration of home monitoring devices in the user interface is meant to enrich their interaction capabilities with the user while maintaining their already available ones.

According to the initial scenario, the user interface can easily capture measurement results since the monitoring devices are equipped with radio transmitters that are used to send these measurements to the medical centre.

It should also be easy to capture the information provided by built-in captors on the patient's behaviour during the measurement procedure as the initial description of the scenario specifies that "voice and light prompts support required behaviour" (see Chapter 9).

The user interface output modalities could then be used to inform patients of their daily results, explain them, compare them with those of the previous day, and with weekly or monthly averages. The dialogue controller could generate this information and tailor its content and presentation according to the user's profile. It would also be possible to assist users in the application of the various measurement procedures by providing them with timely instructions, reminders and explanations while they are carrying out these procedures.

To implement this prospective extension of the initial scenario, and integrate home monitoring devices in the patient's user interface, the most simple and effective approach is to consider them as specific monomodal input devices.

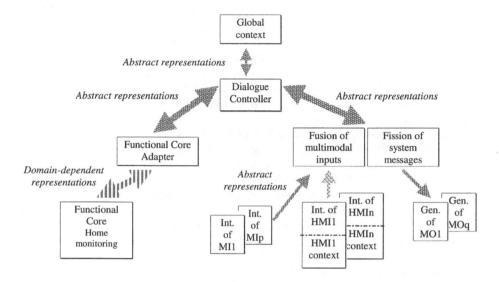

Fig. 2. Overall architecture of the multimodal user interface – Home monitoring application.

- 'Fusion of...' and 'Fission of...': these components represent the multimodal interpreter and generator.
- 'Int.' and 'Gen.' designate interpreters and generators.
- 'MI1',..., 'MIp', 'MO1', ..., 'MOq' designate monomodal input/output data (p/q different modalities).
- HMI1...HMIn designate data and events generated by the n home monitoring devices.

They may be viewed as specific input devices in the sense that the information they generate cannot be combined with information from other input modalities; hence, in Figure 2, the lighter arrow from the HMI boxes to the multimodal interpreter means that this component will just transmit the data coming from the HMI components to the dialogue controller without processing them.

The only processing to be carried out on the raw data generated by the monitoring devices is their translation into abstract representations "understandable" by the dialogue controller. This component will design from them suitable output messages (regarding both information content and presentation) which will be conveyed to the user through the user interface output channels; hence the absence of arrow between the multimodal generator and the set of HMIs in Figure 2.

This flow of input and output information will operate independently of the built-in interaction mechanisms of the monitoring devices. The user interface designer will ensure the necessary consistency between these two information sources and will take care that users are spared perceptual and cognitive overload.

4.2.6 EMMA, a Suitable Language for Expressing Abstract Representations?

As exemplified by this validation exercise, the implementation of sophisticated functionalities in a multimodal user interfaces implies annotating abstract representations of the user's input and the system output with meta-information, such as recognition scores, time stamps, etc. Such meta-information is necessary for translating user input into valid commands/requests to the application core, and system output into calls to appropriate presentation software tools.

EMMA, the Extensible MultiModal Annotation language under development in the W3C Multimodal Interaction Activity (W3C (d), 2003) may provide a satisfactory solution to this issue in the short term.

Although EMMA "is intended as a data format for the interface between input processors and interaction management systems" and may be considered "the markup language used to represent human input to a multimodal application", its usage may be (and, hopefully, will be) extended to annotate system output and information content of messages between system components, since its focus is on meta-information (W3C, (d), 2003).

By way of example, the annotation content for user inputs includes, in particular, the following meta data (grouped thematically):

- lack of input, uninterpretable input,
- identification of input source,
- time stamps, relative positioning of input events,
- human language of input, identification of input modality,
- reference to processing used (e.g., grammars),
- reference to signal, confidence scores of recognition (for signal recognition).

Authors of (W3C (c), 2003) consider wrongly EMMA as "a language for representing the semantics or meaning of data". In fact, the semantics of the data coded using EMMA is implicit; EMMA is simply an annotation code (or notation), but a useful one.

5. Conclusion

The Chapter proposes and describes a generic software architecture for multimodal user interfaces. This architecture represents an attempt to combine the benefits of layered software architectures that are simplicity and reliable development, with those of a component-based design approach, namely easy reuse of available components and plug-ins, incremental development and easy evolution of the application.

This generic architecture model is based on the ARCH metamodel. It also takes account of, and complies with, the emerging requirements, recommendations and standards of the W3C.

To illustrate the advantages of the proposed architecture, validate its appropriateness, and show how to put it into practice, it has been put into practice in the area of home TeleCare, and used to design the overall architecture of a multimodal user interface for patients in the framework of the scenario entitled 'Patients and EHRs: Tele home monitoring reference scenario' (see Chapter 9).

This validation exercise has demonstrated the flexibility of the proposed architecture and its potential to facilitate the implementation of novel concepts and the integration of available plug-ins.

Chapter 18
Role-Adapted Access to Medical Data:
Experiences with Model-Based Development

Christian Stary

University of Linz
Department of Business Information Systems
Communications Engineering
Freistaädterstraße 315
A - 4040 Linz, Austria
christian.stary@jku.at

Abstract. In this Chapter we revisit a task-driven and model-based development technique and show its support for role-specific health-care data processing. We provide a case study that aimed towards role-based adaptation for universal accessible software systems driven by business process definitions and a common set of data and functions for a diverse set of user groups. The tests of the model-based TADEUS framework, its method, and tool enabling adaptability in light of the acquired business processes were performed for an Upper Austrian hospital successfully. The application of the TADEUS technique reveals the benefits of role-based design of universally accessible software systems.

1. Introduction

From a user perspective, universal access to information technologies requires the adaptability of technical systems towards
- individual styles of interaction
- individual views on information
- individual ways to accomplish tasks (cf. Stephanidis, 2001a).

Individual styles of interaction refer to the way and means of human-computer interaction. Humans access and process information individually, at the content, presentation and navigation level, according to their background, preferences and experiences. In addition, humans approach technical systems in different functional roles, such as secretaries and sales persons, even when handling the same type of date, e.g., customer data. Consequently, adaptability has to comprise individual views on information. Finally, when different users perform the same set of tasks, they might accomplish them in different ways. Again, the technical system should provide means to allow different ways for task accomplishment leading to the same results.

A method or tool that should meet the addressed objectives has to enable the mapping of application-domain knowledge (in particular user procedures to accomplish work tasks) to role- and user-specific user interfaces. Unfortunately, the

C. Stephanidis (Ed.): Universal Access Code of Practice in Health Telematics, LNCS 3041, pp. 224-239, 2005.

vast majority of user interface design tools does not support this mapping, either due to the lack of generic specification languages, or due to missing concepts on how to relate task descriptions to presentation and navigation components throughout development (cf. Stary, 2000). The latter, however, is a pre-requisite to dynamically switch between alternate styles of interaction in case of targeting support for a variety of users.

In principle, model-based design techniques enable to keep all design issues apart in the course of development that are essential for adaptation. They accurately implement the idea of keeping particular perspectives on the design knowledge as long as required to develop design alternatives and or adaptable (i.e., flexible) solutions. They may also support prototyping through properly linking runtime environments to task and user specifications. The assumptions here are:

- Universal access might address the style of interaction, data and work processes – which requires keeping different perspectives on design knowledge. The perspectives have to capture all possible elements that might change.
- Designers need support to integrate different perspectives on development knowledge to come up with universally accessible user interfaces.
- Users need hands-on-experiences, i.e., working prototypes, in order to reflect and discuss design ideas with the developers, as well as to initiate adaptation procedures.

The health-care domain is a complex application domain. This is evident from this volume's Chapters devoted on Health Telematics scenarios. Besides a variety of functional roles to be supported in the context of medical record processing (medical doctors, wards etc.) a variety of ways exists to

- accomplish tasks involving medial records
- use interactive appliances
- view data involved.

In the following we present the TADEUS technique (Stary, 2000) and a TADEUS case study as it has been performed for a regional health care provider in Upper Austria. The Chapter concludes with a summary of results.

2. The TADEUS Technique

The technique has the capability to capture different ways of task accomplishment, different styles and devices of interaction, and to enable different views on data. It follows a model-driven approach which keeps perspectives on design knowledge separated and supports the model integration for prototyping. In Table 1, the specific parts of the techniques are summarised and explained briefly.

Table 1. Elements of the TADEUS Technique

Task model	A task model comprises either elements of tasks and/or procedures for accomplishing tasks, such as workflow specifications. In general, it captures the organisation of work tasks and the sequence of activities to be followed for successful work-task accomplishment.
User model	A user model comprises all role-relevant data and behaviour, in order to accomplish the tasks as specified in the task model.
Problem Domain Data model	A problem domain data model captures all structure and behaviour specifications of data required to accomplish the tasks as specified in the task model, according to the roles specified in the user model. The latter provide the role-specific privileges to access and manipulate data.
Interaction model	An interaction model provides a structural and behavioural specification of interaction styles, such as GUIs, as well as devices, such as Personal Digital Assistants (PDAs). Its behaviour specification is relevant to capture (different) navigation paths and patterns.
Prototyping	A prototyping engine executes the specifications (models), and thus, provides designers and users with a user interface prototype following the behaviour specified in the integrated task, user, data, and interaction model
Development Procedure	A development procedure is advised (and finally required for prototyping) to differentiate and integrate the various models.

A developer usually performs the following steps to create user interfaces and adaptation patterns:

Step 1:   Business Process Specification. The units of the organisation at hand, its functional roles, data, activities, and relationships are elicited and represented through a business-process model. Such a model might concern the procedure for operation scheduling in the health care domain.

Step 2:   Model Specification, Refinement, and Adaptation. Several TADEUS models are specified based on the business process specification: Task model, user model, interaction model, data model. The relationships between the models are detailed and checked for task completeness and consistency. As required by the User Interface for All concept, the procedures for task accomplishment are adapted to user needs, following the different perspectives on tasks as applied by users. In addition, the relationship of the task model to the user model has to be adapted to role perspectives, since a user role might require to assign particular sub processes or a set of processes to a workplace represented through that role. The data model has to be adapted to the task and the role perspectives. For instance, in the course of operation planning, a doctor and a ward have different views on the operation data. Finally, the interaction model is adapted to the presentation and navigation requirements stemming from the role-specific task procedures (-> navigation) and the task-specific data (-> presentation).

Step 3:   Prototyping. The TADEUS specification (i.e., the set of integrated models) is executed according to the flow of work specified in the task model. User interface prototypes are generated. Interactive task support is demonstrated in a role- and task-specific way. The style, devices or features of interaction can be adapted further to user needs initially at the specification level, and subsequently at the prototype level, since the prototype and the application model are linked permanently in TADEUS. The diagrams used for specification are supported by most of the object-oriented software development techniques, such as OSA (Embley et al., 1992) and UML (Fowler et al., 1997):

-    ORDs (Object-Relationship Diagrams) describing the structural relationships between classes or objects

-    OBDs (Object-Behaviour Diagrams) describing the behaviour (dynamics) of objects

-    OIDs (Object-Interaction Diagrams) describing the interaction between life cycles of objects (specified through OBDs).

These types of diagrams enriched with highly expressive design elements (for an elaborated description see Stary, 1998) allow for effective integration of context information with user interface specifications, as well as for transforming contextual knowledge to code. The diagrammatic (re)presentation has not only been chosen for the sake of communicating development ideas, user participation, and traceability of the design process, but also to enable prototyping.

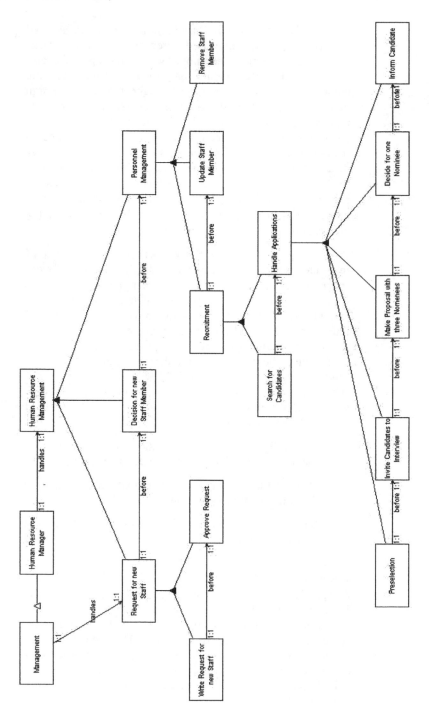

Fig. 1. A Sample Business Intelligence Model

2.1 (Task) Domain Modelling

Based on the business intelligence model, those tasks that are expected to be supported through interactive software are selected. These tasks are refined and related to each other, according to the sequence of accomplishment in an Object Relationship Diagram ORD. The tasks are represented as classes (containing identifiers and descriptions, but no methods and attributes) or objects. The structural and behaviour relationships are represented as links between the classes/objects. For instance, the global task human resource management might be decomposed like shown in Figure 1 (rectangles denote classes, inks relationships – triangles correspond to specialisation, black triangles to aggregation). In case the analysis leads to a representation of sufficient granularity, the task model can directly be extracted from the business intelligence model (as in the sample case). This specification is the starting point for further refinement and the assignment to interaction elements, leading to instances of application specifications, such as shown in Figure 2 for recruitment support. It has been generated using the TADEUS prototyping engine.

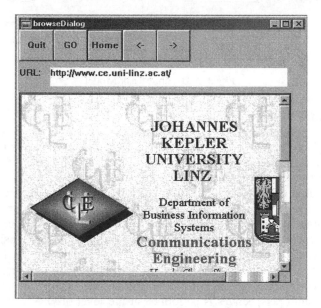

Fig. 2. A Sample Browser Window Prototype

2.1.1 Principal Decomposition of Tasks and Work Procedures

Since User Interfaces for All should allow to adapt to different work scenarios, at this level of design task elements might be added to task or subtasks, in case different human resource managers are assigned to the same task but follow different procedures (i.e., sub tasks related through the 'before' temporal relationship). Adaptability at the work task level is implemented through capturing all subtasks and their relationships that lead to identical results.

For each subtask at the end of an aggregation line of a global task, the procedure to be followed for task accomplishment, including the input/output-behaviour, has to be defined. As a consequence, the ORD of the static task model is related to a set of Object Behaviour Diagrams (OBDs), each corresponding to the accomplishment of a sub task. For instance, in Figure 3 the OBD for candidate search is displayed (the rounded rectangles denote states, the links transitions). The dummy "do nothing"-transition has to be used for the sake of consistency.

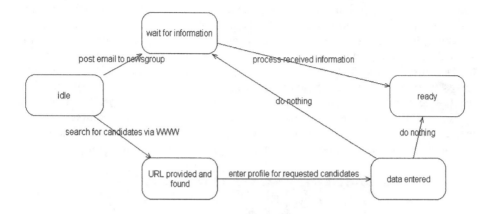

Fig. 3. A Dynamic Task Model

2.1.2 Individual Task Accomplishment

At this stage, again the adaptation to different work scenarios is addressed. Behaviour elements might be added, in case different human resource managers performing an identical subtask follow different action lines. Adaptability at the sub task level is implemented through capturing different state transitions in a task model OBD. Specifically, the static user model comprises user group definitions, as the organisation of tasks requires. There are two ways to define user groups from the perspective of an organisation, namely the functional and the individual perspective. For instance, each department of the organisation in question has a particular set of privileges, such as the right to modify personnel data (functional perspective). Each staff member also has a user profile based on individual skills and preferences, such as using a Web-interface and use of button bars instead of menus. In TADEUS the integration of both perspectives is performed at the level of ORDs. It propagates to the relevant data (in the problem domain data model) and dialog elements (in the interaction model), and finally, to the application model.

Coupling the user context with the task context requires the use of 'handles'-relationships. Since TADEUS displays specifications in a single workspace according to the model-related view concept, the relationships can be set in an effective and efficient way. The dynamic user model captures the work and interaction process from the perspective of a particular role. For instance, a user might be involved in several tasks, such as working as an accountant and controller. Hence, from the task perspective, the dynamic user model is a synchronised combination of task model OBDs under the umbrella of a particular user role. The specification has to show the task-relevant, synchronised involvement of a particular end user group in one or more subtasks. In TADEUS this step does not require additional OBDs, but might require synchronisation of existing OBDs. Setting synchronisation relationships is supported through OIDs. Using them, mutually dependent transitions of the involved OBDs are simply connected by dragging visual relationships denoting the passing of flow control – see, for instance, Figure 5.

2.1.3 Individual Role Interpretation

Besides the assignment of tasks to different functional roles (in this case a particular task, e.g., recruitment, is assigned to a particular role, e.g., human resource manager), as required for task accomplishment, individual work procedures can be designed. Behaviour elements might vary from role instantiation to role instantiation. Similar to the previous stage, different human resource managers performing an identical sub task may follow different action lines, this time, however, within the limits of their role which might only concern subtasks. Adaptability at that level is implemented through different state transitions in a user model OBD. The designer has to define the classes of data required for task accomplishment. Identifiers, attributes, operations and relationships have to be provided. Setting up a data model is also required, in order to provide information for the integration of the data-related functionality with the interaction facilities later on (such as assigning input fields to data that are expected to be entered by the user).

In order to ensure the integrity and completeness with respect to the tasks that are going to be supported, the elements of the static data model have to be put into the context of the task elements of the static task model (ORD). This step is achieved through setting the 'is based on' relationship between (sub) tasks and data specifications. For instance, the task 'search for person' 'is based on' 'person'. Additionally, the relationships to the user model have to be completed. It has to be checked whether the access permits given through the role specification in the user model fit the specified data model elements, and vice versa, whether each of the data classes has been actually assigned to at least one functional role specified in the user model. The behaviour of the problem domain data has to be specified. For instance, the life cycle of 'person' has to be defined, according to the attributes and methods specified in the class 'person'. In case of multiple involvement of a data element in several tasks, such as 'person' in handling human resources, the dynamic specification integrates different behaviour specifications in a single representation capturing all possible states of that data element. Finally, the life cycle has to be synchronised with one or more OBDs of the dynamic task model, since each of the transitions concerning data has to be performed in conformity to at least the tasks specified in the task model. The results of this synchronisation procedure are again OIDs.

2.1.4 Specific Views on Problem Domain Data

The adaptation to different user roles and instances (see previous stage) is propagated to the data required for task accomplishment. According to task- and role-specific requirements the data elements might be assigned in a variety of ways. For instance, a human resource manager might have dedicated work tasks privileges, such as the interactive manipulation of the salary of personnel data records, whereas a workflow controller is allowed to assign work tasks to staff members. Adaptability at the problem domain level is implemented through capturing different data elements in a data model ORD.

Assigning Interactions

The first step in interaction modelling concerns the set up of generic interaction features. In case of platform-specific solutions (e.g., for GUIs) the structure of the elements and styles has to be loaded from resource scripts or similar repositories. In assigning tasks and user actions to presentation elements, a platform-dependent design might, in particular for GUI development, save time and effort for specification.

The second step in interaction modelling concerns the static refinement and adjustment of generic interaction features, such as window management. In particular, platform-specific structures have to be adjusted to particular constellations of the elements and styles, since they provide a variety of arrangements (e.g., through recursive structures, such as container objects). Before the tasks and the problem domain data are assigned to the selection and grouping of the interaction elements and styles, in this step traditionally the fundamental look and feel of the interactive application (for GUIs) is specified.

The third step in interaction modelling can be considered to be the first move towards application-specific design. The selected and pre-arranged interaction elements are further refined and tuned with other application elements, in order to achieve fully customised interaction features. Platform-specific elements and styles are adjusted to particular constellations of task-, user-, and data-specific controls and screen structures. This step leads to object definitions at an abstract level, since these design elements are in a sense unique for the application. For instance, it is specified at this stage of development that the 'human resource management' menu contains the entries 'search', 'modify', 'remove'. The result is a structural specification (i.e., ORD) of the user-interface features that have been specified in the context of the task, user, and data model. The relationships used for assigning interaction elements to task and data elements are TADEUS-specific ones, such as 'is attached to', as well as commonly used ones for object-oriented specification, such as 'has part' and 'is a'. Typically, application elements are added as subclasses to dialog classes, such as group boxes in case of GUI platforms (see Figure 4 for Microsoft MFC).

For each of the elements of the customised interaction ORD, an OBD has to be created to specify the task- and user- conformant interaction. For instance, the life cycle of a form has to be defined, according to the attributes and methods specified in the class 'form'. The life cycle has to be synchronised with one or more OBDs of the other models, since each of the transitions concerning interaction elements has to be performed in conformity to the tasks, user roles, and data specified. The results of this synchronisation process are again OIDs. This way it becomes evident, which of the interaction elements have to be manipulated to accomplish each of the tasks (including the manipulation of data). For instance, by the time personnel data have to be inserted, the OBD for name field has to be synchronised with an input field – see Figure 5 (JF = Jump Forward, JB = Jump Backward).

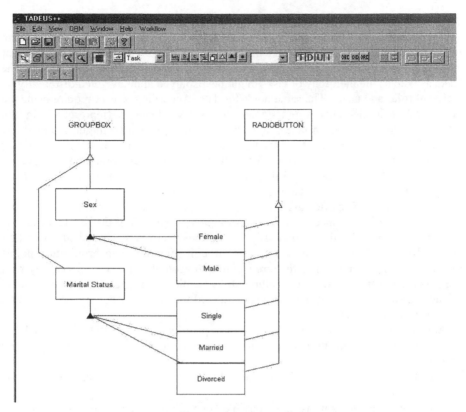

Fig. 4. Refining Generic Interaction Elements in the Structural Interaction Model

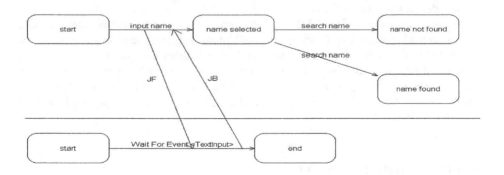

Fig. 5. Relating OBDs for Task-Conform Interaction

2.1.5 Individual Presentation, Navigation, and Manipulation

The adaptation to different interaction styles, and consequently to different presentation media, navigation and manipulation tools is addressed at the level of assigning elements of the interaction model to both the task and the user model. The tasks as well as the hierarchy of tasks might be displayed and navigated differently by different roles and users. The same holds for data. According to user requirements the tasks and data elements are assigned to display elements (represented in the interaction model). For instance, a human resource manager might interactively manipulate salary data in a browser window, whereas a workflow controller views data of staff members in a form. Adaptability at the interaction domain level is implemented through capturing different interaction styles in the interaction ORD and assigning them to elements from the task, user, or data model.

Completing the Specification for Prototyping and Online Adaptation. Contextual, in the sense of role-specific and task-complete application design requires the synchronisation of the previously specified activities involved in task accomplishment. This requirement is met through providing synchronisation points between states and transitions that are required to accomplish tasks successfully with the specified user interface architecture. OIDs enable the diagrammatic specification of the global behaviour of the application according to the business processes to be supported at various levels.

Additional (global) conditions can also be specified through OIDs linking OBDs. In setting up an application model this way, several issues are considered to be crucial:

- Which key events, eventually triggered by users, lead to interactions with the software system?
- All interaction-relevant tasks, actions (i.e., operations on data elements), and data have to be linked to or be a part of the interaction model, since they have to be presented to end-users.
- Every possible interrelationship between interaction elements should be traceable, in order to avoid side effects in behaviour.

Prototyping is enabled in TADEUS based on the application model, and thus, can be performed before the functional specification (of methods) is provided. The TADEUS tool set provides an interpreter and a consistency checker, both required for contextual design and role-specific adaptation. Based on the integrated specification available through the application model, an interaction window, as shown in Figure 2 for the Search for Candidates example, can be directly generated using the TADEUS user interface generator.

3. The Validation Exercise

Role-adapted interaction in the context of universal accessible software systems means that the functionality of a system can be adapted to the roles users have to play when accomplishing work tasks. Consider, for instance, the admission of a patient to an operation. The functional role a user plays in that case is the one of the admission clerk, checking whether all formal requirements are met to schedule the patient for an operation. Role-adaptation follows business processes rather than functions for the manipulation of data, such as insert patient data. It requires a concept to represent the context of operations like insert patient data. As previously discussed, model-based approaches like TADEUS are candidates to meet this requirement. In the following we report on a test case using TADEUS.

The business processes from that case stem from a regional health care provider. They can be decomposed into distinct classes, which comprise the medical, care-taking, and logistic activities with respect to patients (records): Admission, anamnesis, diagnosis, therapy, discharge. Business processes have to be understood as a set of logically arranged tasks that are executed to achieve a defined set of results. A process is characterised by the following properties:

- There exist internal or external customers for whom the set of results has to be achieved.
- A process involves more than one organisational unit – it is a cross-border activity.
- Each process results in the information or physical objects
- A process might involve activities at the management as well as at the operational level.

Of particular interest for the development of universal accessible software systems are those cases where patient data are accessed or manipulated by different users or different functional roles of users. Hence, we look at those processes that involve several different roles, such as the ward and medical experts. The subsequent reference model served as initial framework (Figure 6).

Admission   Anamnesis   Diagnosis   Therapy   Discharge

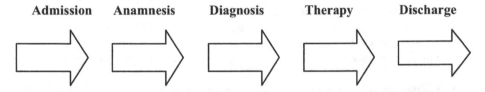

Fig. 6. Fundamental Health-Care Processes

A set of processes have been modelled, involving patient data access and manipulation through different roles: (i) External events and activities (extramural area) for Orthopedia and Coxathrose; (ii) Hospital management for Orthopedia, Coxathrose, Admission, Diagnosis. The processes have been modelled in ARIS©, a business process (re-) engineering language and tool.

Role-based adaptation requires the representation of work context in a variety of models. Based on the process definitions of the case, the TADEUS models could be specified: The task model denotes the workflow specification in terms of ordering the activities to accomplish a medical task successfully. The order the (sub)tasks are listed corresponds to the logical sequence they have to be performed – see the subsequent sample state transition diagram for the treatment of a case (Figure 7).

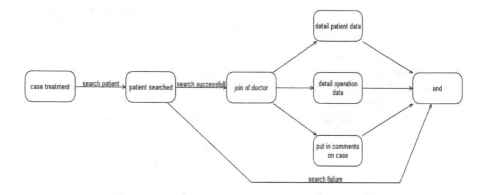

Fig. 7. A Task-Model ORD: Treatment of a Case

The input has been transferred to TADEUS-model specifications (like the behaviour diagram shown in Figure 7). Then, in order to receive role-relevant feedback, several scenarios have been specified with respect to patient-data management:

- The *administration assistant* (located in the application centre) is responsible for acquiring and typying in the personal data of a patient.
- The *operation ward* is responsible for the assignment of operation data (location, time, date, doctor) to the patient data.
- The *doctor* has access to patient data at any time and might access several layers of detail, and add text to personal patient data.

The display of patient data has to be designed in a way specific to each functional role:

- The administration assistant is likely to use one or more forms to be filled in with patient details. A *detailed view of the patient's data* is required.
- The operation ward needs *major patient data* to allocate one or more operation data in the course of scheduling operations, however, not using the entire set of personal data (in contrast to the administration assistant).
- The doctor needs some navigation support when tracing the patient even within a stay at the hospital. In contrast to the others, this role might be supported properly through a browser-like scenario, each perspective (*personal data, operation data, notes*) assigned to a dedicated display area.

Although each role requires access to patient data, the navigation tasks and manipulation capabilities differ significantly. Therefore, for each of the roles a scenario has been designed. Each scenario is in line with the recent developments in Health Telematics. The major application areas of patient-data management have been addressed through the scenarios: (i) Admission, discharge and transfer of patients; (ii) Appointments and scheduling of events (such as operations); (iii) Inclusion of routine clinical notes, e.g., before transferring a patient. Scenario 1 (admission assistant at the application centre) focuses on the admission of patients. Scenario 2 (operation assistant the diagnostic centre) handles the scheduling of operations for a patient. Scenario 3 (doctor at the diagnostic centre) tackles the insertion of clinical notes to a patient record.

Scenario 1: The *administration assistant* files patient data in the information system. The procedure is as follows: Search for patient - In case patient data are already available, the patient data are displayed and can be edited; in case patient data are not available an empty form is displayed and data can be typed in.

Scenario 2: The *operation ward* has to finalise an operation for a certain patient. The procedure is as follows: Search for patient - In case patient data are available the patient data are displayed and operation details (location, time, date, doctor) can be added; in case patient data are not available, an error message, e.g., 'No patient data are available', is displayed and the search might be active again before the ward is able to enter operation details.

Scenario 3: A *doctor* wants to retrieve patient data and eventually add some information about the case. A browser-like navigation allows the display of operation and personal data. In addition, comments on the case might be added.

After scenario definition the TADEUS tool has been used to generate executable user interfaces from application models, and to enable role-adapted interaction. The working user-interface prototypes allow hand-on-experience of interactive work procedures and are exemplified subsequently. For the sake of intelligibility of the control flow, specific interaction elements for user-feedback sessions, so-called handles, as the one shown in Figure 8 when searching for patient data, have been developed.

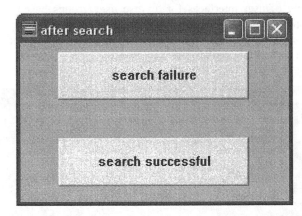

Fig. 8. Navigation Handle for Case-Sensitive Prototyping – Search for Patient Data

The sample TADEUS-prototype shot in Figure 9 displays the selection dialog for the doctor when entering the work process. He/She might edit patient personal data, operation data or want to provide case-sensitive data. This selection handle concerns the (sub)tasks a doctor might perform.

When entering the dialog *comments on case,* TADEUS displays the form for a selected patient as shown in Figure 10, and the doctor might directly enter comments on the selected patient.

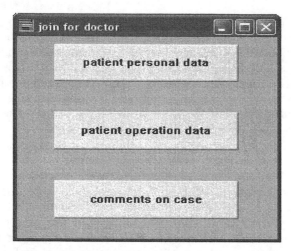

Fig. 9. Selection Handle for Role-Specific Subtasks

Using the handles to navigate through task hierarchies as well as the interactive elements for the presentation and manipulation of data, users in dedicated functional roles can directly experience the look-and-feel for that role. Developers are able to develop a variety of user interfaces for diverse user groups based on a set of core functions and application data dynamically. Through changing the specifications, the user interface can be adapted to other roles or even to individual differences accomplishing a certain task in that role.

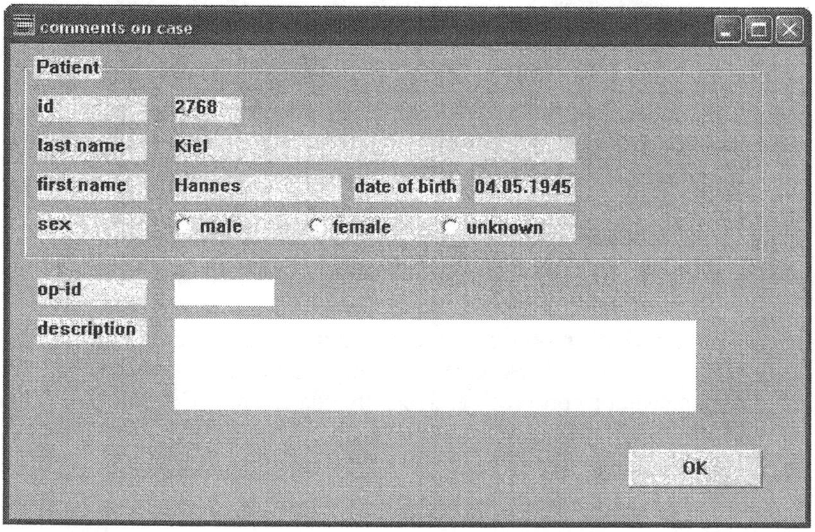

Fig. 10. A Sample Role-Specific View on Data

4. Conclusion

Role-based adaptation enables role-specific access to information systems for a diverse set of users, and can be achieved through model-based methods and tools representing business intelligence, such as TADEUS. The reported case study to achieve role-based interaction has been performed in the domain of a health-care provision. The experiences show the non-linearity of the model-based development procedure. Although in a first step the existing business processes have been specified, the envisioned core processes are not complete at software-design time with respect to the data (required for integrated and mutually tuned task accomplishment). In addition, access and navigation aspects are neither integral part of process nor of software design. Hence, the interaction model (required for user-interface generation) has to be designed in a follow-up activity for the envisioned core processes involving the (patient-)data records.

Another important result concerns the use of prototyping tools when demonstrating design proposals to medical experts and potential end users. The TADEUS prototype had to be enriched with control panels that visualise the flow of control from a user-task perspective for the sake of mutual understanding, such as guiding users through both cases for patient-data search (successful and unsuccessful search procedure for patient data).

However, we advise the use of work process-driven user-interface prototyping tools, such as TADEUS, not only in the area of health-care telematics. The case demonstrated an effective procedure to start re-engineering the (health-care) business in a mutually tuned way involving both technical and organisational issues.

Acknowledgement

Simone Stoiber has established the contact with the health care provider as well as provided the process definitions. Markus Dollhäubl has developed the prototypes.

Chapter 19
MedicSCORE and the Evaluation of ClinicCoach

Elizabeth Hofvenschiöld and Frank Heidmann

Fraunhofer
Institute for Industrial Engineering (IAO)
Nobelstrasse 12
Stuttgart D-70569, Germany
{Elizabeth.Hofvenschiold, Frank.Heidmann}@iao.fhg.de

Abstract. A universally designed system has many and various requisites. The system needs to be accessible and usable by as many users and in as many contexts as possible. To ensure that it adheres to universal design (UD) and accessibility principles, it needs to be tested. The evaluation of such a system must also be multivariate otherwise the many aspects that need to be taken into consideration for a universally designed system will be missed. The MedicSCORE model developed by the usability engineering team at the Fraunhofer IAO aims to provide a multifaceted and holistic framework for the design and evaluation of electronic health records (EHR). The MedicSCORE model is described in this Chapter, as well as the results of an expert evaluation that can be carried out in a relatively short period of time and at low cost. The evaluation, which essentially consists of an expert screening and a user observation, is based on the MedicSCORE framework. The application tested is called ClinicCoach, an electronic patient record (EPR) developed by HIG Coachit (for information, please refer to the ClinicCoach scenario in Chapter 7).

1. Overview of MedicSCORE

MedicSCORE was developed with the aim of designing and testing EHR with reference to UD and universal accessibility (UA) principles. It is based on WebSCORE©, a usability reference model developed by the Fraunhofer IAO for the conception, design and evaluation of web sites. The framework of both models is essentially the same. The major difference is that MedicSCORE was specifically created for the domain of health telematics (in particular for the evaluation of EHRs). The philosophy behind the framework is of implementing UD principles and a holistic approach when designing and evaluating software systems. The model is also based upon the usability principles of the international ergonomic standards ISO 9241, ISO TS 16071 and the international multimedia standards ISO 14915.

C. Stephanidis (Ed.): Universal Access Code of Practice in Health Telematics, LNCS 3041, pp. 240-254, 2005.
© Springer-Verlag Berlin Heidelberg 2005

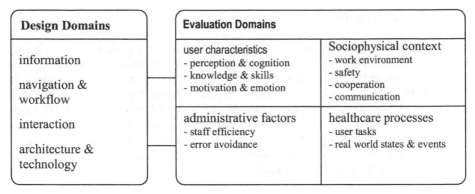

Fig. 1. MedicSCORE Model

The model is comprised of two sets of domains: the design domains and the evaluation domains (see Figure 1). These are described in detail below. The MedicSCORE framework is the basis for the MedicSCORE expert evaluation described later on in this Chapter. The model's domains allow usability experts to evaluate an EHR in a consistent and holistic manner, which is also inexpensive and time-efficient.

1.1 Design Domains

MedicSCORE's four design domains are 'information', 'navigation and workflow', 'interaction' and 'architecture and technology'. For the purposes of this project, only the first three domains are described in this Chapter. The domain 'information' covers all aspects of the information provided by the system. Some of the factors considered in this domain are the quality and quantity of the information, the way in which the information is presented and how the information is expressed. An evaluator can use the following questions to help evaluate this domain: Is the content suitable for the tasks at hand? What kind of font is used? Is the font large enough? Can users make adjustments such as improving the contrast between text and background?

The domain 'navigation and workflow' looks at the navigational aspects of the system. The navigation concept is evaluated, as is the person-system dialogue. For example, does the system support the user in his/her tasks through its clear navigation concept and workflow based on a recognised mental model? Other important questions are: Do the information architecture and navigation concept enable the user to easily and intuitively navigate within the system? Does the system offer adequate orientation help to the users? Is the navigation concept consistent?

The domain 'interaction' addresses the interactive elements of the system. The interactive nature of an application is evaluated, as is the suitability of the interactive elements for the user's tasks. Examples of questions that are posed of the system when evaluating this domain are: Are the interactive elements consistent? When a user interacts with an element, is there sufficient and helpful feedback for the action? Do the interactive elements provide the expected response and are they suitable for the situation?

1.2 Evaluation Domains

Each of the design domains is considered with regard to the set of the evaluation domains, 'user characteristics', 'sociophysical context', 'administrative factors' and 'healthcare processes'. The ergonomic quality of each design domain is defined in terms of its suitability for its target users, their main tasks, the sociophysical context and organisational constraints. For example, the range of perception and cognition among users is taken into consideration during an evaluation. These factors are particularly important for the development of a UD system. Also, the tasks observed or simulated during an evaluation must be relevant otherwise the resulting data may not be valid. It is important to understand the sorts of tasks the users wish to accomplish using the system.

2. Using MedicSCORE

2.1 Overview

The MedicSCORE expert evaluation is ideally carried out with one or two usability experts. It is important that the experts have experience in the field of EHR and are familiar with UA and UD principles. The MedicSCORE expert evaluation described here is comprised of an expert screening and a user observation. It is also possible to incorporate a cognitive walkthrough of the evaluation if the evaluator feels that the user observation and the screening do not provide the depth of detail he or she requires.

2.2 Expert Screening

In the expert screening, the EHR is analysed with regards to the MedicSCORE design and evaluation domains. A list of questions for each design domain (in this case only 'information', 'navigation and workflow' and 'interaction') is developed, and using this list, the evaluator inspects the system in detail. Examples of questions have been given in the previous section of this Chapter. Whilst using the list, the evaluator must always keep in mind the evaluation domains and how they affect each design domain. It is recommended that the evaluator take notes whilst screening the application and later put the results in a table divided according to the three design domains.

2.3 User Observation

To understand the context the users work in and their motivations, it is helpful to observe the users in the environment(s) in which they use the system. If possible, following the users in their tasks making notes on the general nature of the situation and any difficulties that may occur, and asking questions when something is not clear are good ways of gathering in-situ data. The users can also be interviewed after the observation if the evaluator wishes to clarify certain topics or ask for more detailed information on the tasks the user carried out during the observation.

2.4 Outcomes

The outcomes of the MedicSCORE expert evaluation is a list of strengths and weaknesses of the evaluated EHR. Another outcome is a problem severity rating. A criticism of expert screenings is that the potential problems highlighted by the evaluators have no severity ratings. This means that the problems highlighted will probably be relevant to the users but to what extent? The user observation and interviews allow the evaluator to rate the problems and judge how important each one is. This is important because it helps the development team decide which problems have the highest priority (e.g., which problems should be fixed first) and how much effort should be directed into this activity.

3. ClinicCoach Evaluation

An EPR called ClinicCoach was tested using the MedicSCORE model as a basis for evaluation. The user observation carried out for this evaluation entailed a usability expert (also referred to as the evaluator) following hospital staff on their rounds and observing the way in which they interacted with the application. The expert also informally interviewed the staff members after the observations. The screening comprised of the usability expert carrying out typical tasks with ClinicCoach on a PDA and on a PC. Notes were taken on any problematic areas as well as positive findings. The two methods proved a good combination as the expert had a means to rate the severity of usability problems and validate the issues highlighted by the screening.

The results presented in the user observation section are mainly descriptive and are supported with screenshots of the system. This is to provide a context of use and help the reader understand how users interact with the application in one of its actual environments. The expert screening results are presented according to the three MedicSCORE design domains. By doing this, it is hoped that the strengths and weaknesses of the EPR are presented in a clear manner. This technique may also be used as a template for other evaluators wishing to use the MedicSCORE framework and present their findings in a consistent way.

3.1 The Context of the Evaluation

User observation took place at one of the accident surgery wards in the Kassel Clinic, Kassel, Germany. The usability expert observed a nurse and her assistant on one of their afternoon rounds and recorded data on their interaction with the ClinicCoach application. The informal interviews took place at the nurses' station in the ward, in the staff kitchen and outdoor recreational area. The expert screening took place on HIG Coachit's premises in Kassel. One of the application developers demonstrated how the system worked and provided some technical background information, and then the expert proceeded to test the EPR.

3.2 Results of the User Observation

The user observation provided the usability expert with a rich amount of contextual data. It is fortunate that hospital staff are used to working with many people and typically have the ability to communicate clearly. This helps the observation exercise tremendously especially if the staff members are properly briefed before an observation and are then comfortable with the presence of an evaluator. The validity of the results is also likely to increase if the users being observed act as naturally as possible.

The results of the user observation are divided into four parts. The first describes data gathered from the end of one shift and the start of another. The second discusses the observations made on one of the nurse's rounds and the third gives information on the report writing and data transfer activities. The last section briefly describes the data gathered during the informal interviews conducted.

3.2.1 Shift Handover

The usability expert was permitted to join in a handover meeting, which occurs at the end of one shift and the beginning of another. In this meeting, a representative of each nursing team (red, blue and green) gave the incoming nurses and their assistants an overview of their rounds and any new patient information. Each of the team representatives spoke from memory and frequently checked his or her PDA for more detailed information. They easily switched from patient record to patient record. The rest of the staff made notes on a patient list printed shortly before the meeting. The PDA users seemed comfortable with their mobile devices and their communication of experiences and advice flowed smoothly. However, it was observed that once in a while, two of the speakers needed to bring the PDA closer to their eyes or bend their heads toward it so as to read the data on the screen better.

3.2.2 Shift Duties

After the meeting, the staff got ready for their rounds. The usability expert was assigned to the green team (one nurse and her assistant). Before beginning her round, the green team's nurse synchronised the PDA with the ClinicCoach PC to update it and to send any new information it contained to the system's database. She then read a note given to her by one of the ward's interns. The nurse then described that sometimes it was not possible to add information to the PDAs during the rounds or in-between them because, for example, the appropriate PDA could not be found. To remedy this, the ward staff wrote brief notes with the missing information and handed them over to the staff on the next shift.

As the nurse reached her patient's room, she called up the patient's records on ClinicCoach. Having done so, she proceeded with her tasks such as making the patient's bed with her assistant, checking the patient's temperature, inputting the temperature in the system (see Figure 2) and dispensing the medication. After disinfecting her hands, the nurse retrieved her PDA from one of her uniform's pockets and rapidly checked off the tasks that had been completed.

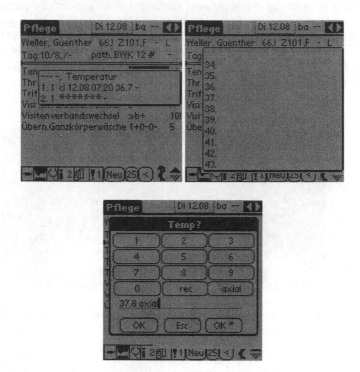

Fig. 2. The first screen shows that the nurse has clicked on Temperature 1+1-

From here she can input the patient's temperature. To do so she clicks on the second line of asterisks and the pop-up menu shown on the second screen appears. Once a temperature is chosen, the nurse can then define the exact temperature (in this case 37.8 degrees Celsius) and click 'OK' ('OK*' is chosen when the patient's temperature is particularly high or unusual for his or her state of health)

The pattern of data entry was basically the same for each of the patients. The usability expert observed that when the nurse had to call a doctor or collect more medicine for a patient, her assistant entered the patient data into the PDA. She was not as familiar with the application but did not seem to have any problems in using it. It was also easy for her and the nurse to pick up and continue a task on the mobile device even if they had been interrupted and had to leave the PDA for some time.

3.2.3 Patient Reports and Care Levels

After finishing their rounds, the nurse and her assistant proceeded to complete certain administrative duties. The nurse mentioned that it was important for her to write patient reports, which described the patients' state of health (see Figure 3). She also remarked that because the PDA was so light and easy to handle in comparison with the A3 size metallic clipboards and paper forms they used to use, she could write the reports wherever she wished.

The nurse showed the evaluator how she could input pre-written phrases so as to save time. The phrases were listed in alphabetical order and the nurse could skip to the one she required by 'scribbling' the first letter of the phrase on the PDA's scribble pad. The nurse could then change some of the wording or add to it by either using the keyboard function or scribble pad. She mentioned that the keyboard was easier to use and preferred it to 'scribbling'.

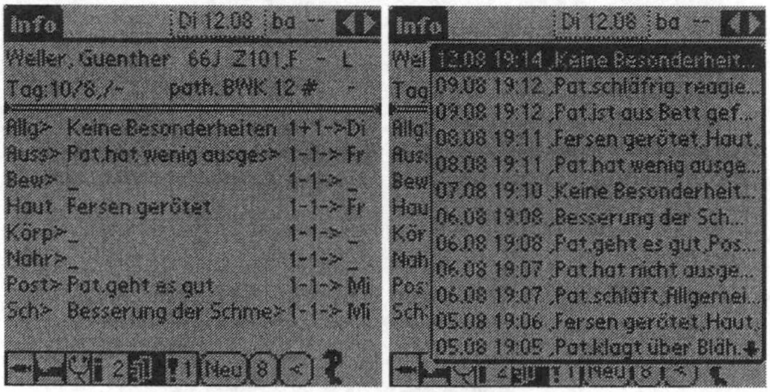

Fig. 3. The first screenshot is of a patient report page. The nurse can also call up list showing a history of general statements on the patient's state of health. The second screenshot illustrates this

After writing the brief patient reports, the nurse proceeded to check the care levels given to each patient. The experience gathered from her rounds allowed her to see if the patients would remain at the care levels assigned to them, needed more care or less care. She was particularly happy to demonstrate to the evaluator the two methods of calling up and then changing the information. The nurse demonstrated that if the person checking and then inputting the data was a novice nurse or carer and was not immediately confident as to what level of care the patient needed, they could cross check with the patient's records and deduce the correct level of care. On the other hand, if the person using the application was experienced and could more or less immediately deduce the patient's level of care, this person had the option to go directly to the care level page and alter the data if needed. The evaluator noted that the system accounts for experienced and novice users and provides the opportunity for expert short cuts. The nurse also mentioned that the ward staff have the chance to erase or correct mistakes for up to two hours after inputting it into the application. However, it would not be possible to correct the mistake if the PDA had been synchronised and the data updated onto the database.

At the nurses' station (or ward office), it was observed that two patient record systems were in use: the ClinicCoach system and an application from the company Siemens. Therefore, the nurse was obligated to input the care level information by hand into the other system. She did not seem bothered by the procedure but did admit that she would prefer it if the data transfer could be done electronically as it is done between the ClinicCoach PDA and PC.

3.2.4 Informal Interviews

Three nurses and two assistants (varying in age from late teens to late forties) were briefly and informally interviewed by the usability expert. They were asked about their experiences with the system, their initial reactions when ClinicCoach was introduced and, if they were part of the green team, the evaluator brought up any outstanding questions about their observed actions.

Almost all of the interviewees stated that they were sceptical about the system when it was first introduced but also admitted that they were sceptical about new technology in general. This ranged from feelings of mild to considerable scepticism. They said that they were given an introductory lesson to ClinicCoach that lasted several hours and then had to use the system alongside the existing form of data collection (paper forms on A3-sized metallic clipboards). This phase was meant to last one month but most of the ward staff discarded the clipboards after two weeks and just used the PDAs. When asked why this was the case, most of the interviewees replied that they had gotten used to the PDAs and found the clipboards cumbersome to work with. The PDAs were much handier, lighter and could be easily slipped into a pocket when visiting patients. However, the deciding factor was the fact that ClinicCoach supported their tasks and provided the functionalities of the clipboard method with added benefits. Four out of the five interviewed also mentioned that the application's ease-of-use made it truly acceptable. When asked about the PC version of ClinicCoach, the interviewees replied that it was fine and that they were happy with the printing functionality. This enabled them to print out patient reports or graphs as needed. It also allowed the nurses to print out patient specifics and give them to a doctor, who then would take it to another ward. Previously, the doctor would take the patient's complete form with clipboard and if a nurse needed a patient's data, she would have to fetch the clipboard or wait until it was returned.

The interviewees did also mention several disadvantages of using ClinicCoach on the PDAs. One nurse was unhappy about the data presentation. She mentioned that the writing was too small and that the contrast was not clear enough. She also stated that she had seen a colleague's personal PDA, which had larger writing and better contrast. The nurse wondered if the option was available to increase the size of the font and determine the contrast according to an individual's requirements. She then mentioned that the size of the device prevented her from having an overview of all of a patient's details. The nature of the paper forms allowed her to briefly glance over them and immediately grasp the patient's general state of health and any important issues. The nurse felt that the PDA did not offer the same quick overview although the same amount of information was available on both systems.

3.3 Results of the Expert Screening

The usability expert screened the PDA and PC versions of ClinicCoach. To do so, a number of tasks were completed using both devices. The evaluator took notes throughout the exercise and highlighted the potential problem areas as well as the positive points of the EPR. The system evaluated was slightly different to the one observed in the Kassel Clinic. The functionality was the same but the designation and the division of the ward were different. For example, instead of dividing up the ward into three colours, it was divided according to room numbers. The results of the PDA screening are presented first. The PDA's screening was more comprehensive than the PC one because it was felt that the users spent more time with the PDA. The time given for the expert evaluation was also a restricting factor. It is also important to state that the evaluator's findings are by no means complete. The aim of the evaluation was to implement and validate the MedicSCORE method and check for general positive and negative features of the system.

3.4 PDA Results

3.4.1 Information

In the information design domain, the usability expert looks at how the information is presented, what kind of information is available and at how it is expressed. The amount of information present in the evaluated application is dependent on what the hospital staff input into the system. They therefore determine its completeness and complexity. Thus the system offers the user the opportunity to enter a great range of data if it is required. This functionality allows the user to make the patient records as complex or a simple as is needed and was perceived by the evaluator as being very positive. Another thing that the expert found user-friendly and appropriate for the user group was the way in which the data was expressed. When possible (i.e., there was enough space), the terms given in the application, which ranged from medicine names to care tasks, were given in whole. This supports novice users as well as experienced users in particular circumstances (e.g., extremely fatigued and stressed) in correctly interpreting the information and accomplishing their tasks. Another positive finding was that the EPR was black and white. This ensured that different categories and highlighted areas were made prominent in a simple but striking way. Software systems often rely heavily and solely on different colours to distinguish between categories and/or highlight different levels of navigation, which is discouraged when implementing a universal design approach.

One negative aspect of the application is the size of the font. As mentioned in the user observation section, one nurse found she had difficulty reading the information because it was too small. The contrast between the background and the different screen elements was also not optimal. Ideally the users should be allowed to change the font size and adjust the contrast of the screen so that they can read the information easily. An inconsistency was also discovered in the placement of certain data. The room numbers of the patient are placed on the right hand side of the complete patient list screen and patient days screen ('Patienten Tage') and on the left hand side of the patient list according to room number (e.g., patient 10 – 18 screen) and on any of the task screens (e.g., ice). The logic behind this is most likely based on the division of the ward based on room numbers – any screen from a category such as rooms 10 –18 and showing the patient room numbers have the room numbers on the left. This might be clear to the developers but not necessarily so to the users.

3.4.2 Navigation and Workflow

In this section, the results relating to the navigation and workflow of the evaluated system are presented. A positive finding of the system is that the main menu is always accessible by clicking on the caduceus symbol. This symbol is also consistently placed on every screen (apart from the Login screen and main menu screen obviously) so that the user can easily find it. Page titles and highlighted buttons (i.e., if a bottom row button is pressed, it is darkened while all others remain light) also contribute to the positive aspects of the application's navigation. These features support the user's navigation through the system and therefore help in the efficient completion of tasks. Another positive finding is the application's clear information architecture. This is reflected in the types of categories available and information available in these categories. For example, the structure of 'Aufgabe' or tasks is wholly relevant to the users. The most common tasks are given and the whole category can be easily reached via the main menu. This finding is supported by the evaluator's experience during the user observation. The navigation concept implemented for the PDA version of ClinicCoach is also consistent. This is also very important if the users are to easily navigate through the application and complete their tasks quickly and easily.

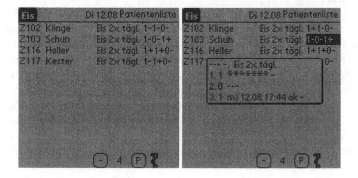

Fig. 4. Screenshot of the 'Ice' page – the user has an overview of all patients who require ice and how often they require it. The second screenshot shows that the user can also confirm that he or she has given a patient ice – it is not necessary to go into the patient's records and confirm there

In general, there were few negative findings related to the navigation and workflow aspects of ClinicCoach. Understandably, due to the size of the PDA screen, an overview of the information architecture is difficult. There is less space to present data and compromises often have to be made. However consistency in the navigation of the system does help to give the user orientation. Despite the page titles, orientation is sometimes difficult. The lower levels of information architecture are quite complex and navigating through them is quite tricky. The absence of a back function also makes moving back one step and checking the previous data difficult. For example, the user decides to go into the 'Eis' (or ice) category given under tasks (see Figure 4) and then wishes to check those patients who are not on the ice list. Once on the screen showing the patients who do not receive any ice, it is not possible to go back one step to the screen showing the patients who do receive ice, which is conceivably a function that users would find useful and meaningful.

3.4.3 Interaction

The findings related to interaction aspects of the system are presented in this section. As in the previous section, the results here are very positive. For example, confirming tasks that have been completed is easy and quick to do. A second positive finding is the design of the interactive elements. They are consistent (with the exception of the small box showing the number of elements or patients on a screen – it looks interactive but is not). A third helpful aspect is that users have two methods of inputting information. They may use the scribble field or the pop-up keyboard available. A fourth positive finding is that the nature of the interactive elements is almost always consistent. For example, clicking on a patient surname will bring the user to the patient list. Another example is the nature of the left and right arrows presented at the top right hand corner on all patient record screens. The user can use these arrows to switch between patients on the list. This functionality is a meaningful and practical digital translation of the previous physical task of flipping through the patient charts.

Despite the intuitive nature of the application, the evaluator did find some negative aspects of the system. The first is the inconsistency of the vertical scrolling elements. Two types of arrows are used – one for pop-up menus and forms and the other for the screens. This is not necessary as their function is the same and should be consistently represented. Another issue is the hidden refresh function. This function is available but not clear. The left and right arrow keys used to switch between patients function as refresh or up-date. Also, the evaluator noticed that when new data is entered into a patient's record; the freshly entered data sometimes appear after the ok button has been clicked on the pop-up menu and sometimes it does not appear. If they do not appear, then the user must refresh the page to see the new or altered information. Another potential problem that users may have is that using the stylus in combination with the small font on the screen requires a certain amount of motor precision. The user needs to use the stylus accurately otherwise a wrong element might be chosen.

3.5 PC Results

3.5.1 Information

The information presented in the PC version is the same as that in the PDA version. The major difference is the way in which it is presented. The font in the PC version is obviously larger and easier to read than that on the PDA. The PC application is also in colour. Few colours are used though and are implemented in a harmonious manner (i.e., they do not distract or disorientate the user when completing tasks). Another positive finding is that an overview of the most important patient data is possible (see Figure 5). The data presented is easy to scan and the graphs are easy to read. Obviously, the screen size of the PC's monitor makes it possible to present larger amounts of data.

On the negative side, the presentation of the data on the general patient data page (or 'Patient Kurve' screen) could be optimised. The data is in a long list and distinction between the different categories is not obvious. It is difficult to see where one category ends and the next one begins.

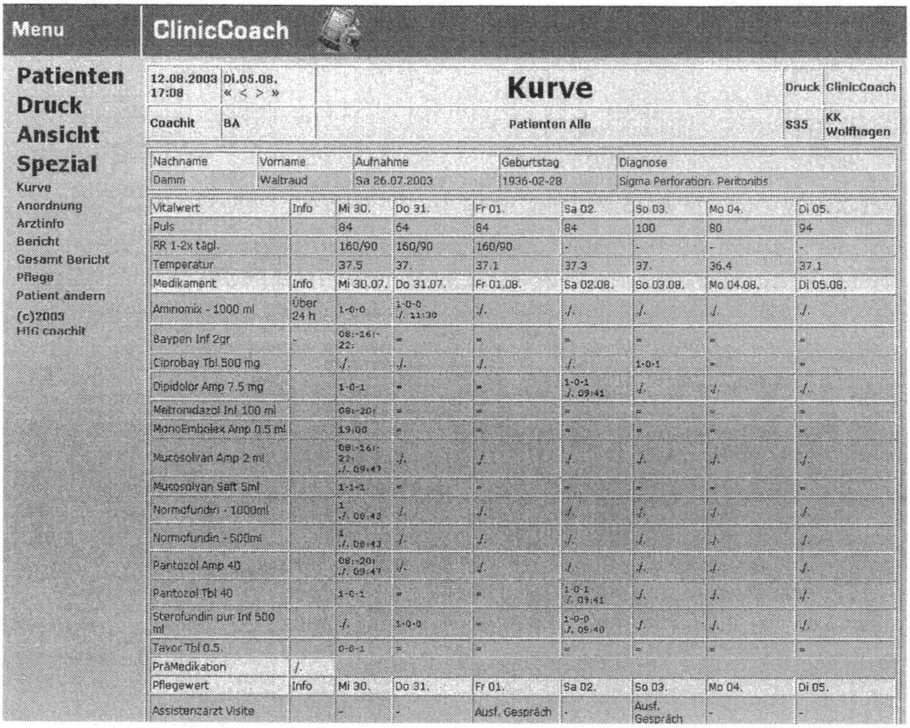

Menu	ClinicCoach

Patienten	12.08.2003 17:08	Di.05.08. « < > »			Kurve			Druck	ClinicCoach
Druck									
Ansicht	Coachit	BA			Patienten Alle			S35	KK Wolfhagen

Spezial	Nachname	Vorname	Aufnahme		Geburtstag	Diagnose		
Kurve	Damm	Waltraud	Sa 26.07.2003		1936-02-28	Sigma Perforation, Peritonitis		

Left menu: Kurve · Anordnung · Arztinfo · Bericht · Gesamt Bericht · Pflege · Patient ändern · (c)2003 · HIG coachit

Vitalwert	Info	Mi 30.	Do 31.	Fr 01.	Sa 02.	So 03.	Mo 04.	Di 05.
Puls		84	64	84	84	100	80	94
RR 1-2x tägl.		160/90	160/90	160/90	-	-	-	-
Temperatur		37.5	37.	37.1	37.3	37.	36.4	37.1
Medikament	Info	Mi 30.07.	Do 31.07.	Fr 01.08.	Sa 02.08.	So 03.08.	Mo 04.08.	Di 05.08.
Amniomix - 1000 ml	Über 24 h	1-0-0	1-0-0 /. 11:30	./.	./.	./.	./.	./.
Baypen Inf 2gr		08/-16/-22:	=	=	=	=	=	=
Ciprobay Tbl 500 mg		./.	./.	./.	./.	1-0-1	=	=
Dipidolor Amp 7.5 mg		1-0-1	=	=	1-0-1 /. 09:41	./.	./.	./.
Metronidazol Inf 100 ml		08/-20/	=	=	=	=	=	=
MonoEmbolex Amp 0.5 ml		19:00	=	=	=	=	=	=
Mucosolvan Amp 2 ml		08/-16/-22: /. 09:42	./.	./.	./.	./.	./.	./.
Mucosolvan Saft 5ml		1-1-1	=	=	=	=	=	=
Normofundin - 1000ml		1 /. 08:42	./.	./.	./.	./.	./.	./.
Normofundin - 500ml		1 /. 08:43	./.	./.	./.	./.	./.	./.
Pantozol Amp 40		08/-20/ /. 09:42	./.	./.	./.	./.	./.	./.
Pantozol Tbl 40		1-0-1	=	=	1-0-1 /. 09:41	./.	./.	./.
Sterofundin pur Inf 500 ml		./.	1-0-0	=	1-0-0 /. 09:40	./.	./.	./.
Tavor Tbl 0.5.		0-0-1	=	=	=	=	=	=
PräMedikation	./.							
Pflegewert	Info	Mi 30.	Do 31.	Fr 01.	Sa 02.	So 03.	Mo 04.	Di 05.
Assistenzarzt Visite		-	-	Ausf. Gespräch	-	Ausf. Gespräch	-	-

Fig. 5. Screenshot of a patient's most important details (overview screen)

3.5.2 Navigation and Workflow

The navigation concept and the information architecture of the PC version are slightly different to those of the PDA version. A positive finding is that page titles are given for each screen and this helps user navigation through the system. Reserving the top and the left hand side of the page for main navigation areas also supports user navigation. Another positive finding is the back function. It is in form of a web browser back button but it is intuitively placed (along with other browser functions such a forward button) at the top left hand corner of the screen.

Despite the clearly designated areas for navigation on the PC version, the evaluator did find several negative aspects of the application. For example, the information architecture is not the same as it is for the PDA version. The opportunity to see an overview of the most important patient data is very helpful (a user would have to switch between the care and medication screens on the PDA) but the difference in information architecture in other areas could make it difficult for users to use the application effectively and quickly. Another negative finding is the difference in navigation concept between the two versions. As mentioned above, the designated navigation areas are clearly marked but navigating on the secondary and tertiary levels of the system is complex and orientation support is lacking. For example, the terms used for the different categories of information are not the same for both versions. What is known as tasks or 'Aufgabe' on the PDA is named 'Ansicht' (overview) on the PC. Also, none of the icons used on the PDA are present on the PC.

Orientation support such as highlighting the category a user has just chosen is also missing on the PC but is available on the mobile version.

3.5.3 Interaction

The nature of the interaction on the PC is also different to that of the PDA. To start with, the PC version is used through a keyboard, mouse and a large monitor whereas the PDA version is used via a stylus and a touch screen. A positive finding is the consistent design of the links (interactive elements). However, if colour is the differentiating factor, then the colour implemented for the links should be distinctly different from the colour of non-interactive elements.

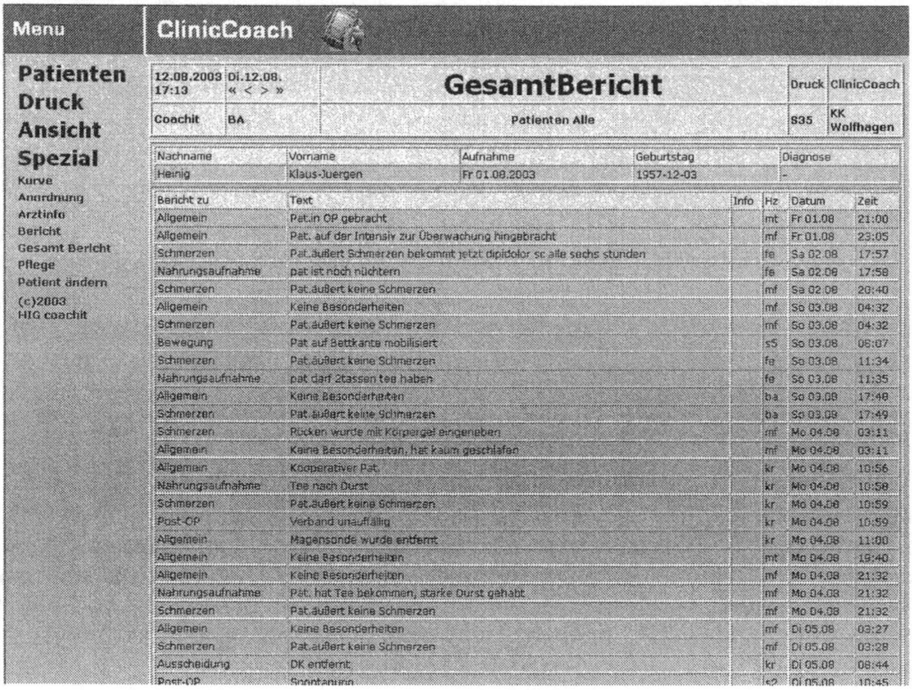

Fig. 6. Screenshot of a patient report page (for the PDA version of this page, please see Figure 2) The items (e.g., 'Kurve', 'Anordnung') underneath the main navigation elements in the left hand column are part of the category 'Patienten' or Patients. This is not clear – it seems that they belong to the 'Spezial' or Special category

One negative aspect of the PC version is inappropriate placement of certain interactive elements. When a category in the left-hand column is clicked, then a set of sub-categories appears under the last main category (see Figure 6). It is common and good practice to place interactive elements that are directly related to each other, next to each other. This principle is implemented widely in the PDA version of ClinicCoach but not in the PC version. The nature of the interactive elements is also inconsistent in the PC version. In the PDA application, the surname of a patient can be clicked to access either the patient list or the chosen patient's records. On the PC version, the patients' surnames are non-interactive and therefore cannot be clicked. Another negative finding is the use of arrows under the current date in the top part of the screen. The arrows are remarkably similar to the arrows used on the PDA to jump between the patients. The interactive elements look the same but have different functions, which do not support the fluid and easy transition from the mobile version to the stationary one.

3.6 Recommendations for Optimisation

Several recommendations for the optimisation of both ClinicCoach versions can be made from the information gathered during the user observation and the findings discovered in the screening. Comments on the optimisation of the system have also been made in previous sections; it is the aim of this section to consolidate these and present the most important ones here.

3.6.1 PDA Version

The severity of the issues found on the PDA version of ClinicCoach range from mild to important. An important issue that appeared in the evaluation of the PDA version is the small font size of the text. The screen size of the mobile device limits what can be shown at one time. However, users should have the option to increase the size of the font and alter the contrast if they feel it is necessary.

The PDA version of ClinicCoach could also benefit from a more consistent layout and representation of interactive elements. For example, the placement of the patients' room numbers varies on different screens. Also, there are two types of scroll arrows for the pages (e.g., patient list page) and pop-up menus. If two elements have the same function, they should be consistent in appearance. This issue is important but does not have to be addressed immediately. The application would also benefit from a back function; again this is a relatively important issue but one, which also does not have to be immediately addressed. As mentioned in the 'navigation & workflow' section, user orientation should be supported by a back function. This is because it is tricky to go back one step on the secondary or tertiary levels of the system.

3.6.2 PC Version

The issues highlighted on the PC version are more severe than their PDA counterparts. The PC version of ClinicCoach would benefit from improvements in the information architecture, navigation concept and consistency of interactive elements. It is unfortunate that the information architecture and to an extent, the navigation concept of the PC are not as good as those of the PDA version. It is understood that they cannot be entirely the same due the nature of the devices but the stationary version needs to be improved. Firstly, the wording of the main, secondary and tertiary navigation levels should be the same for both versions. This is an important issue that should be addressed as soon as possible. Secondly, the layout of elements should be as similar as possible to the PDA version. In effect, the closer in appearance the PC version is to the PDA, the more it will support the effective and efficient use of ClinicCoach on both devices. For example, the icons used on the mobile version could also be used on the PC. Again, this issue is also important but need not be immediately addressed. It is also possible to interpret the PDA layout and make it work for the PC. The main navigation areas could be moved to the top and the bottom of the screen on the PC version just as it is on the PDA. Such measures would increase the quality of the navigation and workflow aspects of the stationary application.

The PC version would also benefit from an improvement in the 'interaction' domain. In the PDA version, interactive elements that are related to each other are placed next to each other. This is not always the case for the PC. The nature of the interactive elements must also be consistent. If patient surnames are interactive on the mobile version, then they should also be clickable and lead to same area on the stationary version. This is also a rather important issue and should also be addressed as soon as is possible.

4. Discussion and Conclusion

The MedicSCORE model provides a framework for the expert evaluation of a EHR. The design domains are described but a long list of relevant questions is not provided. Guidance is only given because the nature of health telematic applications is multifarious and complex. Usability experts familiar in the field should be experienced enough to develop their own lists of questions based on the design and evaluation domains. The questions can also naturally be based on standards, guidelines and heuristic evaluation criteria.

The expert evaluation described here also assumes that the evaluators have access to users working in context. If this is not the case, a cognitive walkthrough can replace the user observation and supplement the expert screening. However, as mentioned in the previous section, a disadvantage of an expert screening and a cognitive walkthrough is that they cannot validate the severity of the problems found.

This Chapter has also illustrated how a MedicSCORE expert evaluation can be carried out and describes the results of such an evaluation on ClinicCoach, an EPR developed by the company HIG Coachit. The methods implemented for the MedicSCORE expert evaluation proved to be useful, practical and efficient. In a relatively short period of time, one usability expert could highlight the major strengths and weaknesses of an EPR. This is of course dependent upon many factors. It is important to stress that an expert evaluation, although valuable, is no substitute for a thorough usability test with representative users.

The results of the evaluation show ClinicCoach to have many strengths and some weaknesses. Most of the positive findings were admittedly found in the PDA version of the application. When the evaluator spoke with developers, they intended for the primary device to be the PDA and therefore concentrated most of their efforts on it. However, it is the opinion of the evaluator that even if the PC is the secondary device, the application running on it should still be as supportive and intuitive as possible. This can be achieved through consistent design and the implementation of a very similar (if not the same) information architecture and navigation concept. The recommendations described in the previous section and the MedicSCORE model as a whole may be used as a foundation for EPR developers when aiming to create universally designed and accessible applications for the future.

Chapter 20
Standards Adherence and Compliance

Elizabeth Hofvenschiöld and Frank Heidmann

Fraunhofer
Institute for Industrial Engineering (IAO)
Nobelstrasse 12
Stuttgart D-70569, Germany
{Elizabeth.Hofvenschiold, Frank.Heidmann}@iao.fhg.de

Abstract. Universally accessible design aims to eliminate the barriers that standard design often presents to many groups in the world's population. In this Chapter, we look at how standards can promote universal access and design for the field of health telematics. We first discuss why standards are important and essential in the successful implementation of a universal access and design approach. Following this, the challenges that many application and system developers face in their attempts to apply standards to the design process are highlighted. The appropriate standards for the IS4ALL project are identified and a set of project standards for it are developed by selecting them from the larger group of identified standards and by tailoring them as needed. Strategies for implementing the project standard in a project will be described, as will the outcomes of the process. Finally, we will illustrate how an audit can be organised to assess the compliance of a health telematic application using the project standard set.

1. Can Standards Promote Universal Access and Design?

Standards can do so if used in the correct manner and if their limitations are recognised. Standardisation can contribute to the increased usability and accessibility of using information and communication technologies. According to Ziegler (2001) three areas have implications for the accessibility of information technology. These areas are the usability of a system (effectiveness, efficiency and user satisfaction), personal characteristics and cultural and social factors. Standards can help to reduce the effect that these areas would have on the accessibility and usability of a system. However, before we can apply standards to the IS4ALL efforts, we need to understand their possibilities and limitations for information and communication technologies in general. The descriptions of the benefits and shortcomings discussed here are essentially based on the works of Buie (1999) and Stewart (2000).

So what exactly are the advantages of using standards when developing information and communication technologies? The advantages of standards are numerous. Incorporated into standards are the best practices in HCI, which help to ensure the quality of the standards. Most obviously they standardise the look and feel of an interface. Standards also help developers achieve the mandatory compliance and can

C. Stephanidis (Ed.): Universal Access Code of Practice in Health Telematics, LNCS 3041, pp. 255-270, 2005.

help to facilitate the design process. Standards essentially represent a simplified view of the world and this is helpful when you need a clear and straightforward structure in the development phase.

However, standards should not be perceived as a complete solution to addressing accessibility and universal design issues. Standards are sometimes relied upon to solve all the HCI problems that come to the surface and more often than not, developers discover that the standards are vague and do not cover the difficult aspects (e.g., design decisions) of the design process. The impact of standards on the usability of a system can also be misinterpreted. Many software houses believe that standard compliance equates usability and therefore certifies their applications as user-friendly. This is misleading. Standards are only part of the solution – essential but not the complete answer.

2. Project Standards

2.1 Overview

In order to make standards work for a project, it is helpful to develop a project standard. A project standard is comprised of standards specifically suited to the project and which are often tailor-fitted. The foundation of the project standard here is comprised of three sets of international standards. These standards are ISO 13407, ISO 9241-10, ISO 9241-11 and ISO TS 16071 (not officially an international standard but a technical specification, which is widely used). Obviously these standards encompass large amounts of information and not all recommendations are directly relevant to IS4ALL and future developers of accessible health telematic applications. A brief description of each standard will be presented in this section and the parts particularly relevant to the project will be highlighted. These highlighted parts will form the basis for the project standard (see Table 1).

Table 1. International standards that comprise the project standard for IS4ALL. (N.B. It is not the objective of this Chapter to provide complete lists of the international standards but to provide a framework for the implementation of standards. It is assumed that the reader will have access to the relevant standards discussed and it is highly recommended that the above standards be studied and applied as instructed.)

ISO 13407	Human-centred process	High Level
ISO 9241-11	Specification and evaluation of usability	Middle Level
ISO 9241-10	Specifications of general dialogue principles	
ISO TS 16071	Detailed specifications for accessibility for users with special requirements	Low Level

Other relevant sources are ISO 23973 Working Draft Software Ergonomics for World Wide Web user interfaces and Technical Report 19764 Guidelines, methodology, and reference criteria for cultural and linguistic adaptability in information technology products. It is important to note that these are not ISO international standards and are subject to review. However, they do include useful guidelines and advice that are helpful to developers of health telematic applications when creating universally designed and accessible products.

2.2 ISO 13407

ISO 13407 Human-centred design processes for interactive systems describes the generic HCI design process and promotes human-centred design. Such an approach is essential if a system is to be truly accessible and usable by as many people as possible. A process standard helps to cover the hard parts of HCI design but it is very general and still needs to be tailored to this project's needs. It is important to understand that a specific project process is necessary, as a general process standard cannot guarantee a good interface (Buie 1999). ISO 13407 should be used in combination with other standards. This is because although ISO 13407 aims to address technical human factors and ergonomic issues, it does so in a general manner. In summary, ISO 13407 prescribes four human-centred design activities that should take place at all stages of a project (see Figure 1). These are to:

- Understand and specify the context of use;
- Specify the user and organisational requirements;
- Produce design solutions
- Evaluate designs against requirements.

The following sections describe in more detail what ISO 13407 recommends for system developers and project managers. Most of the information is summarised as only the most pertinent parts for use in IS4ALL and future health telematic projects are presented here.

2.2.1 Active User Involvement and Understanding User and Task Requirements
This section describes one of the first principles defined in the standard. It is essential that users be included in the development process. The target user population and the tasks involved can be linked to the whole design cycle, as can the organisation purchasing the system. Users who will eventually use the system can be called in to evaluate prototypes thereby increasing acceptance and commitment at a later stage

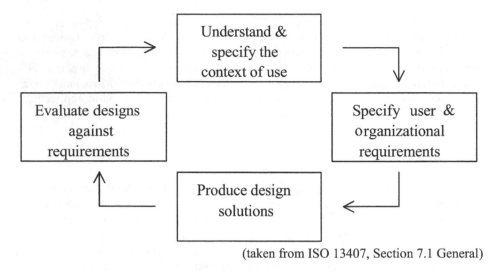

(taken from ISO 13407, Section 7.1 General)

Fig. 1. The interdependence of human-computer design activities according to ISO 13407

2.2.2 Understand and Specify the Context of Use
ISO 13407 states that the context of a system is identified in terms of:
- characteristics of intended users,
- tasks the users are to perform,
- environment in which the users are to use the system.

For IS4ALL the most important of these three are the first two. If an accessible and universal design approach is to be implemented, then all characteristics of all users (or at least those of the elderly and users with disabilities) must be considered. The tasks that the users shall perform when using an electronic health record application are multifarious as there are all sorts of users. The last is also important but essentially the environment of use need not be specified because the idea behind a truly accessible and usable system is that it can be used in all contexts.

2.2.3 Specify the User and Organisational Requirements
The users' as well as the organisation's requirements must be specified if the process is to be human-centred. The specification of requirements should provide quantifiable levels against which the emerging design can be tested, set appropriate priorities for different requirements and be confirmed by the users.

2.2.4 Prototyping and Iterative Testing
Models or prototypes allow the early testing of design ideas and also helps the development team members to communicate early on in the process. Prototyping can be done at any stage in the process and users can be asked to test them. The results from the evaluation can then be fed back into the design cycle ensuring that the human-centred approach drives the design process. It is essential that users get involved at an early stage so that the process is as iterative as possible in order to achieve the design objectives. This is particularly valid for universal design approach.

And in order to apply the information gathered in one project to another, good documentation practices must be implemented so that others can learn from what you have discovered.

2.2.5 Evaluation: Planning and Assessment

The evaluation process must be planned. What are the features to be tested? Who is going to run the evaluation? When are the tests to be scheduled and what are the resources required for them? These are some of the questions that must be answered to develop a test plan for a project. It is also important to plan evaluation for as many stages of the project as possible. An expert evaluation is a fast and economical way of identifying major problems. However, it must be remembered that this is not a substitute for user testing.

Evaluation is used to check if a design has met the human-centred requirements and to assess conformity to international, national or statutory standards. ISO 9241-11 and ISO 9241-10 provide some important advice on specifying and measuring usability. Field validation ensures that the system meets the requirements of the users, tasks and the environment. For IS4ALL this would entail testing the various applications on various devices in different contexts. As in the previous section, the documentation and communication of results are very important. If questions arise about certain design decisions, the team can always go back and check why a certain solution was chosen instead of another.

2.3 ISO 9241-11

There are seventeen parts of ISO 9241 Ergonomic requirements for office work with visual display terminals (VDTs). We will concentrate on Parts 10 `Dialogue Principles' and 11 `Guidance on Usability'. Many other parts of ISO 9241, such as Part 12 `Presentation of Information', are relevant to IS4ALL as well but will not be discussed here. It was felt that ISO 9241-10 and 11 were the most appropriate parts out of the seventeen for application to this project. However, not all of Part 11 is presented in this section (Part 10 is presented in section 3.5). As with ISO 13407, some areas are more pertinent than others for IS4ALL. The areas described here are the explanations of how the usability of a product can be specified and evaluated as part of a quality system.

2.4 Specification and Evaluation of Usability in the Development Process

There are various situations in which usability may be evaluated, for example in product development, procurement or in product certification. For this Chapter, the specification and evaluation of usability in the development process is described. The recommendations are general and can be useful in all situations.

2.4.1 Specification of the Intended Context of Use
Information about the user characteristics, their goals and tasks as well as the environment should be considered when the specific system/product requirements are defined.

2.4.2 Specification of the Usability Requirements for a Product
ISO 9241-11 can be used as a framework for the specification of the usability requirements of the system or product. Measures of effectiveness, efficiency and satisfaction can be selected and from this, the acceptance criterion can be determined (for later evaluation).

2.4.3 Product Development
The definition and framework for usability can be used by the whole development team to arrive at a common understanding of the concept of usability. All team members need to understand what it is if they are to successfully develop a highly usable and acceptable product. The usability requirements specified can then be used to evaluate the product's usability at any stage in the development process.

2.4.4 Measurement of Usability
ISO 9241 contains all sorts of information on the evaluation of a product's usability. For example, the determination of the user's goals can aid in the choice of tasks that are suitable for a usability test. Appendix B in ISO 9241-11 provides a list of factors that could be measured. It is beyond the scope of this Chapter to present the information here and it is recommended that the reader go to ISO 9241-11 Appendix B directly for further details.

2.4.5 Usability as a Framework for a Quality Plan
The previous subsections (3.4.1- 3.4.4) can be used as a framework for a quality plan to define, document and verify the usability of a system or product. Figure 2 illustrates the relationships between the activities and documents arising from them, or the type of result.

2.4.6 Use / Application in Conjunction with Other Norms and Standards
ISO 9241-11 can be used in conjunction with other ISO 9241 standards. The reader is directed to Appendix D in the ISO 9241-11, which provides information on the use of the standard in combination with other standards.

Activities   Document / Result

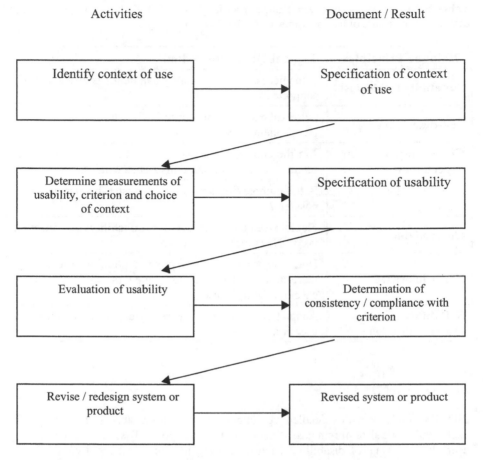

Fig. 2. Illustrations of the relationship between activities and documents according to ISO 9241-11

2.5 ISO 9241-10

Part 10 of ISO 9241 describes seven general principles for the ergonomic design of interactive software systems for visual display terminals. These principles and accompanying recommendations are totally relevant for any application developed in IS4ALL or in the general field of health telematics. Table 2 presents the dialogue principles and some of the questions that developers should be asking themselves about the application being designed or evaluated. The information is taken directly from ISO 9241-10 and the reader is encouraged to consult the standard for more details.

Table 2. Table showing the seven dialogue principles from ISO 9241-10 and questions that developers could pose of the application being developed or evaluated

Dialogue Principles	Typical Questions Asked
Suitability for the task	Is the necessary functionality available? Is efficient work supported?
Self-descriptiveness	Self-explanatory and intuitive? Clear and context-independent help functions?
Conformity with user expectations	Are the concepts used familiar to the application field? Internal consistence and consistence with other systems?
Suitability for learning	Is the complexity controllable? Is step-by-step learning possible?
Controllability	Flexible sequence of events? Suitability for different tasks? No (time) restrictions?
Error tolerance	Does the system design prevent possible errors? Are there any Irreversible consequences without double-checking with the user?
Suitability for individualisation	Adaptation to different work styles, work contexts and user preferences?

2.6 ISO TS 16071

ISO TS 16071 provides detailed guidelines on developing accessible systems for users with special requirements. It also outlines the types of issues encountered by users with a range of disabilities such as hearing loss or blindness. ISO TS 16071 should be used in combination with other standards such as ISO 13407 (to ensure not only an accessible system but a human-centred one) and various parts of ISO 9241. In this Chapter, ISO TS 16071 rounds off the IS4ALL project standard set as part of the implemented accessible and universal design approach.

It is difficult to choose only certain parts of the standard for description that would apply to the development of universally accessible health telemetric application. Almost all of the standards are applicable to the creation of such applications. It is therefore recommended that the reader go directly to ISO TS 16071 and refer to the standard when developing and evaluating a system, which needs to be accessible and acceptable. The standard also provides a set of impact categories, which rank the different recommendations. A recommendation can either be core, primary or secondary and refers to either the operating system or application. Detailed descriptions of these categories are provided in the standard.

3. Using the Project Standard Set

Standards can be implemented at all stages of the development process by using various means. The standards described in the previous section contain recommendations for their use at various steps in the design cycle. With reference to Table 1, it depends on the types of standard and the level of guidance provided. For example, the ideal implementation of ISO 13407 would be at the beginning of a project to determine the overall human-centred design strategy. ISO 924-111 provides a more detailed guideline of specifying and evaluating the usability of a system or product. It also provides tables and checklists that a developer could use to help evaluate a product. ISO TS 16071 gives detailed specifications for the accessible design of human-computer interfaces. These detailed recommendations offer the developer the opportunity to make an application or system as accessible as possible. The procedure for using the project standard follows the process recommended by ISO 13407. Table 3 illustrates this.

Table 3. Table showing general development cycle categories and accompanying standards (ISO 13407 dictates the stages in the process)

Stage in the Process	Standard(s)
Understand and specify context of use	ISO 9241-11
Specify the user and organisational requirements	ISO 9241-11 ISO TS 16071
Produce design solutions	ISO TS 16071
Evaluate designs against requirements and dialogue principles	ISO 9241-10 ISO 9241-11

4. The Audit Process

This section illustrates how an audit can be organised to assess the compliance of a product to a particular standard or parts of it. The standard being implemented for this audit is the project standard presented in the previous sections. In particular, Parts 10 and 11 of ISO 9241 from the project standard will be specifically applied to this assessment. The reference scenario used for the audit is WardInHand, an electronic patient record application that runs on a PDA (for more information about WardInHand, please refer to the corresponding Chapter in this book).

An outline for the auditing process is described in some detail. It is important to remember that the process varies according to the stage in the development cycle where it occurs. Illustrated here is the process developed for implementation at the evaluation stage of the design cycle. However, it is generally applicable for all areas of the design process and can be adjusted for use at different stages. A representative sample of the results of the compliance audit is also presented.

4.1 Overview

The process of this audit is essentially taken from ISO 9241-11. This is because Part 11 of the standard provides a good framework for an evaluation strategy. There are four stages in the process. The first step is the determination of the measurements of usability. The first half of the second step is the evaluation of WardInHand against the measurements. The second half of the step is the determination of the application's consistency with the standards. At the third stage, recommendations for improvement are given. The fourth and final step is comprised of long-term recommendations for redesign.

4.2 Determination of Usability Measurements

ISO 9241-10 and ISO TS 16071 dictate the usability measurements for this audit but only the use of ISO 924-10 will be discussed in more detail here. Using the seven dialogue principles given in Part 10 is a good way of assessing the general effectiveness, efficiency and potential acceptance of an application (see Table 1). They are also particularly handy when there is not much time for a complete and detailed standards compliance audit in a project. This is not to say that the use of more detailed standards such as the technical specifications in ISO TS 16071 should be ignored. Indeed, the recommendations for the design of accessible systems are very important and should be used in the development of inclusive products. The reader is directed to ISO TS 16071 for the complete list of technical specifications, which can be used as a checklist for a system evaluation or as guidelines for the design of a new application. For this particular audit, the seven design dialogues from ISO 9241-10 (see Table 2) and only a select amount of recommendations from ISO TS 16071 are to be used.

4.3 Evaluation of WardInHand: Combined Results from a Pluralistic Walkthrough and Expert Screening

There are a number of ways in which you can check an application for standards compliance and adherence. For this audit, the results of a pluralistic walkthrough and expert evaluation were used. The prototype used was made up of over seventy screen shots of the WardInHand application (see Chapter 8). There was no clickable prototype available for the test and it was therefore difficult to determine if the application complied with certain dialogue principles such as controllability and error tolerance. Presented below are examples of the detailed audit. Beneath each screenshot is a table, which shows problematic issues with the application, the dialogue principle it does not comply with, and a 16071 specification that could help solve the problem.

4.3.1 Personal Data Screen

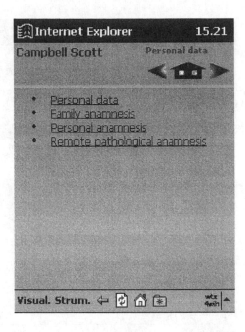

Problem	9241-10 Dialogue Principle	16071 Specification
Very small font	Suitability for the task (e.g., Can the task be completed successfully regardless of the small font?)	Enable font customisation and legibility
Colours implemented are not ideal	---	Provide colour palettes designed for people who have visual impairments
Unexpected grouping of information and use of terminology	Conformity with user expectations	Clarify natural language usage
Icons used were ambiguous	Self-descriptiveness	Provide object labels

4.3.2 Pulse Rate Screen

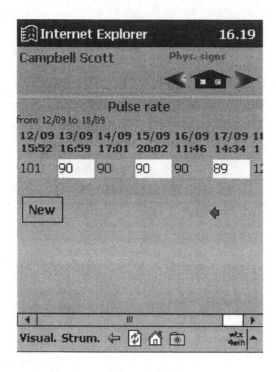

Problem	9241-10 Dialogue Principle	16071 Specification
Unexpected and inappropriate display of pulse rate data	Conformity with user expectations	Enable users to customise viewing attributes (secondary issue)

4.3.3 Blood Pressure Screen

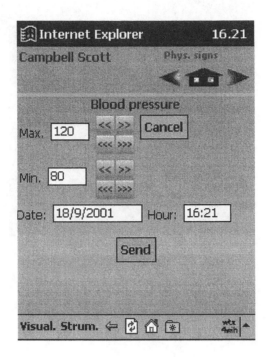

Problem	9241-10 Dialogue Principle	16071 Specification
Arrow symbols on buttons not understood	Self-descriptiveness	Provide object labels
'Maximum' and 'minimum' are not the proper clinical terms – systolic and diastolic are	Conformity with user expectations	Provide object labels
Some medical staff find it important to indicate the area from which the blood pressure was taken (e.g., right arm)	Suitability for individualisation	Enable customisation of user preferences

4.3.4 Drugs Screen

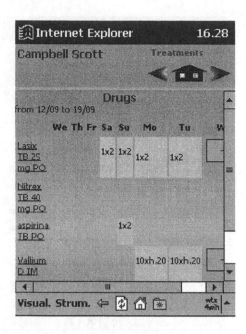

Problem	9241-10 Dialogue Principle(s)	16071 Specification
Screen layout disliked by user as information is not clearly presented and may lead to misunderstanding	Suitability for the task	Enable appropriate presentation of tables
Medication timing is different from country to country – in some countries it is not enough to say 'twice a day' for example – the instructions must be more explicit (e.g., once in the morning and once in the afternoon)	Conformity with user expectations Suitability for individualisation	Enable customisation of user preferences

4.4 Summary of Results

The summary of the audit findings is presented in this section. The results are in table format (see Table 4) and categorised using the seven dialogue principles of ISO 9241-10.

Table 4. Summary of results of audit with dialogue principles from ISO 9241-10

Criteria	Comments
Suitability for the task	The task of the reference scenario was to use a PDA to access an electronic patient record. The application was generally usable but the information architecture was not clear. There were inconsistencies in the navigation concept as well. For example, there were at least four different ways in which you could input patient information.
Self-descriptiveness	There were discrepancies in the self-descriptiveness of the application. There were spelling mistakes, which led to confusion, and the units of measurement next to input fields were not given. For example, it was not clear whether the user had to enter the patient's body weight in kilos or pounds. Some of the icons used were also misleading.
Conformity with user expectations	The use of drop-down menus and underlined words as links was conformist. However, the use of other elements was misleading, as it was not clear which actions they would trigger. For example, the use of double or triple arrows on buttons was not understood. Some of the icons used did not correspond with the user's expectations (e.g., Home icon was not understood).
Suitability for learning	It would be challenging for a user to learn how to use the application in a short period of time. The information architecture is relatively complex and as mentioned earlier, the navigation concept is inconsistent. Some of the functions are easy to learn such as the patient's personal anamnesis information. In general, the user would need to use the application for some time to become familiar with it. It does not afford immediate accessibility to all user groups.
Controllability	The application was relatively easy to control. However, the layout of certain screens was not optimal and was confusing. Having no time restrictions when using the application was positive.
Error Tolerance	It was challenging to determine the degree to which the application was tolerant of errors. This was because a paper prototype consisting of over seventy different screen shots was used. On some screens, there was the opportunity to confirm or cancel a particular input.
Suitability for individualisation	It is assumed that at Log-in (first screen), the user's profile is determined and the preferred or allowed information is presented. On all other screens, it was possible to see if there was the opportunity for individualisation.

4.5 Recommendations for Optimisation

ISO TS 16071 provides good recommendations on overcoming accessibility issues. The specifications given in the screen shot tables (see Section 5.3) were essentially the most appropriate solutions given for the problems encountered. It is important to remember that the specifications are not the only possible solutions. For some issues, such as ambiguous icons, other measures should be implemented as well. Using universally acceptable icons and/or running several user tests with different types of icons are ways in which a solution can be found.

4.6 Long-Term Design Recommendations

The long-term recommendations are based on all of the dialogue principles from ISO 9241-10 and the specifications of ISO TS 16071. The reader is directed to these and other standards (e.g., ISO 9241-11 and 12) for detailed information and guidelines as to making an application as universally accessible and usable as possible.

5. Summary

This Chapter illustrates how international standards can contribute to developing universally accessible and inclusive products with specific reference to the health telematic applications. There are challenges in using standards as they are often rather broad and seemingly general. One method of dealing with some of these challenges is to develop a project standard set to help focus the development effort and encourage a user-centred design approach. A project standard set developed for IS4ALL and comprised of ISO 13407, 9241-10, 9241-11 and ISO TS 16071 is described, and an accompanying audit process is also presented.

Chapter 21
Participatory Insight to Universal Access:
Methods and Validation Exercises

Michael Pieper[1] and Karl Stroetmann[2]

[1]Fraunhofer - FIT
Schloss Birlinghoven
Sankt Augustin 53754, Germany
michael.pieper@fit.fraunhofer.de
[2]empirica
Oxfordstr. 2
D-53111 Bonn, Germany
Karl.Stroetmann@empirica.com

Abstract. Participatory methods can, in principle, be applied for a variety of purposes to gain insight into the context of use of an artefact or the way in which tasks are performed by end users. Consequently, participatory methods are equally valid for problem identification, clarification of the issues relevant to a particular topic, but also for the detailed evaluation of devices, products and interfaces. Typically, participatory methods facilitate rich empirical data sets useful for design teams and evaluators. In our case, participatory methods have been used to facilitate access to medical data by patients at home. To this end, a variety of participatory approaches are available, the more important ones being: questionnaires, face-to-face or telephone interviews based on a formal questionnaire or on an interview guide, user trials, task analysis and group discussions such as brainstorming sessions or focus group meetings.

1. Involving End-User Communities

Participatory usability inspection takes as its basic premise the view that product developments should be driven from user requirements rather than from technological capabilities. End users should be encouraged to participate in design wherever possible. Thus the starting point for usability evaluation and systems design is to understand the user population in some detail, and understand what they may need from products before going too far down the path of deciding about specific design solutions. Design is often driven by technical feasibility that can lead to a poor match to users' needs. Participatory approaches are conversely concerned with ensuring that products:
- have real value for end users
- are matched to user capabilities
- are fit for the purpose for which they were designed

C. Stephanidis (Ed.): Universal Access Code of Practice in Health Telematics, LNCS 3041, pp. 271-296, 2005.
© Springer-Verlag Berlin Heidelberg 2005

From this perspective, participatory approaches place emphasis on tools and techniques that assist developers in understanding more clearly the end-user demands they are designing for and the attributes of those people who will be influenced by a design. However, involving patients who are elderly, frail or suffering from certain illnesses in participatory usability inspections and systems design requires some degree of sensitivity on the part of evaluators and designers, and an awareness of the way in which most cultures stigmatise health problems. These cultural factors in turn influence the way information is captured. For example, self reports from patients often underestimate their difficulties, as problems in coping are seen as being a reflection on oneself rather than being due to a poorly designed system environment.

Since many requirements for products emerge out of direct experience of using prototypes or mock-ups, these problems can at best be dealt with by an iterative methodology rather than a linear evaluation and design approach which moves directly from requirements capture through specification and implementation. For that reason participatory approaches support iterative design, recognising that in many cases developers may have to enter several cycles of "development and evaluation" before a satisfactory solution is reached. Participatory approaches emphasise the importance of obtaining good feedback about how products perform in actual use, and it is noted that this is often a lacking in design activities. Many design solutions have previously failed to gain information about how the final product will be used and consequently they are not sufficiently sensitive to the changing and developing needs of different end-users. Unlike other approaches, participatory approaches cover not only the design of the product itself but also other, wider factors that can dramatically affect the success or failure of a product - for example, factors such as the environmental context in which the product will be used, etc.

At the heart of participatory end-user involvement is thus the concept of usability. If products and services do not have the necessary usability characteristics they are unlikely to be successfully applied. In consequence, it is very important for developers to take into account the characteristics of different end-users, the things they do and want to do differently, and where and when they want to do them. This Chapter offers advice on how to get the relevant design knowledge about these issues.

2. Description of the Participatory Approach and Methods

The key concept of participatory approaches is a design for all philosophy or strategy, based upon the principle that products should be usable by as wide a range of the population as possible. Design for all is based on the notion that by ensuring that the least able can use a product, one maximises the numbers of potential users, and also creates products which can be easier for the more able to use as well.

2.1 Problem Being Addressed

The concept has much to offer, as by designing for less able groups it becomes possible to accommodate larger numbers of able people as well. For example, ensuring that health care information is accessible not only for medical practitioners but for their patients as well allows for appropriate lifestyle accommodation of the patients and at the same time makes it easier for practitioners to tele-monitor patients' health status from distance, unless excess of certain threshold values calls for professional intervention. Therefore, most generally participatory approaches allow user-involved and consensus-based design of systems to be used by different end-user communities.

2.2 Devices / Techniques Used

There are a variety of instruments or devices that can be used to plan and organise a participatory inquiry. Some of them are described below.

2.2.1 Short Visits to End-User Sites

Description
Generally visits aim at some kind of contextual inquiry. They are best carried out by a group of researchers who develop a medium- to long-term relationship with an end-user target group (i.e., physicians and patients) who are interested in providing data. Holtzblatt and Jones (1993) have identified the following steps to organise visits for contextual inquiry:

- Identifying the customer: identify the groups that will be using the new technology or are using similar technology, and arrange to access organisations within the groups that give a cross section of the overall target population
- Arranging the visit: write to the targeted organisations identifying the purpose of the visit, a rough time-table, and how long of the visiting time the exercise will take. Ensure that some feedback from the visit is possible before leaving. Ensure that the participating end-users understand how many visits evaluators intend to make over the time period of the evaluations.
- Identifying the users: a software product will affect many people not just the patient as end user, but also presumably his family, relatives and friends. Evaluators should ensure that they understand the key persons in this context who will additionally be affected by a new system or changes in the current one.
- Setting the focus: Evaluators should beforehand select what aspects of the users' usage problems they wish to make the focus of each visit, and write down their starting assumptions. They should make a statement of purpose for each visit, and after the visit, evaluate to what extent they have achieved their purpose.
- Carrying out the interview / observation: Evaluators should stay with the selected users until they have managed to answer the questions they have raised in 'setting the focus'. Very often this may involve inviting the user to directly share and comment on the evaluator's notes and assumptions.
- Analysing the data: the process of analysis is interpretative and constructive. Conclusions and ideas from one round of observations have to be input to the next round, and an evaluation of the results so far should be one of the purposes of subsequent visits.

When to use it

Short visits for contextual inquiry is one of the best methods to use when evaluators really need to understand the patients' usage context. The environment in which people make use of a system or a service really influences how they use the product. Thus, this technique is highly effective for finding out about usage practices in domains evaluators know nothing about. The technique is best used in the early stages of development, since a lot of the information the evaluator will get is subjective, e.g., how people feel about their health problems, how they deal with it by using technological means, etc. In conclusion, short visits as a complete micro-method is summarised in Table 1.

Table 1. Short visits for contextual inquiry

Name of method	Short visits for contextual inquiry
Problem being addressed	Gain a better understanding of the relationship physician/patient, their respective expectations, interactions, attitudes and views
Device/technique used to address the challenge	Open, unstructured interviews/discussions
Procedure	Gain confidence of the person to be visited, explain relevance of the research, arrange an appointment
Outcomes	Better understanding of the specific situation of the patient, gain trust of both physicians and patients re further questioning and for pilot experiments, first hypotheses to be pursued in further research
Assumptions	Only a stepwise approach fully involving physicians and patients will motivate them to participate in such research

2.2.2 Questionnaires

Description

The questionnaire provides a structured way of gathering information. It allows for the same question to be asked in the same way to a number of informants. This enables statistical analysis of the data to be used, which allows a large amount of information to be summarised in a convenient form. A questionnaire can be constructed to investigate user experience with a product, their need for a new product, identification of how well they do with the technology they use etc. A typical questionnaire consists of a limited number of questions with pre–defined answer categories, focused on the topic of interest. It can also consist of some more open questions where the informants need to write in answers in their own words. Questionnaires are usually distributed to a sample of the target population and the responses are collected and then summarised using statistical analysis. Such a questionnaire can also be used in an interview situation where an interviewer reads the questions and fills in the answers on behalf of the subject.

When to use it

Questionnaires are often used when there is a potentially large number of users of a product, and a developer wants to obtain information from as large a sample of these as possible. Questionnaires can be a cost effective way of obtaining background information, as the use of postal questionnaires is much less resource intensive than conducting large numbers of personal interviews, and is particularly useful when informants live some distance from each other. Postal questionnaires can be used to collect a wide range of information, including background information about the persons themselves, and their opinions regarding existing equipment and future design options. One advantage of questionnaires is that the informant can spend all the time they want in filling out the form, allowing them to make up their mind without any external pressure. For some disabled informants, this might ensure responses that would not come out in an interview or group discussion. Postal questionnaires, which do not require the respondent to identify him/herself, may also make it easier for the respondent to answer personal or potentially embarrassing questions, due to the anonymity which such techniques may provide, compared with other methods. Questionnaires can vary in the degree to which they are structured, and for postal use structured questionnaires are likely to be of most value. Structured questionnaires are useful for obtaining simple factual information, rather than complex opinions however, as respondents are forced to make simple answers to questions or to chose from limited sets of options. More open questions can be used to some extent in postal questionnaires, but as there is no opportunity to discuss the question and answers with respondents, their use in these cases is limited. Less structured questionnaires are more appropriate for use as part of personal interviews, where any ambiguity in question and answer can be resolved. In addition, less structured questionnaires are more appropriate for addressing issues, which are inherently complex e.g., the requirements that a person may have for products in the future.

2.2.3 Interviews

Description

Interviews are conducted talking to an informant, either directly or on the telephone. Individual opinions and subjective preferences about products can be collected. The interview can be performed in a structured manner using a questionnaire which is filled in by the interviewer (see previous section) or it can be more open ended using an interview guide that describes the areas the interview should cover. Since the interview is conducted on a one–to–one manner, it should be possible to create an atmosphere that facilitates good responses, which clears up misunderstandings about the questions and ensures that the informant expresses what he/she really means. It can also be performed in the informant's home or workplace. People who also have problems in expressing their opinions in groups should be interviewed instead.

When to use it

Interviews can be carried out at any stage of the design process as a means to gather information. They can be used to identify detailed user requirements and to be informed about the user's experience with a particular product. In the user requirements stage, unstructured or semi–structured interviews should be used to allow the process to be user led. In later phases of design more structured forms, such as an administered questionnaire may be used. The interview is especially appropriate when questions are of a sensitive nature, or complex information is involved, as is often the case in the Assistive Technology area. It is also suitable when it is suspected that the interviewees might be low on motivation to participate or give information. Interviews are a more time consuming method to use than questionnaires, particularly if data are collected from a large number of informants. However, if the number of informants is small (and especially if the informants have problems filling in a questionnaire) the interview is the most cost efficient method. If the information is recorded using a tape recorder, a considerable amount of time is used transcribing the tape. It is often more efficient to use two interviewers, and let one take notes throughout the interview whilst the other asks the questions. Finally, Table 2 describes interviewing, as a complete micro-method.

Table 2. Interviews

Name of method:	Formal, partially structured interviews (patients)
Problem being addressed	Gaining a better understanding of specific design issues and identification of patient priorities, capabilities and needs
Device/technique used to address the challenge	Structured questionnaires, paper copies of screen shots
Procedure	Mailing of explanatory letter and questionnaire, screen shots; arrangement by telephone of a time slot for a more detailed telephone interview or for a visit to the patient's home; realisation of the interview and writing a record of the results; integration of results from all interviews
Outcomes	Structured assessment and record of design issues, priorities, solutions preferred, etc.
Assumptions	Patient involvement and knowledge of their expectations, attitudes and experiences are key ingredients for developing guidelines for design-for-all access by patients to their EHR

2.2.4 Brainstorming

Description

Brainstorming is one of several techniques to facilitate group creativity and is one of the oldest and best known. The idea is to let people come together and inspire each other in the creative, idea generation phase of the problem solving process. Brainstorming is used to generate new ideas by freeing the mind to accept or criticise any idea that is suggested, allowing freedom for creativity. The tool has been broadly used in design. However, there has been a wide range of studies intended to evaluate the efficiency of the technique, and the majority of these studies shows that people who is working in isolation produce more and better ideas than when working as a group. So, why is brainstorming still so popular? One important reason is probably that the group process as such is rewarding and creates a feeling of ownership of the result. In the brainstorming process everybody in the group can take credit for good ideas. The result of a brainstorming session is hopefully a couple of good ideas, and a general feel for the solution area.

Table 3. Brainstorming

Name of method:	Focus groups, brainstorming with care personnel, experts
Problem being addressed	Obtaining a more detached, objective assessment of patients' situations, needs and capabilities re accessing their EHR
Device/technique used to address the challenge	Semi-structured, open discussions
Procedure	Meeting in a pleasant environment, creation of an open, trustful atmosphere, provision of lists of potential access forms/devices; copies of screen shots; list of issues and topics to be covered
Outcomes	Structured lists of issues and problems, suggestions for solutions, generalisable assessments of priority issues, of patients' capabilities and needs, recommendations for seamless integration into the overall care process
Assumptions	People who regularly care for and have contact with these patients are in a better, more neutral position to assess universal access and interface design issues than individual patients who can only report about their individual experience and expectations and who may under- or overestimate their capabilities, may be too shy to admit their real access problems etc.

When to use it
Brainstorming is usually applied in the very early stages of design. Especially when there are people with different backgrounds that can give different input to the design process, brainstorming may be a good start. Table 3 summarises the method described above as a complete micro-method.

2.2.5 User Trials

Description
In user trials, "real users" test a product trying it out in a relatively controlled or experimental setting, where they are given a standardised set of tasks to perform. The result can be a "problem list" which contains valuable information for designers regarding the potential for improving the usability of a product. Time spent completing a task or the number and types of errors made in use, is information that can be used to compare two different products or two versions of the same user interface. Subjective statements about acceptance are normally part of the results of such trials. The testing procedure originates from experimental psychology, and may be performed in a very formal way, performing controlled experiments and using statistical analysis techniques. However, in this section we will describe a simpler or more "qualitative" approach to such trials, requiring that observers have an understanding of the system to be tested so that they can easily deduct from the user's behavior that a problem has been encountered. In doing this, knowledge of the user group is, of course, also very valuable in interpreting the results of such trials. In this situation, the observer must however, be aware that there is always a possibility of "seeing what you want to see". Using more than one observer will minimise this problem and is to be encouraged as a general procedure to follow. In usability laboratories, it is also common to videotape users interactions with the system being evaluated, as this allows particular events to be reviewed after the trials are completed, and also acts as a useful record of problem interactions. This also can be particularly useful as a medium of communication, allowing others to see the problems experienced by users in the trials. For a more detailed guide to usability testing see Dumas and Redish (1993).

When to use it
User trials are normally applied when a prototype product is running, or when a complete product is to be evaluated. Low-tech mock-ups and prototypes may also be used. They are often used before a final product design has been agreed on, and are commonly used on pre-production prototypes. They are often used as a simpler way of evaluating products compared to more extensive field trials, which commonly take place when a more completed product is to be evaluated prior to market release. Table 4 summarises the method in terms of the criteria applicable to complete micro-methods.

Table 4. User trials

Name of method:	User trials in controlled or experimental settings
Problem being addressed	Trying out a product or service with targeted end-users in a relatively controlled experimental setting, where they are given a standardised set of tasks to perform.
Device/technique used to address the challenge	Observation of prototype or mock-up application by targeted end-users/ Evaluation of appropriate thinking aloud protocols'
Procedure	Compare usage of different system versions or different versions of the same user interface.
Outcomes	"problem list" which contains valuable information for designers regarding the potential for improving the usability of a product or service.
Assumptions	When using such techniques with frail or severely ill patients, it is important to take into account, that such users may require long periods of time to become comfortable using a new alternative products and services , and in addition some of the problems users are likely to experience with new products will only manifest themselves after extended periods of use.

2.2.6 Task Analysis

Description

Task analysis can be defined as the study of what a user is required to do, in terms of actions and/or cognitive processes, to achieve a task objective. The idea is that task analysis provides some structure for the description of tasks or activities, which then makes it easier to describe how activities fit together, and to explore what the implications of this may be for the design of products. This can be particularly useful when considering the design of interfaces to products, and how users interact with them. Task analysis can be applied to studying how users use existing products, and such an analysis will assist in the process of understanding the difficulties they face in using existing products, and improvements that might be needed. Task analysis techniques can also be used in a predictive fashion to represent how users may operate products that are being developed. Such representations can act as a vehicle for communication between developers and others involved in the development process e.g., end users or their representatives. Task analysis techniques can also assist in the development of training manuals for products, as the structure that is implicit within the design of an interface is more easily revealed when represented in such a way. Task analysis techniques can also be used in the development of evaluation plans, as an understanding of what activities are the most important to the user or have critical consequences for their safety helps place priorities on any evaluation studies planned. Information on how often different activities need to be performed is also particularly useful to have for these purposes.

An important point to be made is that in order to be maximally effective, such an analysis should be extended to encompass all of the user's interactions with a product or device. In addition to everyday tasks, more infrequent tasks such as maintenance and cleaning, as well as known types of misuse, should be included in the analysis. All forms of task analysis are concerned with the description and representation of tasks or activities, and provide organisation and structure to that description. This can be useful when describing an existing set of activities performed by a person, but also is of value when trying to design a new product. Thinking through the sequences of activities that a person would need to go through to use a product can assist in identifying whether these are organised logically or not, and can assist in designing and redesigning the operations needed to use a product. Two processes are usually followed when a task analysis is conducted. The first of these is some understanding of sequence or dependency between different activities. Thus it is important to understand a particular activity in the wider context. For example, a person using a communication aid may want to communicate hunger, but first needs to attract the attention of the person with whom they want to communicate. After they have communicated hunger, there is a need for them to be fed. The second process is one of representing how activities or tasks fit together. This is a process of representing how large tasks can be decomposed into smaller components, and the logical relationship between these. A common technique used is called hierarchical decomposition, which means breaking larger activities into smaller activities until a sufficient level of detail is reached. A good way of achieving such decomposition is to repeatedly ask the question "how" to break activities into smaller units. For example in a communication aid where an identified activity is to attract the attention of the teacher, this might be further de-composed into the child having to press a specific button on the communication aid, repeating the key press in the event of no response by the teacher etc. One well-known approach, which breaks tasks or activities down into smaller units, is the Hierarchical Task Analysis (HTA) technique developed by Shepherd (1989). In addition to decomposition it is also common when using task analysis to explore how activities fit into a wider context. It can be useful to repeatedly ask the question "WHY" in order to assist in this process, with activities becoming increasingly more abstract.

When to use it
The technique should be used during the analysis phase of design to ensure proper description of user activities. It can be used to analyse interactions with an existing system or as a means to structure discussions about a hypothetical product. Task analysis data can be used as input to the detailed design of interfaces to products, and can also be used in planning evaluation studies. In later stages of the development the current solution can be checked against the original task or activity analysis to see how the design deviates from the intended solution, and what consequences this leads to. Table 5 summarises task analysis as a complete micro-method.

Table 5. Task analysis

Name of method:	Task analysis (patients)
Problem being addressed	Gaining a better understanding of what a patient is required to do, in terms of actions and/or cognitive processes, to achieve a task objective
Device/technique used to address the challenge	Interviewing or observing patients and taking notes
Procedure	The first part of the analysis is to understand the activities to be represented by interviewing or observing patients and taking notes. This is followed by the representation of the activities in some way (e.g., flow charts, hierarchical decomposition and state transition diagrams), and a process of verification to confirm that the representations are correct reflections on the state of affairs.
Outcomes	Structured description of how activities fit together, what activities are the most important to the user or have critical consequences for their safety
Assumptions	Task analytical annotations act as a suitable vehicle for communication with patients, thus helping place priorities on developing guidelines for EHR product design

3. Method Validation

In this part of the Chapter we will describe how some of the above methods have been used in the context of the reference scenario of Chapter 9 to facilitate insight to universal access. Our collection of data and information relied on a variety of these methodological approaches appropriate for the question(s) under consideration, the respective situation of the persons involved, and their adequacy to elicit the information required for our research:

- Informal, only slightly structured interviews and (sometimes very intensive) discussions with physicians in their offices and patients in their homes.
- Interviews based on formal, partially structured questionnaires (using predefined questions with a limited number of response options as well as open questions), conducted face-to-face and over the telephone with patients.
- Focus group meetings with care personnel and people involved in providing telecare and social services.

3.1 Visits (Informal Interviews / Discussions)

Before undertaking any validation exercise of this kind, it is important to establish a well-founded rapport with all persons involved, be they physicians, nurses, care takers, patients or family members. The purpose is to gain their acceptance and to obtain their trust and confidence. It was expected that this would indeed help to motivate them to participate.

Unless a contact exists already in some other context, initial approaches can be made by letter (perhaps with a short written note about the purpose of the exercise), or by phone asking for an initial telephone exchange of 10 to 15 minutes at a time convenient to the other party. The purpose is to present the project and the objectives of contacting the physician and to allow him/her to ask questions etc.

If the response is positive and the physician signals enough interest, a face-to-face meeting lasting 30 to 60 minutes should be agreed upon. Considering the usual time burden on most medical professionals, these and the following contacts/steps should be planned carefully with sufficient lead and follow-up time.

Patients or their family members should always only be approached after their physician or care personnel have agreed to this, and perhaps only after they have introduced their patients to the researcher. Involving a project participant who is a medical doctor and therefore has professional experience in dealing with both sides is definitely an asset. A short list of discussion points with the physician may include the topics listed in Figure 1:

1.   Context of the research project/exercise, participants, funding
2.   Purpose and objectives to be achieved, next steps and overall work process, timetable
3.   Workload/demand on time anticipated for the physician, for the patients
4.   Selection criteria for participating patients, support in contacting the patients, next steps and time frame
5.   Ethical issues and their formal solution, confidentiality issues concerning patients
6.   Research methods and tools, analysis, expected results
7.   Expected benefits/utility for physician, his/her patients, society, ...
8.   Devices to be used, technical prerequisites and support, costs and their reimbursement
9.   Authorship of research results, potential publications in medical journals etc.
10. Any open questions, unsolved issues, formal agreements as needed
11. Exchange of telephone numbers, formal points of contacts in case questions or problems surface, or when emergency support is needed, etc.

Fig. 1. Informal interviews - discussion points for physicians

With patients, only a selection of such points should initially be discussed so that information is adequate and comprehensive, but not beyond their comprehension. Participation of a nurse or a first contact in the doctor's office will be helpful to faster gain their trust and motivation to participate. One or, at most, two researchers should participate in such informal interviews so that the other party is not overwhelmed. Observing these points and approaching carefully selected physicians known to be open to new approaches, experiments or research, we usually encountered interest and openness to participate. Once their doctor was convinced of the benefits of the project, patients - with rare exceptions - were usually more than happy to participate, too.

It turned out that visits and slightly structured interviews with physicians and patients are a time consuming, but extremely useful procedure to much better understand the application context, the relationships and interactions between physician and patient, their attitudes, expectations, problems, or non-verbal issues which may support (or interfere with) the consensual sharing of patient vital data and information, and access to the EHR by both physician and patient. At the same time, this helps to gain acceptance by these actors, to obtain their trust and confidence, to motivate them to participate, and thereby to prepare the ground for more formal analyses to follow.

3.2 Interviews

More formal, structured interviews, which contained both closed and open questions were devised, based on earlier experience as well as on questionnaires available from other research projects and the literature. In order not to overtax the time of the physicians or the patients, they focused on the primary objectives of the study and key assessment questions derived there from. As only a small sample of persons was interviewed, the demographics section was short - a detailed analysis, by, e.g., social status, is not warranted with a very small sample.

Of course, such questionnaires have to be in native language, and words used have to be at a linguistic level appropriate for the person interviewed. They were applied to the same persons with whom - at the start of the exercise - informal discussions as described above were undertaken. In the Appendix to this Chapter, excerpts from patient questionnaires translated into English are presented to stimulate the development of related questions in similar situations.

Formal, partially structured questionnaires proved very valuable to obtain a more in-depth understanding of specific issues of patient access to their EHR. An important aspect was that in such an interview situation each patient was 'alone' and could freely speak about his or her attitudes and expectations, but also about their computer literacy (or illiteracy), their individual interests and preferences in accessing their own data, the implications perceived for their relationship with the physician, etc.

3.3 Focus Group Meetings

Attempts to discuss such issues in a focus group/group discussion setting failed. Contrary to reports by others about discussion groups, there did not exist much interest in sharing such opinions with other patients. In view of the wide differences in individual interests, capabilities and experience with computers and the Internet, involvement in handling their disease and motivation to take an active part in managing it, and in the socioeconomic environment and education/income situation of patients, this result is not surprising. We observed this also in other contexts; this may be different with respect to the "average" citizens not suffering from any specific, severe chronic disease (with which some patients have already lived for many years) or for patients with an acute disease with which they have no experience and about which they have no knowledge, or for family members "only" interested in helping somebody, learning more about a certain disease etc.

On the other hand group discussions lead to a multitude of very useful and interesting suggestions and hints with respect to another group of concern for our research, namely care providers or other professional people who have considerable experience with such patients and their socioeconomic environment and their usage of ICT. Here our concern is a relatively homogeneous group of persons who are experienced in sharing knowledge and experience, who are used to observing activities of other persons and to supporting them in performing such activities, who can interact and are prepared to accept different opinions, to elaborate on ideas presented by others, to be constructive and helpful in improving the situation of patients and frail people at home. It turned out that meetings with a clearly defined focus and purpose, pre-structured by providing topics and issues for discussion, lists of concerns, examples or pictures of potential access devices, print-outs of screen shots etc. to support some kind of "artificial walkthrough" were much more fruitful than open brainstorming sessions without such prompts.

Because physicians as well as individual patients may have very specific and individualistic observations and suggestions (depending on former experience, personal situation, individual preferences and habits, etc.), focus group discussions may prove very useful in providing a broader, more generic perspective, and also lead to useful assessment results otherwise more difficult to attain. They were undertaken with two groups: On the one hand with a small group of carers and nurses involved in directly dealing with individual patients, on the other hand with a few selected professionals involved with, or planning to deliver, telecare services to older people. This provided us with more generic insights from the perspective of both patients in their respective individual settings and providers marketing and sustaining such services and their perceptions of user needs, attitudes and expectations. The Appendix to this Chapter presents excerpts from a focus group discussion guideline translated into English:

Introductory items:

Welcome
Introduction of each participant
Context of research, study or exercise
Objectives and purpose of meeting
Duration of meeting, procedural rules etc.
Expected outcomes, benefits

Generic issues:

Role and relevance of patient access to their EHR data

Set of data most relevant/useful for patients (in different situations)

Generic issues of data access and presentation (i.e., selection of data for presentation, flexibility of selection and presentation format, level of competence of patients, technical versatility and computer literacy, etc).

Motivation of patients and their involvement in the management of their disease

Etc.

Specific topics:

A) Access devices

Available in patient home (paper/fax, telephone, TV, desktop computer, etc)

New types (cellular phones, PDAs, tablet PC/mobile pads, etc)

Appearance (size, weight, signals for status, etc)

Menu/general presentation issues

Usability

Quality (waterproof, sensitivity to falls, etc)

Reliability

General functionality (battery life, buttons, key board, acoustic signals, etc)

B) Presentation of EHR data

(Discussion may be supported by pictures/copies of screen shots, etc. The following items may be discussed repeatedly for each screen shot)

Selection mode for desired data/access interface

Type of presentation (graphical, tabular, etc)

Quantity of data presented, time frame (day, week, etc)

One data set at a time, or two or more sets in parallel

Naming of graphs, data points etc.

Size and type of letters and numbers

Use of colours

Identification of upper and lower bounds/limits

Simplicity/complexity of overall presentation

Etc.

Outlook:

Feedback, next steps, etc.

Thank you!

Fig. 2. Excerpts from a focus group discussion guideline

The results of these meetings were recorded in short written notes and annotations (in native language) based on the numbering of the discussion guideline and amended/complemented with new headings/key words as new topics arose from the discussions which were deemed relevant to the assessment.

Unfortunately, at the present stage of development, concrete user trials and specific task analyses could not yet be performed. However, in case further resources should allow progress to the stage of a simple prototype application to be demonstrated to patients, it is expected that these methods will be indispensable to further develop universal access criteria for patient access to their EHR.

4. Discussion

As indicated above, research based on these methodologies is of a preliminary, rather exploratory nature, and the sample of patients involved is both small in numbers and concerns a very specific group. As a consequence, findings cannot be generalised in any quantitative sense; rather, they should be regarded as a first indication of the variety and breadth of issues to be taken into account when seriously considering access for patients to their EHR. Key generic results of the participatory methodology used to elicit Universal Usability recommendations relate to general conclusions, access devices, and presentation of EHR contents.

Generally only those data of particular importance for most patients, which they can understand, interpret in their relevance and assess with regard to their implications for lifestyle, behaviour and medication, should be pre-selectable for access by the patient. In other words, as a first important step, only a (flexible) subset needs to be easily accessible in a different non-physician/care provider mode by the patient. This patient subsystem should be flexible with respect to the data to be selected for inclusion, the set available for viewing by patients, the range of access devices used for viewing the data, and the modes of presenting the data and adjusting their presentation.

Generally patients must have access rights to their whole medical history, i.e., to all data any doctor has about them on file. However, adequate presentation of any and all of this data can only be accomplished in the longer term. A priori, it must be taken into account that even for a very specific, chronic situation affecting several patients at the same time, patient access and viewing must be adjustable to their individual situation. As already mentioned above, even those patients are very different with respect to their computer literacy (or illiteracy) and experience of the Internet and various access devices, their individual interests and preferences in accessing their own data, their personal involvement in handling their disease and motivation to take an active part in this, and also in the socio-economic environment and education/income situation.

To initiate the concept of patient access to their EHR and support its diffusion, those modes of access and access devices which patients are familiar with should be used, and where the probability that it is available in their household or can easily be implemented is high:

Paper:	Most patients state as first priority a presentation of their weekly or monthly data on a piece of paper. This is a mode they are used to, and which sometimes already today can be accessed, albeit cumbersome, by asking their physician for a print-out during a visit or by postal mail. Easy, flexible, on demand access would be via a telefax machine attached to their telephone, a printer connected to the PC or laptop available in the household (with a connection to a telecom network), or as an extension to a TV set-top-box.
Telephone:	It is the most widely used and familiar access device and a 'must' for severely ill chronic patients. But even modern ISDN telephones do not have displays suited for presenting the type of data under discussion. So far, a telephone is only suited as an 'intermediate' access device for other modes of presentations via a fax machine or a screen.
PC/laptop:	A computer is not unusual in the household these days, and even elderly people are getting more and more into using them, also for accessing the Internet and its Web services. One of our patients, who is almost 80 years old, turned out to be very computer literate, and, not surprisingly, his preferred access medium is his PC. And with younger patients having relevant experience at the workplace, this will become more and more familiar.
TV:	Accessing their EHR via a TV screen is still a new idea for most patients. But as a TV set is available in all households and more than 40% of older people are used to accessing information via teletext, it is not surprising that they would, in principle, very much favour such an access device (except for those used to a computer). Indeed, it is to be expected that this would be the preferred means of access if the technology to achieve this were available. In this sense, the TV screen and technologies adapted from the ones people are used to when accessing different TV programmes, and Teletext would be the most "universal" ones from the point of view of the majority of patients.

Other access devices such as mobile telephones are not favoured; those who have some experience with them regarded them as too complex and difficult to use, and the screen is simply too small at present (similar considerations would apply to using PDAs - but children probably would favour such devices). Mobile access beyond the home is also no issue because these high-risk patients do not travel much and have to be close to some sort of storage for their dialysate fluid several times a day. Whether mobile Web pads used within the home would be an interesting alternative remained unclear; people are not yet familiar with this technology.

Briefly summarised the results obtained when presenting and discussing appropriate screen shots, at the generic level some general observations are particularly relevant. Patients must be able to carry out amongst other tasks, the following:

- Select those data from the universe of information which are particularly relevant for their very specific situation

- Access these data any time they want
- Switch from a graphical to a tabular presentation format
- Change the time period shown (weekly, bi-weekly, monthly)
- Switch from seeing only one data set to two or three shown in parallel

Since patients have very heterogeneous preferences, some prefer to see only one data set at a time (more is too complex for them), others insist on at least two in parallel to get a "feeling" for the correlation between these vital data. Depending on their subjective health status or changes in it, they want to look at the data immediately rather than in a more usual weekly or even bi-weekly rhythm. And although a graphical presentation of time series data is clearly the preferred mode, one patient would rather look at the more familiar tabular form in which he was used to seeing similar data.

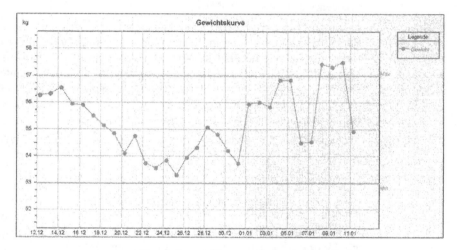

Graph 1: weight measures for one month

Graph 1, a graphical presentation of the daily weight of the patient, identifies a presentation format approved by all. This basic type of graphical presentation of time series data by a line connecting the daily values, and thereby allowing easy identification of changes in the value, was favoured also for all other relevant patient vital data. However, some detailed suggestions for improvement were made for easier comprehension by patients:

- Larger type of letters for heading of the graph, numbers on the axes, and legend.
- Clearer identification and naming of axes
- more contrasting colours and a thicker line to identify the upper and lower bounds of the values pre-set for the patient's weight by the nephrologist
- more prominent identification of values lying outside of the pre-set boundaries (e.g., by a red flag, a flashing signal or similar).

In addition, patients very clearly voted for an option to have these data presented for different lengths of time periods and for earlier time periods.

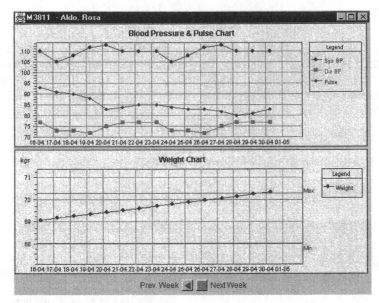

Graph 2: Combination of blood pressure, pulse and weight chart on one screen

The same basic considerations apply to Graph 2, although here the heading of the graph is much more prominent and readable. Integrating the value for "pulse" into the upper graph was not regarded as useful, and this line should be deleted. Whereas some patients preferred the simplicity of to the more complex combined presentation of several vital data in, others voiced a very strong preference for having these data presented in tandem. This assessment strongly correlates with the age and activity level of the respective patient and his self-assessment as to whether he can use these data for himself to adjust behaviour, diet and even medication to return the measured data to the optimal level prescribed by the physician.

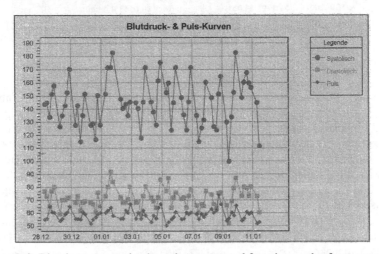

Graph 3: Blood pressure and pulse values, measured four times a day for two weeks

Graph 3 presents four daily measurement values for blood pressure and pulse. Again, the value for pulse was regarded as disturbing rather than supporting comprehension of these vital data. An option to stretch or draw out the values for the same time period over a greater width would be useful, and an option to somehow "relate" the respective systolic to the diastolic value was identified as perhaps useful to better understand the meaning of these data. Again, whereas some patients assessed this graph as very helpful, others were overwhelmed by its complexity and preferred the presentation of only the daily mean values as in the two preceding graphs.

Table 6. Blood pressure and pulse values, measured four times a day for two weeks

Trends für

Telefon: Alter: 56 Jahre   Pat.-Nr.: Dias 1

Datum	Gewicht	Sys/Dia(Mitt)		Puls	
22.07.2001	95.8 kg 10:56	161 / 92 (150)	00:44	75	00:44
		170 / 97 (155)	10:58	68	10:58
		159 / 90 (136)	13:44	69	13:44
		156 / 93 (131)	18:27	66	18:27
21.07.2001	95.8 kg 10:45	148 / 88 (119)	00:55	78	00:55
		155 / 92 (138)	10:46	68	10:46
		155 / 87 (107)	12:36	73	12:36
		156 / 84 (132)	16:52	72	16:52
20.07.2001	95.20 kg 10:47	165 / 92 (144)	20:56	69	20:56
		163 / 92 (147)	00:44	72	00:44
		152 / 96 (129)	10:49	72	10:49
		156 / 87 (126)	13:16	72	13:16
19.07.2001	94.87 kg 10:13	146 / 85 (118)	21:15	80	21:15
		159 / 91 (130)	00:51	76	00:51
		150 / 92 (137)	10:16	68	10:16
		151 / 91 (134)	13:04	66	13:04
		156 / 89 (137)	17:16	68	17:16
18.07.2001	94.33 kg 10:14	154 / 88 (136)	21:45	69	21:45
		160 / 94 (131)	00:59	72	00:59
		156 / 95 (134)	10:17	70	10:17
		145 / 92 (124)	13:58	65	13:58
17.07.2001	95.20 kg 11:08	153 / 90 (132)	19:11	66	19:11
		184 / 98 (143)	11:10	67	11:10
		145 / 90 (120)	13:16	69	13:16
		152 / 90 (121)	17:37	68	17:37
		152 / 87 (127)	21:37	75	21:37

Although PD patients are used to seeing their data in tabular form, Table 6 was heavily criticised. The following recommendations were made: a better separation of the daily blocks of values (e.g., by a horizontal line or a gap); a clear identification of the meaning of each value (time is not identified as such); no abbreviations; deletion of the mean blood pressure value (which patients cannot put a meaning to); data measured at the same point in time should be on the same line. Data for a longer time period and mean daily values would also be helpful. But as mentioned earlier, most patients prefer a graphical presentation to such tabular presentations because it allows them to more easily and quickly identify trends over time which would indicate that some change in behaviour or medication is needed, and which identify critical values in an easy manner.

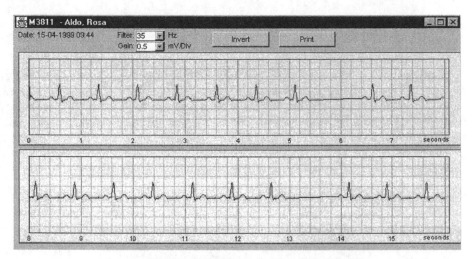

Graph 4: 16 second rhythm strip (one-lead ECG)

Graph 4 was rejected by all patients as not useful for them. This is the type of data they cannot make sense of, and experts were afraid that small irregularities like the one seen in this graph, but which - according to physicians - does not signal a real problem, would only unnecessarily disturb patients and even lead to bothersome phone calls to the physician.

5. Concluding Remarks

Having access to their EHR and being able to see selected vital data in such an improved form was highly welcomed by all patients. Although some preferred access in paper form, e.g., via a fax machine at home, others would welcome access via a standard computer and an easy to use, but flexible interface they are already used to, or on a TV screen with an easy to handle, very simple remote control[1]. Amongst the patients interviewed, there was none for whom this would not be a realistic option as long as the interface is easy to handle, uses large buttons and large characters etc. as outlined above. But of course, for severely disabled persons such as blind patients, this access mode would break down and a different interface had to be used.

---

[1] Already in the early 90s pilot applications showed that even very frail old (90) ladies can operate such a system, see Stroetmann and Erkert (1999).

Appendix – Excerpt from the Patient Questionnaire

Dear patient,
Your opinion is important to us and will help to improve our tele-monitoring devices and the presentation of your vital data on a computer or TV screen or paper, and to design them to your needs. We will visit you in person / call you to discuss the following questions / issues with you. We expect that this will take about 20 – 30 minutes of your time.
Thank you !

Study-No.: _____   installation date: _____

Investigator: _____ current date: _____

Was the installation made punctually according to your appointment ?

   O   O   O   O   O
   Yes   No   greater than: 15 min.   30 min.   60 min.
   delay

Are you satisfied in the way devices have been installed and explained to you ?

Installation: O   O
                    Yes   No   if No:

Explanation: O   O
                    Yes   No   if No:

Are the user-manuals and descriptions of the devices easy to understand ?

           O   O   O
      not read   Yes   No   if No:

Are you satisfied with the in-home placement/mobility of the devices ?

Weighing: O   O
                    Yes   No   if No:

Home Hub: O   O
                    Yes   No   if No:

Blood Pressure-Unit: O   O
                    Yes   No   if No:

Heart Rhythm-Unit: O   O
                    Yes   No   if No:

Do you feel comfortable using the Blood Pressure-cuff and Heart Rhythm-Unit-wrist bands ?

Blood Pressure-cuff: O   O
                    Yes   No   if No:

wrist bands: O   O
                    Yes   No   if No:

Are you satisfied with the way measurements are displayed and/or announced ?

Weighing:

Display:	O	O	
	Yes	No	if No:

announcement:	O	O	
	Yes	No	if No:

Blood Pressure-Unit:

Display:	O	O	
	Yes	No	if No:

Heart Rhythm-Unit:

Light & Sound	O	O	
	Yes	No	if No:

According to your experience, how easy are the devices to use ?

Weighing:	O	O	O	O	
	very easy	easy	not easy	difficult	because:

Blood Pressure-Unit:	O	O	O	O	
	very easy	easy	not easy	difficult	because:

Heart Rhythm-Unit:	O	O	O	O	
	very easy	easy	not easy	difficult	because:

Overall, are you satisfied with the Home-Telemonitoring-Devices and how would you rate your satisfaction ?

Weighing:	O	O	O	O	O
	very good	good	average	below average	worse

Blood Pressure-Unit:	O	O	O	O	O
	very good	good	average	below average	worse

Heart Rhythm-Unit:	O	O	O	O	O
	very good	good	average	below average	worse

overall impression:	O	O	O	O	O
	very good	good	average	below average	worse

Would you like to have access personally to your data (chart and/or diagram) ?

	O	O	O
	Yes	sometimes	No

Remarks:

....

Note for the interviewer: **As required, you may repeat some or all of the following questions for each chart/mock-up:**
With respect to having access to your own data, please have a look at the following graph/table/... (read the name/heading of the graph/table/... to the patient). We would like to have your opinion and discuss with you the following points:

which type of presentation do you prefer, which one is more readable for you?

....

....

What about the overall quantity of data presented in this graph (or table)?

....

....

Would you prefer to have these data only for a day, or rather for a week, or for a month, or ...?

O   O   O   O

1 day   1 week   1 month   other, specify:

....

....

Do you want data on each of your relevant vital data at a time, or do you think, for yourself it would be more helpful to have two or more sets of data shown in parallel?

....

....

What about the naming of the graph, of the data points etc. - would this be ok for you, or what would you suggest to be changed/improved?

....

....

May we also ask you how you assess the size and type of letters used in this chart?

....

....

And what about the use of colours to highlight some of the data or information?

....

....

Is it easy for you to identify the upper and lower bounds/limits set by your doctor for your vital data in the chart? Is it helpful for you?

....

....

How would you rate the overall presentation of data in the chart, is the overall presentation easy to understand, does it help you to guide yourself in better dealing with your chronic disease?

....

....

Are there any other comments, suggestions for improvement you could make?

....

....

....

....

After having discussed all charts with the patient:

To sum up our discussion of accessing your own health data, let me ask you three more questions:

If you could chose how to obtain your data, would you prefer the data on paper (e.g., via a fax machine), on your TV screen, via a computer screen, a mobile phone, or ...???

O   Paper (by mail) _____

O   Paper (by fax) _____

O   TV screen _____

O   Computer screen _____

O   Mobile phone _____

O   Other _____

Would you prefer to receive them daily, weekly, or in a different interval? Or would you rather chose yourself?

O	O	O	O
daily	weekly	different interval	chose myself

If different interval, please specify: _____

Would you like to make any other suggestions or remarks helpful for you to better look after yourself?

....

....

Last but not least: Do you have further comments not covered by the questions, or any remark you would like to mention here?

....

....

In your household, do you personally access/use regularly:

TV	O	O	O
	Yes	sometimes	No

If yes, do you use teletext?	O	O	O	
		Yes	sometimes	No

Fax machine	O	O	O
	Yes	sometimes	No

Mobile phone	O	O	O
	Yes	sometimes	No

Computer	O	O	O
(PC, laptop or similar)	Yes	sometimes	No

Please provide us with some information on your personal situation:

Your age: _____ years   **Gender:**   Male O   Female O

Primary (chronic) disease:

....

Any secondary disease: ....

....

New technologies can be complex and demand perfect vision or nimble fingers. What has your experience been? First, ...

..on some machines you have to touch on a screen. Do you find using touch-screens easy, somewhat difficult or very difficult - or have you not tried?

O	O	O	O
easy	*somewhat difficult*	very difficult	*Has not tried / no experience*

What about using your fingers to use a credit or similar card, when using a cash point, making a phone call, or paying for goods?

O	O	O	O
easy	*somewhat difficult*	very difficult	*Has not tried / no experience*

...and typing, say, your name, on a keyboard?

O	O	O	O
easy	*somewhat difficult*	very difficult	*Has not tried / no experience*

Thank you very much for your co-operation!

Chapter 22
IS4ALL Method Base: Choosing Micro-methods and Tailoring to Custom Practices

Demosthenes Akoumianakis[1] and Constantine Stephanidis[1,2]

[1] Foundation for Research and Technology – Hellas (FORTH)
Institute of Computer Science
Heraklion, Crete, GR-70013, Greece
cs@ics.forth.gr
[2] University of Crete
Department of Computer Science, Greece

Abstract. This Chapter provides a guide for choosing and tailoring methods from the IS4ALL method base. The Chapter provides an account of the scope of the methods in the development life cycle and an overview of the criteria to be considered in order for an organisation to make informed and effective choices. To this end, an attempt is made to present (examples of) alternative regimes for using the methods and thereby offering insight into the choice of relevant techniques.

1. Scope of Methods

In Figure 1, a summary is provided of the methods considered by IS4ALL and the specific stages in the software development life cycle. Each method listed in the right hand column is associated with a certain design target, which in turn falls in with a specific development stage. Thus for example, NFR analysis (see Chapter 13) can be used to identify relevant quality attributes to be supported by the system and which influence the system's requirements specification. An alternative view on the methods in the context of software development life cycle is to assess their relative input and / or output in relation to specific stages. As shown, for example, Non-Functional Requirements Analysis (NFRA) can be used to provide input to understanding the business needs, requirements elicitation and detailed design activities, while it can also lead to the identification (output) of a certain set of desirable or relevant quality attributes to be addressed in the course of design and development.

C. Stephanidis (Ed.): Universal Access Code of Practice in Health Telematics, LNCS 3041, pp. 297-309, 2005.
© Springer-Verlag Berlin Heidelberg 2005

	Understanding business needs	Eliciting requirements	Detailed design	Prototyping / Development	Assessment / Evaluation
Universal Access Assessment Workshop	Input	Input / Output	Input/ Output		
Unified User Interface Design		Input	Input	Input	Input
Non-functional Requirements Analysis	Input	Input/ Output	Input		
Screening		Input	Input/ Output		
W3C-WAI Content Accessibility Auditing		Input	Input/ Output		Input
Usability Inspection				Input	Input
Multimodal Interfaces			Input	Input	
Model-based development	Input			Input/ Output	
MedicSCORE		Input			Input
Standards adherence & Compliance			Input		Input/ Output
Participatory Methods		Input/ Output	Input		Input

Fig. 1. IS4ALL methods and software development lifecycle

Phase	Micro-design target	Method
Requirements engineering	• **Quality attributes** • **User interface requirements**	▪ **Universal Access Assessment Workshop** ▪ **Non-functional Requirements Analysis** ▪ **Unified User Interface Design** ▪ **Participatory Methods**
Concept formation & Design	• **Designing artifacts** • **Building design representations** • **Capturing design rationale** • **Low-fidelity prototypes**	▪ **Unified User Interface Design** ▪ **Model-based development** ▪ **Screening** ▪ **Participatory Methods**
Prototyping & Development	• **Supporting adaptation** • **Accessibility** • **Architectures for universal access**	▪ **Multimodal Interfaces** ▪ **Unified User Interface Design** ▪ **Model-based development**
Evaluation	• **Standards conformity** • **Usability** • **Benchmarking**	▪ **W3C-WAI Content Accessibility Auditing** ▪ **MedicSCORE** ▪ **Standards adherence & Compliance** ▪ **Usability Inspection**

Fig. 2. Method input / output in the context of software development stages

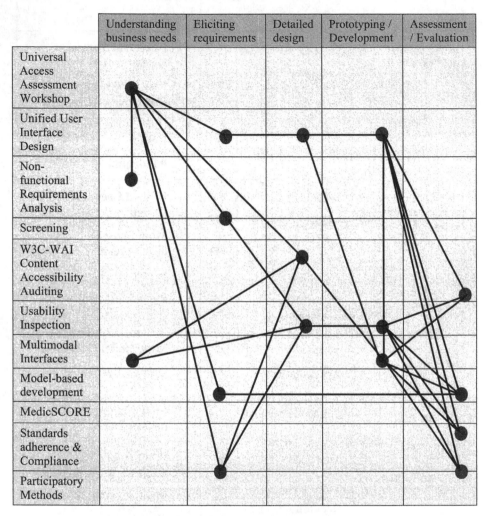

Fig. 3. Portfolios of IS4ALL methods

It is worth pointing out that the method grid presented in Figure 2 conveys clearly the broad scope of the methods and their capability to support most stages in a software development life cycle. Another important issue relates to the combination of methods. Figure 3 describes the links between the methods aiming to provide examples of potential method portfolios. The lines establishing links between methods provide an indication of method complementarity. Each line links one method used in a certain stage with other methods relevant to another stage of the software development life cycle. In this manner, one can obtain an overview of the alternative pathways through which an enterprise or a design team can progress across stages to attain specific targets. It is also evident that there is no best method or pathway since different design teams or enterprises may choose alternatives method portfolios depending on internal codes of practice (see section later on in this Chapter).

2. Examples of Alternatives Regimes for Using the Methods

To exemplify the above, let us assume the potential contribution of the IS4ALL method base under specific circumstances and design cases. We propose to address this by considering the following regimes:

- Starting a new project recognising that adaptability, scalability, platform independence and ubiquitous access constitute important qualities to be addressed
- Revising an early design concept so as to make it universally accessible
- Specifying requirements and undertaking detailed design work
- Building prototypes and computer mock-ups
- Improving the accessibility of an existing system

The above are representative of critical stages in a project's lifecycle, while illustrating alternative contributions of the universal access code of practice.

2.1 Staring a New Project

When starting a new project in which universal access is an important consideration, there are a series of considerations to be taken into account. A primary concern is the scope of universal access to be considered. It has been pointed out several times in the project's deliverables that universal access may imply different issues for different projects. For example, when the priority is to allow access to the broadest possible target user community then it is of paramount importance to provide a system that meets the requirements of all target user communities. In other words, adaptability to user groups becomes the primary consideration streamlining the design inquiry towards identifying alternative interaction styles, which may be appropriate for each different target user group.

In other projects, universal access may be relevant because of the long lifecycle of the product or service to be developed. For example, systems for managing electronic patient records or digital libraries are two examples of systems which are indended for long-term use irrespective of the prevailing technological paradigm. Long-term use in this context means continued use over a long period of time. For such systems, clearly an important concern is to ensure *scalability* across technological regimes of the same or different technological trajectories. For instance, in the current technological trajectory of internet-based services, one can identify alternative regimes, some being carried over from previous trajectories (i.e., desktop computer connected to the internet), while others are novel or forthcoming (next generation of cellular telephony, network attachable devices, ubiquitous computing).

To address requirements such as the above, IS4ALL has described a technique called non-functional requirements analysis (see Figure 4), which serves a two-fold purpose, namely identification of critical non-functional requirements (e.g., adaptability, scalability, personalisation, interoperability) for universal access and analysis of how these critical non-functional requirements are intertwined.

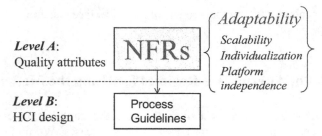

Fig. 4. NfRs and corresponding process-oriented design guideline

Using a suitable reference scenario (i.e., on-line management of pharmaceutical prescription orders), the project has exemplified the application of the non-functional requirement of adaptability and how the technique can be used to derive alternative design artefacts (see Figure 5). The outcomes of such a process provide designers with a concrete design space of competing alternatives, as well as a clear specification of what developers need to account when building the system.

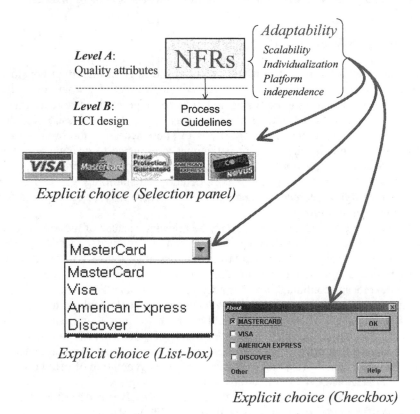

Fig. 5. Non-functional requirements and design artefacts

2.2 Revising an Early Design Concept

A common stage in re-engineering existing products or building new ones is the development of a design mock-up to provide a reference point for design deliberations between developers and end users. However, it is frequently difficult to plan and organise a such a process. IS4ALL has described how a technique called Universal Access Assessment Workshop (UA²W) can help define shortcomings in the design concept, as well as envision new contexts of use and corresponding design mock-ups (see Figure 6) by consensus. The technique makes use of a range of informal (or semi-formal) instruments to capture deliberations amongst design teams and to facilitate agreement on revised design concepts and artefacts. In this manner, design teams can use consensus creation methods to agree on the range of artefacts to be implemented, as well as to build the accompanying rationale for each alternative option. Figure 6, describes the outcome of this method for the case of making the on-line management of pharmaceutical orders accessible to a wider community including elderly at home, pharmaceutical professional on the road, etc. Similar validation exercises have been conducted with reference to the HYGEIAnet and WardInHand reference scenarios.

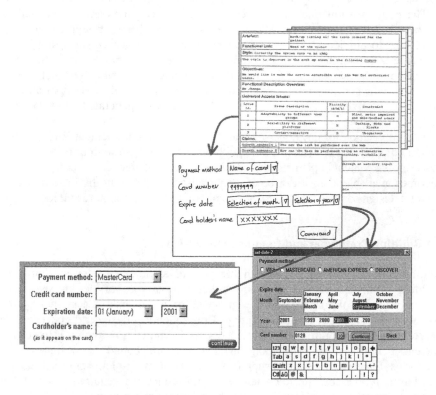

Fig. 6. Revising and extending design concepts to depict alternative use patterns

2.3 From Requirements to Detailed Design Work

The previous examples have illustrated the use of techniques to elicit requirements for universal access and translate these new requirements into concrete design alternatives. However, the methods did not address whether the alternatives should be lead to separate versions of a product or whether all alternative concepts should co-exist within the same implementation of the product. Clearly, such a consideration has impact not only on the technical approach to be followed by the development team, but also on the economics of universal access. Sometimes, it may be possible and indeed appropriate to consider maintaining two parallel versions of a product (i.e., one for desktop environments and one for WWW access). However, this is not necessarily a representative case of universal access. On the other hand, it is also hard to envisage as many different versions of the same product as the potential target user groups or the intended execution contexts. Consequently, the question of fusing alternatives into a common and extensible implementation becomes of paramount importance. IS4ALL has considered and detailed the application of a design method called unified user interface design, which allows designers to encapsulate design alternatives through abstractions. In the example depicted in Figure 7, this issue is illustrated by reference to our case study of on-line management of pharmaceutical orders.

The diagram shows how a concrete artefact (upper part) can be modelled as an abstract design component (middle part) and how this abstract design component can be refined to provide alternative implemented user interface versions to accomplish the same task though through different styles. Thus, one style has been devised for execution of the task on a small screen devise such as PDAs while yet another style is presented which allows text entry through a virtual keyboard. It is important to note that all three styles (including the original one) can be generated from the abstract design component.

The implication for developers is that they will need to implement only the abstract design component and establish links with other low-level resources (e.g., libraries or other tools), which implement the specified styles. Moreover, in case a new style becomes available, then it can be directly utilised by updating the links between the abstract design component and the physically realised interaction resources.

2.4 Building Prototypes and Computer Mock-Ups

Another critical point in the design lifecycle of an interactive system amounts to building computer mock-ups of low fidelity prototypes or design sketches. As discussed earlier the size of the design space of a universal access inquiry makes compelling the need for prototyping. Consequently, designers concerned with universal access require appropriate tools to facilitate prototyping. However, the current generation of prototyping tools today are bound to designated target platforms, thus offering limited support for cross- or multi-platform prototyping. The problem is further complicated when certain non-functional requirements pertinent to universal access (i.e., platform interoperability) are considered.

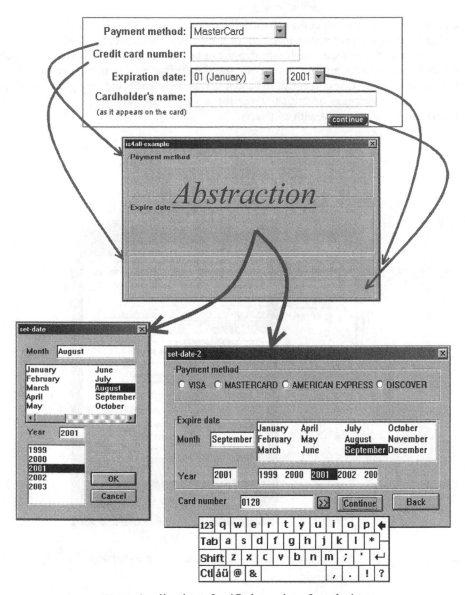

Fig. 7. Application of unified user interface design

To this effect, IS4ALL has explored model-based user interface development and has demonstrated the application of the technique across several application examples and design case studies. Some of the case studies considered prototyping of user-adapted interfaces, automatically generated from various models (i.e., user, interaction, dialogue, business, etc). Other examples have focused on developing prototypes to depict changes in the scope of use of a system (i.e., making a system available over a new platform). For example, Figure 8 depicts a version of the desktop user interface to the electronic patient record of HYGEIAnet, illustrated in the background, and a prototyped mock-up of a user interface running on the iPAQ. In model-based development, such prototypes can be easily compiled provided that the model for the target platform (in this case the iPAQ) is available to the user interface generation engine. Consequently, it becomes relatively easy and straightforward to build system mock-ups of critical tasks for a variety of purposes, including their evaluation and assessment with end users.

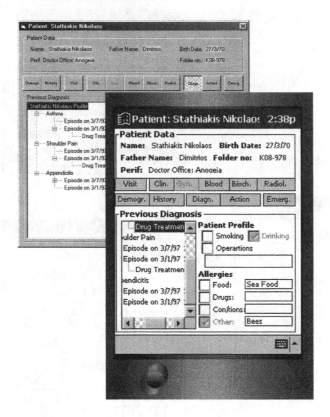

Fig. 8. Example of a task's interfaces on different platforms

2.5 Focusing on Accessibility

Finally, IS4ALL has addressed the issue of W3C-WAI guidelines compliance, which has recently received substantial attention. W3C-WAI guidelines seek to improve the accessibility of web sites and web-based information systems focusing primarily on disability access. The use of the guidelines can be two-fold. The first is in the context of a WCAG compliance audit to assess the degree to which an existing web site complies with the specifications suggested by the guidelines. The second potential use of the guidelines is to provide a means for formative design input, towards improving the final accessibility of the web site or service being developed. IS4ALL has addressed both these uses of the guidelines in separate accounts of the SPERIGEST reference scenarios depicting the practicalities involved in each form of inquiry.

One case study was devised with reference to the SPERIGEST initiative in Italy, where CNR-IFAC explored the use of the W3C Content Accessibility Guidelines for assessing and improving the accessibility of Web-based health services. A second case study dealt with accessibility of the HERMES platform empowering the D4ALLnet portal (see Figure 9).

1.1 Provide a text equivalent for every non-text element (e.g., via "alt", "longdesc", or in element content).

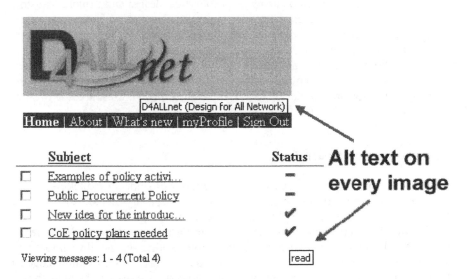

Fig. 9. Examples of embedding accessibility features in Web applications

3. Qualitative Criteria

In addition to the scope of the various methods, which determines method choice and use, there are also some qualitative criteria to be observed and which frequently constitute either impeding of facilitating factors. These are briefly discussed below in an attempt to unfold additional considerations involved in making informed and effective use of methods.

3.1 Gaining the Commitment of Management

An important influential factor in the choice of methods relates to the commitment of management to universal access. As in the case of usability engineering the higher the commitment of management the more complete and involved the design process will be. Completeness of the design approach means that the design team will pay the attention needed to all stages of design and make use of suitable methods to facilitate the objectives of each stage. This may entail a choice of user-based or participatory methods to gather functional and non-functional requirements (e.g., UA^{2}Ws), more demanding design techniques (e.g., unified design) to facilitate artefact representations and mock-ups, and advanced prototyping tools (e.g., TADEUS) which allow quick prototyping of design concepts and assessment of end users' feedback regarding the system being developed. However, all these methods would incur a cost, as they do not constitute typical design practice in prevalent software development paradigms.

Absence of management commitment to universal access will most likely hinder the willingness of the design team to engage in analytical design and explore plausible options. In this case, the universal access inquiry is likely to be limited in scope, resulting in ad hoc selection of methods. It is therefore important for the design team to realise and, if necessary, seek to obtain management commitment to universal access, as this is likely to act as catalyst and a driving force of design activities. Nevertheless, to gain this commitment, the design team should be able to justify the technical approach towards universal access, the claims made on resources as well as the expected / resulting benefits.

3.2 Competence of the Design Team

Finally, effective use of universal access methods requires some special skills, which should be available in the design team. These skills are typically method-specific. For example, seeking to assess compliance to a standard requires knowledge of the standard in question and experience in auditing. Similarly, assessment of the system's accessibility will require experience in using and interpreting accessibility guidelines, competence in the use of tools for carrying out such assessments and knowledge of the limits of these tools. However, one can expect that such skills will be available to the design team or could be easily acquired through external sources.

In addition to the above, there are methods, which can be effectively used only by specialised designers possessing detailed knowledge of certain design domains. Examples of such methods include the UA^{2}W, Non-functional requirements analysis, screening artifacts and model-based development methods for prototyping. Effective use of these methods typically requires prior experience in planning and conducting the design inquiry, and the capability to synthesise results of analytical inquiries. Moreover, the experience gained through the IS4ALL seminars reveals that training to use these methods in practical settings is important and necessary for designers to gain competence. Such training sessions do not need to be extensive but they do require detailed planning and execution to allow designers to gain hands-on experience in the use of specialised instruments for conducting the method. For instance, completing a UA^{2}F or compiling the UAQM require an understanding of the UA^{2}W method, the processes involved and the way in which the designer can move from the concrete to the abstract level.

4. Concluding Remarks

It is widely acknowledged in the international literature that providing clear and concise criteria for selecting design methods is not a trivial task, as much depends on the experience of the design team, the resources available, the specific needs of an enterprise, etc. Moreover, it is also common for organisations to tailor the methods chosen so that they can best fit with a certain organisational culture and pool of competencies. Consequently, organisations that wish to include universal access requirements in their software development life cycles will be best served if they can do so "organically." This means that the steps and artifacts of the methods presented in the IS4ALL code of practice, will require critical review, tailoring, blending, and, in some cases, refinement when integrated into an existing life cycle.

This Chapter provides some general criteria and guidelines for enterprises and professionals in an attempt to clarify the scope and intended use of the methods. From the previous discussion of the methods, their scope and intended use, several conclusions can be drawn. First, all the methods are scenario driven, with the scenarios serving as the "engine" for directing and focusing the methods' activities. This was a case peculiar to IS4ALL, but need not be a precondition for using the methods. Second, the methods focus on documenting the rationale behind the decisions made; in this way, the rationale serves as a knowledge base for both existing and future decisions. Third, they all involve different stakeholders, so that multiple views of universal access quality are elicited, prioritised, and embodied in the system being considered. Fourth, the methods can be tailored to the requirements and internal codes of practice of an enterprise or research group to ensure maximum benefit. Last, the methods exhibit a high degree of complementarity, in the sense that a consultant, a quality assurance group, or a research team can select the specific portfolio of methods to guide their development process.

References

Akoumianakis, D., & Stephanidis, C. (1997). Supporting user adapted interface design: The USE-IT system. *Interacting with Computers*, 9 (1), 73-104.

Akoumianakis, D., & Stephanidis, C. (2001). USE-IT: A Tool for Lexical Design Assistance. In C. Stephanidis (Ed.), *User Interfaces for All - Concepts, Methods, and Tools* (pp. 469-487). Mahwah, NJ: Lawrence Erlbaum Associates (ISBN 0-8058-2967-9, 760 pages).

Akoumianakis, D., & Stephanidis, C. (2003a). Blending scenarios of use and informal argumentation to facilitate universal access: Experience with the Universal Access Assessment Workshop method. *Behaviour & Information Technology*, 22 (4), 227-244.

Akoumianakis, D., & Stephanidis, C. (2003b). Scenario-based argumentation for universal access. In N. Carbonell, & C. Stephanidis, C. (Eds.), *Universal Access: Theoretical Perspectives, Practise and Experience - Proceedings of the 7th ERCIM Workshop "User Interfaces for All"*, Paris (Chantilly), France, 24-25 October (pp. 118 - 128). Berlin: Lecture Notes on Computer Science Series of Springer (LNCS 2615, ISBN 3-540-00855-1).

Akoumianakis, D., Savidis, A., & Stephanidis, C. (2000). Encapsulating intelligent interaction behaviour in unified user interface artefacts. *Interacting with Computers*, 12, 383-408.

Alspaugh, T., & Antón, A.I. (2001). *Scenario Networks for Software Specification and Scenario Management*. Computer Science Technical Report TR-2001-15, North Carolina State University, Raleigh, NC. [On-line]. Available at: http://www.ics.uci.edu/~alspaugh/pubs/alspaugh-tr15-2001.pdf

Balas, E.A., & Iakovidis, I. (1999). Distance Technologies for Patient Monitoring. *BJM*, 319 (7220), 1309-1311.

Barbacci, M., Ellison, R., Lattanze, A., Stafford, J., Weinstock, C., & Wood, W. (2002). *Quality Attribute Workshops (2nd Edition)*. Technical Report CMU/SEI-2002-TR-019 ESC-TR-2002-019.

Barbacci, M., Klein, M., Longstaff, T., & Weinstock, C. (1995). *Quality Attributes*. Technical Report CMU/SEI-95-TR-021 ESC-TR-95-021.

Bass, L., Clements, P., Kazman, R. (1998). *Software Architecture in practice*. Boston, MA: Addison Wesley Longman Publishing Co., Inc. (2nd Edition, 2003).

Bellotti, V., MacLean, A., & Moran, T. (1991). *Generating good design questions*. EuroPARC Technical Report EPC-91-136.

Bernsen, N-O. (1994). Foundations of multimodal representations, a taxonomy of representational modalities. *Interacting with Computers*, 6 (4), 347-371.

Beyer, H., & Holzblatt, K. (1998). *Contextual Design: Defining Customer-Centred Systems*. London: Morgan Kaufmann.

Bias, R.G., & Mayhew, D. J. (Eds.). (1994). *Cost justifying usability*. Orlando: Academic Press.

Boehm, B. (1978). *Characteristics of Software Quality*. New York: Elsevier North Holland Publishing Company, Inc.

Bolt, R.A. (1980). "Put-That-There": Voice and gesture at the graphics interface. *Computer Graphics*, 14(3), 262-270.

Buchanan, G., & Jones, M. (2000). Search interfaces for handheld Web browsers. In *Poster Proceedings of the 9th World Wide Web Conference* (pp. 86-87). [On-line]. Available at: http://www9.org/final-posters/48/poster48.html

Buie, E. (1999). HCI Standards: A Mixed Blessing. *Interactions*, 6 (2), 36-42.

Burzagli, L., & Emiliani, P-L. (2003). W3C-WAI Content Guidelines: application in a health scenario. In C. Stephanidis (Ed.), *Universal Access in HCI: Inclusive Design in the Information Society - Volume 4 of the Proceedings of the 10th International Conference on Human-Computer Interaction (HCI International 2003)*, Crete, Greece, 22-27 June (pp. 1078 - 1082). Mahwah, New Jersey: Lawrence Erlbaum Associates (ISBN: 0-8058-4933-5).

Buyukkokten, O., Molina, H.G., Paepcke, A., & Winograd, T. (2000). Power Browser: Efficient Web Browsing for PDAs. In *Proceedings of the SIGCHI Conference on Human Factors in Computing Systems* (pp. 430 - 437). New York: ACM Press.

Carrière, J., & Kazman, R. (1997). *Assessing Design Quality from a Software Architectural Perspective*. Technical Report, Software Engineering Institute, Carnegie Mellon University, Pittsburgh, PA.

Carroll, J. (Ed.). (1995). *Scenario-based Design: Envisioning Work and Technology in System Development*. New York: John Wiley & Sons, Inc.

Carroll, J. (Ed.) (2001). *Making Use: Scenario-Based Design Human-Computer Interactions*. Cambridge: MIT Press.

Carroll, J. & Rosson, M. B. (1992). Getting around the task-artefact cycle: how to make claims and design by scenario. *ACM transactions of Information Systems*, 10 (2), 181-212.

Ceusters, W., Smith, B., Kumar, A., & Dhaen, C., (2004) Mistakes in Medical Ontologies: Where do they come from and how can they be detected? In D. Pisanelli (Ed): *Ontologies in Medicine*. Proceedings of the Workshop on Medical Ontologies. Amsterdam: IOS Press.

Chung, L., Nixon, B., Yu, E., & Mylopoulos, J. (1999). *Non-Functional Requirements in Software Engineering*. Boston: Kluwer Publishing.

Cimino, J.J., Patel V.L., & Kushniruk A.W. (2001). What do patients do with access to their medical records? In V. Patel, R. Rogers, & R. Haux (Eds.): *MEDINFO 2001* (pp. 1440-1444). Amsterdam: IOS Press.

Clements, P., Kazman, R., & Klein, M. (2001). *Evaluating Software Architecture: Methods and Case Studies*. Boston, MA: Addison Wesley Longman Publishing Co., Inc.

Coutaz, J., & Caelen, J. (1991). A taxonomy for multimedia and multimodal user interfaces. In *Proceedings of the 1ˢᵗ ERCIM Workshop on Multimodal HCI* (pp. 143-148). Lisbon: INESC.

Danzon, P.M., & Furukawa, M.F. (2001). Health Care: Competition and Productivity. In R. Litan & A. Rivlin (Eds), *The Economic Payoff from the Internet Revolution. Brookings Task Force on the Internet* (p. 195). Washington, D.C.: The Internet Policy Institute, Brookings Institute Press.

De Moor, G. (1998) Towards Global Consensus and Co-Operation In Health Informatics and Telematics Standardisation. *International Journal of Medical Informatics*, 48, 1-3.

De Moor, G. (2003) Towards Individualized Health Management: the Importance of Bio-Medical Information Sciences. *Methods of Information in Medicine*; 42 (2), 4-6.

Dix, A., Finlay, J., Abowd, G., & Beale, R. (1998). *Human-Computer Interaction*. NJ, USA: Prentice-Hall, Inc., ISBN 0-13-239864-8.

Dumas, J.S. & Redish, J.C. (1993). *A practical guide to usability testing*. Norwood, NJ: Ablex Publishing.

Dunlop, M.D., & Davidson, N. (2000). Visual information seeking on palmtop devices. In *Proceedings of HCI 2000*, Vol. 2, pp. 19-20.

Embley, D.W., Kurtz, B.D., & Woodfield, S.N. (1992). *Object-Oriented Systems Analysis. A Model-Driven Approach*. Englewood Cliffs, NJ: Yourdon Press.

Erskine, L. Carter-Tod, D., & Burton, J. (1997). Dialogical techniques for the design of web sites. *International Journal of Human-Computer Studies*, 47, 169-195.

Fowler, M., & Kendall S. (1997). *UML Distilled - Applying the Standard Object Modeling Language*. Reading, Massachusetts: Addison Wesley.

Hall JA, Roter DL, & Katz NR. (1988). Meta-analysis of correlated provider behavior in medical encounters. *Medical Care*; 26, 657-675.

Hartson, H.R., Siochi, A.C., & Hix, D. (1990). The UAN: A User-Oriented Representation for Direct Manipulation Interface Design. *ACM Transactions on Information Systems,* 8 (3), 181-203.

Hoare, C.A.R. (1978). Communicating Sequential Processes. *Communications of the ACM*, 21 (8), 666-677.

Holtzblatt, K., & Jones, S. (1993). Contextual Inquiry: A Participatory Technique for System Design.' In D. Schuler & A. Namioka (Eds.), *Participatory Design: Principles and Practice* (pp. 180-193). Hillsdale, NJ: Lawrence Erlbaum Associates.

Iacucci, G., & Kuutti, K. (2002). Everyday life as a stage in creating and performing scenarios for wireless devices. *Personal and Ubiquitous Computing*, 6, 299-306.

Jarke, M., Tung Bui, X., & Carroll, J. (1998). Scenario management: An interdisciplinary approach. *Requirements Engineering*, 3, 155-173.

Johnson, P., Johnson, H., Waddington, P., & Shouls, A. (1988). Task-related knowledge structures: analysis, modeling, and applications. In D.M. Jones, & R. Winder (Eds.), *People and computers: from research to implementation - Proceedings of HCI '88* (pp. 35-62). Manchester: Cambridge University Press.

Kaplan, SH, Greenfield, S, & Ware, JE. (1989). Assessing the effects of physician-patient interactions on the outcomes of chronic disease. *Medical Care*, 27, S110-27.

Karampelas, P., Akoumianakis, D., & Stephanidis, C. (2003). User interface design for PDAs: Lessons and experience with the WARD-IN-HAND prototype. In N. Carbonell, & C. Stephanidis, C. (Eds.), *Universal Access: Theoretical Perspectives, Practise and Experience - Proceedings of the 7th ERCIM Workshop "User Interfaces for All"*, Paris (Chantilly), France, 24-25 October (pp. 474 - 485). Berlin: Lecture Notes on Computer Science Series of Springer (LNCS 2615, ISBN 3-540-00855-1).

Kirwan, B., & Ainsworth, LK. (1992). *A guide to task analysis*. London: Tayler & Francis.

Korn, P., & Walker, W. (2001). Accessibility in the Java™ Platform. In C. Stephanidis (Ed.), *User Interfaces for All - Concepts, Methods, and Tools* (pp. 319-338). Mahwah, NJ: Lawrence Erlbaum Associates (ISBN 0-8058-2967-9, 760 pages).

Kotonya, G., & Sommerville, I. (1998). *Requirements Engineering: Process and Techniques*. USA: John Wiley & Sons, Inc (8, 190-213).

Mace, R.L. (1998). Universal Design in Housing. *Assistive Technology*, 10, 21-28.

Mace, R.L., Hardie, G.J., & Plaice, J.P. (1991). Accessible environments: Toward universal design. In W. Preiser, J. Vischer and E. White (Eds.), *Design interventions: Toward a more human architecture* (pp. 156). New York: Van Nostrand Reinhold.

MacLean, A., Young, R., Bellotti, V., & Moran, T. (1991). Questions, options, and criteria: elements of design space analysis. *Human-Computer Interaction*, 6 (3&4), 201-250. Reprinted (1996) in T.P. Moran & J.M. Carroll (Eds.), *Design Rationale: Concepts, Techniques, and Use*. Hillsdale: Lawrence Erlbaum Associates.

Maybury, M. (Ed.) (1993). *Intelligent Multimedia Interfaces*. Memlo Park, (CA): AAAI/MIT Press.

Maybury, M. (2001). Universal multimedia information access. In C. Stephanidis (Ed.), *Universal Access in HCI: Towards an Information Society for All - Volume 3 of the Proceedings of the 9th International Conference on Human-Computer Interaction (HCI International 2001)* (pp. 382-386). Mahwah, New Jersey: Lawrence Erlbaum Associates (ISBN: 0-8058-3609-8).

Mechanic, D. (1998). Public trust and initiatives for new health care partnerships. *Millbank Quarterly*; 76, 281-302

Miller, EA. (2001). Telemedicine and doctor-patient communication: an analytical survey of the literature. *Journal of Telemedicine and Telecare*, 7, 1-17

Moran, T.P. & Carroll J.M. (Eds.). (1996). *Design Rationale: Concepts, Techniques, and Use*. Hillsdale: Lawrence Erlbaum Associates.

Mueller, J. (1998). Assistive Technology and Universal Design in the Workplace. *Assistive Technology*, 10, 37-43.

Mylopoulos, J., Chung, L., & Nixon, B. (1992). Representing and using Non-Functional requirements: A process-oriented approach. *Software Engineering*, 18 (6), 483-497.

Nardi, B. (1992). The use of scenarios in design. *SIGCHI Bulletin,* 24 (3), 13-14.

Nesbat, S. (2003). A System for Fast, Full-Text Entry for Small Electronic Devices. In *Proceedings of the 5th International Conference on Multimodal Interfaces (ICMI'03)*, Vancouver, BC (pp. 4-11). New York: ACM Press.

Nicolle, C., & Abascal, J. (Eds.). (2001). *Inclusive Design Guidelines for HCI*. London: Taylor & Francis (ISBN 0-7484-0948-3).

Nielsen, J. (1992). Finding usability problems through heuristic evaluation. In *Proceedings of the SIGCHI conference on Human factors in computing systems* (pp. 373-380). New York: ACM Press.

Oliver, N., & Horvitz, E. (2003). Selective Perception Policies for Guiding Sensing and Computation in Multimodal Systems: A Comparative Analysis. In *Proceedings of the5th International Conference on Multimodal Interfaces (ICMI'03)* (pp. 36-43). New York: ACM Press

Olsen, D. (1999). Interacting in Chaos. *Interactions* (September & October), 6 (5), 43-54.

Olson, J.S., & Moran, T.P. (1996). Mapping the method muddle: Guidance in using methods for user interface design. In M. Rudisill, C. Lewis, P.B. Polson, & T.D. McKay (Eds.), *Human-computer interface design: Success stories, emerging methods, and real-world context* (pp. 101-121). San Francisco, CA: Morgan Kaufmann Publishers.

Oviatt, S. (2003). Flexible and robust multimodal interfaces for universal access. *Universal Access in the Information Society, Special issue on multimodality: a step towards universal access*, 2(2), 91-95.

Pfaff, G., & Hagen, P.J.W. (Eds). (1985). *Seeheim Workshop on User Interface Management Systems*. Berlin: Springer Verlag.

Polson, P.G., & Lewis, C. (1990). Theory-Based Design for Easily Learned Interfaces. *Human Computer Interaction*, 5 (2 & 3), 191-220.

Porteus, J., & Brownsell, S. (2000). *Using telecare - Exploring technologies for independent living for older people*. Kidlington, UK: Anchor Trust.

Rahman, M., & Sprigle, S. (1997). Physical Accessibility Guidelines of consumer product controls. *Assistive Technology*, 9, 3-14.

Rieman, J., Franzke, M., & Redmiles, D. (1995). Usability Evaluation with the Cognitive Walkthrough. In *Conference companion on Human factors in computing systems* (pp. 387 - 388). New York: ACM Press.

Rittel, H.W.J. (1972). Second Generation Design Methods. In N. Cross (Ed.), *Developments in Design Methodology* (pp. 317-327). Chichester: J. Wiley & Sons.

Savidis, A., Akoumianakis, D., & Stephanidis, C. (2001). The Unified User Interface Design Method. In C. Stephanidis (Ed.), *User Interfaces for All - Concepts, Methods, and Tools* (pp. 417-440). Mahwah, NJ: Lawrence Erlbaum Associates (ISBN 0-8058-2967-9, 760 pages).

Savidis, A., & Stephanidis, C. (2001a). The Unified User Interface Software Architecture. In C. Stephanidis (Ed.), *User Interfaces for All - Concepts, Methods, and Tools* (pp. 389-415). Mahwah, NJ: Lawrence Erlbaum Associates (ISBN 0-8058-2967-9, 760 pages).

Savidis, A., & Stephanidis, C. (2001b). Development Requirements for Implementing Unified User Interfaces. In C. Stephanidis (Ed.), *User Interfaces for All - Concepts, Methods, and Tools* (pp. 441-468). Mahwah, NJ: Lawrence Erlbaum Associates (ISBN 0-8058-2967-9, 760 pages).

Savidis, A., & Stephanidis, C. (2001c). The I-GET UIMS for Unified User Interface Implementation. In C. Stephanidis (Ed.), *User Interfaces for All - Concepts, Methods, and Tools* (pp. 489-523). Mahwah, NJ: Lawrence Erlbaum Associates (ISBN 0-8058-2967-9, 760 pages).

Savidis, A., & Stephanidis, C. (2001d). Designing with varying design parameters: The Unified Design process. In *Proceedings of the Workshop No. 14 "Universal design: Towards universal access in the info society", organised in the context of the ACM Conference on Human Factors in Computing Systems (CHI 2001)*. [On-line]. Available at: http://www.ics.forth.gr/hci/files/chi2001/savidis.pdf

Savidis, A., & Stephanidis, C. (2004a). Unified User Interface Design: Designing Universally Accessible Interactions. International Journal of Interacting with Computers, 16 (2), 243-270.

Savidis, A., & Stephanidis, C. (2004b). Unified User Interface Development: Software Engineering of Universally Accessible Interactions. *Universal Access in the Information Society*, 3 (3), 165-193. (Managing Editor: Alfred Kobsa, University of California, Irvine, USA).

Savidis, A., Stephanidis, C., & Akoumianakis, D. (1997). Unifying Toolkit Programming Layers: a Multi-Purpose Toolkit Integration Module. In M.D. Harrison, & J.C. Torres (Eds.), *Proceedings of the 4th Eurographics Workshop on Design, Specification and Verification of Interactive Systems (DSV-IS '97)*, Granada, Spain, 4-6 June (pp 177-192). Berlin: Springer-Verlag.

Shepherd, A. (1989). Analysis and training in information technology tasks. In D. Diaper (Ed.), *Task Analysis for Human-Computer Interaction* (pp. 15-55). Chichester: Ellis Horwood.

Shneiderman, B. (1993). Direct manipulation: a step beyond programming languages. In B. Shneiderman (Ed.), *Sparks of Innovation in Human-Computer Interaction* (pp. 13-37). Norwood, NJ: Ablex Publishing Corporation.

Shneiderman, B. (2000). Universal Usability: pushing human computer interaction research to empower every citizen. *Communications of the ACM*, 43, 84-91.

Shneiderman, B., & Hochheiser, H. (2001). Universal usability as a stimulus to advanced interface design. *Behaviour & Information Technology*, 20(5), 367-376.

Stanberry, B. (2000). Telemedicine: barriers and opportunities in the 21st century. *Journal of Internal Medicine.* 247, 615-628.

Stary, C. (1998). Task- and Model-based Development of User Interfaces. In: Proceedings of *IT & KNOW'98*, IFIP World Conference..

Stary, C. (2000). TADEUS: Seamless Development of Task-Based and User-Oriented Interfaces. In *IEEE Transactions on Systems, Man, and Cybernetics*, 30, 509-525.

Stary, C. (2003). Model-Based Role-Adapted Interaction – A Health-Care Case, In C. Stephanidis, (Ed.), Universal Access in HCI: Inclusive Design in the Information Society - Volume 4 of the Proceedings of the 10th International Conference on Human-Computer Interaction (HCI International 2003), Crete, Greece, 22-27 June (pp. 1208 - 1212). Mahwah, New Jersey: Lawrence Erlbaum Associates (ISBN: 0-8058-4933-5).

Stephanidis, C. (1995). Towards User Interfaces for All: Some Critical Issues. Parallel *Session "User Interfaces for All - Everybody, Everywhere, and Anytime"*. In Y. Anzai, K. Ogawa & H. Mori (Eds.), *Symbiosis of Human and Artifact - Future Computing and Design for Human-Computer Interaction [Proceedings of the 6th International Conference on Human-Computer Interaction (HCI International '95)]*, Tokyo, Japan, 9-14 July (vol. 1, pp. 137-142). Amsterdam: Elsevier, Elsevier Science.

Stephanidis, C. (2001a). Adaptive techniques for Universal Access. *User Modelling and User Adapted Interaction International Journal*, 11 (1/2), 159-179. [On-line]. Available at: http://www.wkap.nl/issuetoc.htm/0924-1868+11+1/2+2001

Stephanidis, C. (2001b). The concept of Unified User Interfaces. In C. Stephanidis (Ed.), *User Interfaces for All - Concepts, Methods, and Tools* (pp. 371-388). Mahwah, NJ: Lawrence Erlbaum Associates (ISBN 0-8058-2967-9, 760 pages).

Stephanidis, C. (Ed.) (2001c). *User Interfaces for All - Concepts Methods, and Tools*. Mahwah, NJ: Lawrence Erlbaum Associates (ISBN 0-8058-2967-9, 760 pages).

Stephanidis, C. (Ed.). (2003). *Universal Access Code in Health Telematics Applications and Services*. Deliverable D.3.3 of the IST-1999-14101 IS4All project.

Stephanidis, C., & Akoumianakis, D. (2002): Towards a design code of practice for universal access in Health Telematics. *Universal Access in the Information Society*, 1 (3), pp. 223-226.

Stephanidis, C., & Emiliani, P.L. (1999). Connecting to the Information Society: a European Perspective. *Technology and Disability Journal*, 10 (1), 21-44. [On-line]. Available at: http://www.ics.forth.gr/hci/html/files/TDJ_paper.PDF

Stephanidis, C., & Savidis, A. (2003). Unified User Interface Development. In J. Jacko & A. Sears (Eds.), *The Human-Computer Interaction Handbook – Fundamentals, Evolving Technologies and Emerging Applications* (pp. 1069-1089). Mahwah, New Jersey: Lawrence Erlbaum Associates.

Stephanidis, C., Paramythis, A., Sfyrakis, M., & Savidis, A. (2001). A Case Study in Unified User Interface Development: The AVANTI Web Browser. In C. Stephanidis (Ed.), *User Interfaces for All - Concepts, Methods, and Tools* (pp. 525-568). Mahwah, NJ: Lawrence Erlbaum Associates (ISBN 0-8058-2967-9, 760 pages).

Stephanidis, C., Paramythis, A., Zarikas, V., & Savidis, A. (2004). The PALIO Framework for Adaptive Information Services. In A. Seffah & H. Javahery (Eds.), *Multiple User Interfaces: Cross-Platform Applications and Context-Aware Interfaces* (pp. 69-92). Chichester, UK: John Wiley & Sons, Ltd.

Stephanidis, C., Antona, M. Savidis, A. (2005, in print). Design for All: Computer assisted design of user interface adaptation. In G. Salvendy (Ed.). Handbook of Human Factors & Ergonomics, 3rd Edition. John Wiley & Sons, Ltd.

Stephanidis, C. (Ed.), Salvendy, G., Akoumianakis, D., Arnold, A., Bevan, N., Dardailler, D., Emiliani, P.L., Iakovidis, I., Jenkins, P., Karshmer, A., Korn, P., Marcus, A., Murphy, H., Oppermann, C., Stary, C., Tamura, H., Tscheligi, M., Ueda, H., Weber, G., & Ziegler, J. (1999). Toward an Information Society for All: HCI challenges and R&D recommendations. *International Journal of Human-Computer Interaction*, 11 (1), 1-28. [On-line]. Available at: http://www.ics.forth.gr/hci/html/files/ white_paper_1999.pdf.

Stephanidis C. (Ed.), Salvendy, G., Akoumianakis, D., Bevan, N., Brewer, J., Emiliani, P.L., Galetsas, A., Haataja, S., Iakovidis, I., Jacko, J., Jenkins, P., Karshmer, A., Korn, P., Marcus, A., Murphy, H., Stary, C., Vanderheiden, G., Weber, G., & Ziegler, J. (1998). Toward an Information Society for All: An International R&D Agenda. *International Journal of Human-Computer Interaction*, 10 (2), 107-134. [On-line]. Available at: http://www.ics.forth.gr/hci/html/files/white_paper_1998.pdf.

Stephanidis, C., Savidis, A., & Akoumianakis, D. (2001a). Tutorial on "Engineering Universal Access: Unified User Interfaces". Tutorial in the *1st Universal Access in Human-Computer Interaction Conference (UAHCI 2001), jointly with the 9th International Conference on Human-Computer Interaction (HCI International 2001)*, New Orleans, Louisiana, USA, 5-10 August. [On-line]. Available: http://www.ics.forth.gr/hci/html/files/uahci_2001.pdf

Stephanidis, C., Savidis, A., & Akoumianakis, D. (2001b). Tutorial on "Universally accessible UIs: The unified user interface development". Tutorial in the ACM *CHI 2001*, Seattle, Washington, 31 March - 5 April. [On-line]. Available at: http://www.ics.forth.gr/hci/html/files/CHI_Tutorial.pdf

Stewart, T. (2000). *Ergonomics user interface standards: are they more trouble than they are worth?* Special report. [On-line]. Available at: http://www.system-concepts.com/images/ uploaded/documents/standards.pdf (This paper was originally published in the Taylor & Francis journal, *Ergonomics*).

Story, M.F. (1998). Maximising Usability: The Principles of Universal Design. *The Assistive Technology Journal*, vol. 10(1), pp. 4-12.

Stowe, R. (2001a). *A New Era of Economic Frailty? - A White Paper on the Macroeconomic Impact of Population Aging*. Washington, DC: Center for Strategic and International Studies - Global Aging Initiative.

Stowe, R. (2001b). *The Fiscal Challenge of an Aging Industrial World - A White Paper on Demographics and Medical Technology*. Washington, DC: Center for Strategic and International Studies - Global Aging Initiative.

Stroetmann, KA, & Erkert, T. (1999). "HausTeleDienst"-A CATV-based interactive video service for elderly people. In: M. Nerlich & R. Kretschmar (Eds.), *The impact of Telemedicine on Health Care Management* (pp. 245-252). Amsterdam: IOS Press.

Stroetmann, K.A., & Pieper, M. (2003). Participatory Approaches towards Universal Access - Results of a Case Study in the Healthcare Domain. In C. Stephanidis, (Ed.), *Universal Access in HCI: Inclusive Design in the Information Society - Volume 4 of the Proceedings of the 10th International Conference on Human-Computer Interaction (HCI International 2003)*, Crete, Greece, 22-27 June (pp. 1213 - 1217). Mahwah, New Jersey: Lawrence Erlbaum Associates (ISBN: 0-8058-4933-5).

Stroetmann, K.A., & Stroetmann, V.N. (2002). *E-business sector report no. 7: Health and Social services* - A contribution to the Quarterly Report 2[June]/2002 of the *e-business w@tch* project for the CEC, Brussels (forthcoming).

Subramanian, N., & Chung, L. (2003). Towards standardization of adaptable software architectures. *Computer Standards & Interfaces*, 25 (3), 211-213.

Suri, J., & Marsh, M. (2002). Scenario building as an ergonomics method in consumer product design. *Applied Ergonomics*, 31 (151-157).

Tang, P, & Venables, T. (2000). 'Smart' homes and telecare for independent living. *Journal of Telemedicine and Telecare*, 6, 8-14.

Tognazzini, B. (1995). *Tog on Software Design*. Addison Wesley.

Tsiknakis, M., Chronaki, C.E., Kapidakis, S., Nikolaou, C., & Orphanoudakis, S.C. (1997). An integrated architecture for the provision of health telematic services based on digital library technologies. *International Journal on Digital Libraries, Special Issue on "Digital Libraries in Medicine"*, 1 (3), 257-277.

Ueda, H. (2001). The FRIEND21 Framework for human Interface Architectures. In C. Stephanidis (Ed.), *User Interfaces for All - Concepts, Methods, and Tools* (pp. 245-270). Mahwah, NJ: Lawrence Erlbaum Associates.

UIMS Tool Developers Workshop (1992). A Metamodel for the Runtime Architecture of an Interactive System. *SIGCHI Bulletin*, 24(1), 32-37 (January).

Virtuoso, S., & Dodero, G. (2001): WARD-IN-HAND: an user interface implementation on a PDA platform. Electronically available at: http://www.disi.unige.it/person/DoderoG/wihpaper.htm

W3C (2003a). Multimodal Interaction Requirements - W3C Note, 8 January 2003. http://www.w3.org/TR/2003/NOTE-mmi-reqs-20030108

W3C (2003b). SOAP Version 1.2 Part 0: Primer - W3C Recommendation, 24 June 2003. http://www.w3.org/TR/2003/REC-soap12-part0-20030624/

W3C (2003c). Multimodal Interaction Framework - W3C Note, 6 May 2003. http://www.w3.org/TR/2003/NOTE-mmi-framework-20030506

W3C (2003d). Requirements for EMMA - W3C Note, 13 January 2003. http://www.w3.org/TR/2003/NOTE-EMMAreqs-20030113

Weidenhaupt, K., Pohl, K., Jarke, M., & Haumer P. (1998). Scenarios in system development: current practice. *IEEE Software*, 15 (2), 34-45.

Wootton, R. (2001). Recent advances - Telemedicine. *BMJ*, 323, 557-560.

Yu, C., & Balland, D.H. (2003). A Multimodal Learning Interface for Grounding Spoken Language in Sensory Perceptions. In *Proceedings of the 5th International Conference on Multimodal Interfaces (ICMI'03)* (pp. 164-171), New York: ACM Press.

Ziegler, J. (2001) Can Standards and Guidelines Promote Universal Access? In C. Stephanidis (Ed.), *Universal Access in HCI: Towards an Information Society for All - Volume 3 of the Proceedings of the 9th International Conference on Human-Computer Interaction (HCI International 2001)* (pp. 640-644). Mahwah, New Jersey: Lawrence Erlbaum Associates (ISBN: 0-8058-3609-8).